全国高等学校临床医学专业卫生部规划教材英文版

案例分析系列

Case Files™ Pharmacology

药 理 学

原　著　Eugene C. Toy，MD
Gary C. Rosenfeld，PHD
David S. Loose，PHD
Donald Briscoe，MD

中文主编　周宏灏

编　者（按姓氏笔画排序）

王冠蕾　中山大学基础医学院
包定元　四川大学华西医学中心
关永源　中山大学基础医学院
张　伟　中南大学湘雅医学院
李元建　中南大学湘雅医学院
李　清　中南大学湘雅医学院
陈红专　上海交通大学基础医学院
陈建国　华中科技大学同济医学院
周宏灏　中南大学湘雅医学院
周黎明　四川大学华西医学中心
林志彬　北京大学医学部
姚明辉　复旦大学医学院
魏敏杰　中国医科大学药学院

人 民 卫 生 出 版 社

人民卫生出版社

McGraw-Hill

A Division of The McGraw-Hill Companies

Eugene C. Toy, et al.
Case Files: Pharmacology
ISBN: 0-07-144573-0

Simplified Chinese translation edition jointly published by McGraw-Hill Education (Asia) Co. and People's Medical Publishing House.

案例分析系列 药理学

敬告：本书的译者及出版者已尽力使书中出现的药物剂量和治疗方法准确，并符合本书出版时国内普遍接受的标准。但随着医学的发展，药物的使用方法应随时作相应的改变。建议读者在使用本书涉及的药物时，认真研读药物使用说明书，尤其对于新药或不常用药更应如此。出版者拒绝对因参照本书任何内容而直接或间接导致的事故与损失负责。

图书在版编目(CIP)数据

药理学/周宏灏中文主编. —北京：人民卫生出版社，2008.6
(案例分析系列)
ISBN 978-7-117-09891-5

Ⅰ. 药… Ⅱ. 周… Ⅲ. 药理学—病案—分析—英、汉 Ⅳ. R96

中国版本图书馆 CIP 数据核字(2008)第 017097 号

图字：01-2006-6096

案 例 分 析 系 列
药 理 学

中文主编：周宏灏
出版发行：人民卫生出版社(中继线 010-67616688)
地　　址：北京市丰台区方庄芳群园 3 区 3 号楼
邮　　编：100078
网　　址：http://www.pmph.com
E - mail：pmph @ pmph.com
购书热线：010-67605754　010-65264830
印　　刷：北京智力达印刷有限公司
经　　销：新华书店
开　　本：787×1092　1/16　**印张：**29
字　　数：600 千字
版　　次：2008 年 6 月第 1 版　2008 年 6 月第 1 版第 1 次印刷
标准书号：ISBN 978-7-117-09891-5/R·9892
定　　价：56.00元

全国高等学校临床医学专业卫生部规划教材英文版

案例分析系列

出 版 说 明

为贯彻教育部、卫生部关于加强双语教学的精神，配合全国各医学院校开展双语教学的需要以及适应以问题为中心的教学发展趋势，人民卫生出版社特引进了本套案例分析系列英文教材。该教材原版由美国麦格劳希尔教育出版集团出版，在美国各大医学院使用后反响良好。

书中通过剖析临床实例对相关的临床或基础知识进行回顾和复习，有助于医学生将医学基础知识和临床实践相结合。这种以问题为中心的学习(PBL)模式强调发挥学生主动思考的潜力，培养其自我学习能力。在编排上，作者有意将案例顺序随机化，目的是模拟真正的患者就医情景。为方便查询，书后附有以字母为序的案例排列索引。

加入中文编注后的案例分析系列基本保持原书风貌，并根据我国国内教学情况对重要知识点和词汇进行了点评和加注。本套教材语言叙述通俗、简练，既可加强读者对医学知识的理解，又可学习医学英语。

本系列首批教材包括12本：临床医学6本(内科学、外科学、妇产科学、儿科学、精神病学、急诊医学)，基础医学6本(解剖学、生理学、生物化学、微生物学、病理学、药理学)，将于近期全部推出。

前　言

本书是美国 McGraw-Hill 公司出版的案例分析系列丛书中的药理学分册。它与传统的药理学教材不同，作者精心挑选了 52 个病例展开讨论，从中阐述药理学相关的基本知识。通过分析每一病例的临床症状，提出药理学相关问题，在讨论的基础上归结出要掌握的药理学知识点。这种以问题为中心的学习(PBL)模式强调发挥读者主动思考的潜力，培养其自学能力。读者可在临床作业的情景中学习到药理学的基本知识，这是本书有别于其他药理学教科书的最大特点。本书可以让读者找到理论知识与临床实践的衔接点，消除了单纯理论学习的枯燥。本书不但适合刚进医学殿堂的医学生，同样也适合具有一定实践经验的临床医生；亦可作为其他医务工作人员的参考用书。

为了使得国内读者更好的掌握这本经典教材，我们对其进行了注释，供读者阅读时参考。每个案例的注释包括三个部分：①我们对一些专业的和生僻的词汇做了中文翻译，以方便阅读；②局部内容注解；③对每一病例进行点评。

本书在注释过程中得到了人民卫生出版社和参与注释的作者的大力支持，同时也得到了中南大学临床药理研究所的老师和研究生的协助，特别是我的研究生陶共由同学自始至终做了大量的工作，在此一并致谢。

参与本书注释的作者虽多系国内从事药理学教学多年的资深教授，但毕竟囿于知识水平和时间、精力，疏忽、错漏在所难免，敬请关心和使用本注释本的同行、读者、老师和同学批评指正。

周宏灏

2008 年 5 月 29 日于长沙

❖ INTRODUCTION

Often, the medical student will cringe at the "drudgery" of the basic science courses and see little connection between a field such as pharmacology and clinical problems. Clinicians, however, often wish they knew more about the basic sciences, because it is through the science that we can begin to understand the complexities of the human body and thus have rational methods of diagnosis and treatment.

Mastering the knowledge in a discipline such as pharmacology is a formidable task. It is even more difficult to retain this information and to recall it when the clinical setting is encountered. To accomplish this synthesis, pharmacology is optimally taught in the context of medical situations, and this is reinforced later during the clinical rotations. The gulf between the basic sciences and the patient arena is wide. Perhaps one way to bridge this gulf is with carefully constructed clinical cases that ask basic science-oriented questions. In an attempt to achieve this goal, we have designed a collection of patient cases to teach pharmacology-related points. More importantly, the explanations for these cases emphasize the underlying mechanisms and relate the clinical setting to the basic science data. The principles are explored rather than overemphasizing rote memorization.

This book is organized for versatility: to allow the student "in a rush" to go quickly through the scenarios and check the corresponding answers, and to provide more detailed information for the student who wants thought-provoking explanations. The answers are arranged from simple to complex: a summary of the pertinent points, the bare answers, a clinical correlation, an approach to the pharmacology topic, a comprehension test at the end for reinforcement or emphasis, and a list of references for further reading. The clinical cases are arranged by system to better reflect the organization within the basic science. Finally, to encourage thinking about mechanisms and relationships, we used open-ended questions in the clinical cases. Nevertheless, several multiplechoice questions are included at the end of each scenario to reinforce concepts or introduce related topics.

HOW TO GET THE MOST OUT OF THIS BOOK

Each case is designed to introduce a clinically related issue and includes openended questions usually asking a basic science question, but at times, to break up the monotony, there will be a clinical question. The answers are organized into four different parts:

PART I

1. **Summary**
2. A **straightforward answer** is given for each open-ended question.
3. **Clinical Correlation**—A discussion of the relevant points relating the basic science to the clinical manifestations, and perhaps introducing the student to issues such as diagnosis and treatment

PART II

An **approach to the basic science concept** consisting of three parts:

1. **Objectives**—A listing of the two to four main knowledge objectives that are critical for understanding the underlying pharmacology to answer the question and relate to the clinical situation.
2. **Definitions of basic terminology**
3. **Discussion of the specific class of agents**

PART III

Comprehension Questions—Each case includes several multiple-choice questions that reinforce the material or introduces new and related concepts. Questions about the material not found in the text are explained in the answers.

PART IV

Pharmacology Pearls—A listing of several important points, many clinically relevant, reiterated as a summation of the text and to allow for easy review, such as before an examination

CONTENTS

SECTION I

Applying the Basic Sciences to Clinical Medicine

PART 1. APPROACH TO LEARNING PHARMACOLOGY

Pharmacology is best learned by a systematic approach, understanding the physiology of the body, recognizing that **every medication has desirable and undesirable effects**, and being aware that the biochemical and pharmacological properties of a drug affects its characteristics such as duration of action, volume of distribution, passage through the blood-brain barrier, mechanism of elimination, and route of administration. Rather than memorizing the characteristics of a medication, the student should strive to learn the underlying rationale such as, "Second-generation antihistamine agents are less lipid soluble than first-generation antihistamines and therefore do not cross the blood-brain barrier as readily; thus, second-generation antihistamines are not as sedating. Because they both bind the histamine H_1 receptor, the efficacy is the same."

KEY TERMS

Pharmacology: The study of substances that interact with living systems through biochemical processes.

Drug: A substance used in the prevention, diagnosis, or treatment of disease.

Toxicology: A branch of pharmacology that studies the undesirable effects of chemicals on living organisms.

Food and Drug Administration (FDA): The federal agency responsible for the safety and efficacy of all drugs in the United States, as well as food and cosmetics.

Adverse effect: Also known as side effect; all unintended actions of a drug that result from the lack of specificity of drug action. All drugs are capable of producing adverse effects.

Pharmacodynamics: The actions of a drug on a living organism, including mechanisms of action and receptor interaction.

Pharmacokinetics: The actions of the living organism on the drug, including absorption, distribution, and elimination.

Volume of distribution (V_d): The size the "compartment" into which a drug is distributed following absorption and is determined by the equation:

$$V_d = \text{Dose(mg) drug administered} / \text{Initial plasma concentration(mg/L)}$$

Potency of drug: Relative amount of drug needed to produce a given response, determined largely by the amount of drug that reaches the site of action and by the affinity of the drug for the receptor.

Efficacy: Drug effect as the maximum response it is able to produce and is determined by the number of drug-receptor complexes and the ability of the receptor to be activated once bound. **EC-50** refers to the drug concentration that produces

50% of the maximal response, whereas **ED-50** refers to the drug dose that is pharmacologically effective in 50% of the population.

Absorption: The movement of a drug from the administration site into the bloodstream, usually requiring the crossing of one or more biological membranes. Important parameters include lipid solubility, ionization, size of the molecule, and presence of a transport mechanism.

Elimination: Process by which a drug is removed from the body, generally by either metabolism or excretion. Elimination follows various kinetic models. For example, **first-order kinetics** describes most circumstances, and means that the rate of drug elimination depends on the concentration of the drug in the plasma as described by the equation:

Rate of elimination from body = Constant × drug concentration

Zero-order kinetics is less common and means that the rate of elimination is constant and does not depend on the plasma drug concentration. This may be a consequence of a circumstance such as saturation of liver enzymes or saturation of the kidney transport mechanisms.

Bioavailability: The percentage of an ingested drug that is actually absorbed into the bloodstream.

Route of administration: Drug may be delivered **intravenously** (IV or iv) for delivery directly into the bloodstream, **intramuscularly** (IM) and **subcutaneously** (SC). The medication may be depot and slow release, **inhalant** for rapid absorption and delivery to the bronchi and lungs, **sublingual** to bypass the first-pass effect, **intrathecal** for agents that penetrate the blood-brain barrier poorly, **rectal** to avoid hepatic firstpass effect and for nausea, and **topical** administration when local effect is desired such as dermatological or ophthalmic agents.

PART 2. APPROACH TO DISEASE

Physicians usually tackle clinical situations by taking a history (asking questions), performing a physical examination, obtaining selective laboratory and imaging tests, and then formulating a diagnosis. The synthesis of the history, physical examination, and imaging or lab tests is called the **clinical database**. After reaching a diagnosis, a treatment plan is usually initiated, and the patient is followed for a clinical response. Rational understanding of disease and plans for treatment are best acquired by learning about the normal human processes on a basic science level; likewise, being aware of how disease alters the normal physiological processes is also best understood on a basic science level. Pharmacology and therapeutics requires also the ability to tailor the correct medication to the patient's situation and awareness of the medication's adverse effect profile. Sometimes, the patient has an adverse reaction to a medication as the chief complaint, and the physician must be able to identify the medication as the culprit. An understanding of the underlying basic science allows for more rational analysis and medication choices.

PART 3. APPROACH TO READING

There are seven key questions that help to stimulate the application of basic science information to the clinical setting. These are:

1. **Which of the available medications is most likely to achieve the desired therapeutic effect and/or is responsible for the described symptoms or signs?**
2. **What is the likely mechanism for the clinical effect(s) and adverse effect(s) of the medication?**
3. **What is the basic pharmacologic profile (e. g., absorption, elimination) for medications in a certain class, and what are the differences among the agents within the class?**
4. **Given basic pharmacological definitions such as therapeutic index (TI) or certain safety factor (TD_1/ED_{99}), or median lethal dose (LD_{50}), how do medications compare in their safety profile?**
5. **Given a particular clinical situation with described unique patient characteristics, which medication is most appropriate?**
6. **What is the best treatment for the toxic effect of a medication?**
7. **What are the drug-drug interactions to be cautious about regarding a particular medication?**

1. Which of the following medications is most likely to be responsible for the described symptoms or signs?

The student must be aware of the various effects, both desirable and undesirable, produced by particular medications. Knowledge of desirable therapeutic effects is essential in selecting the appropriate drug for the particular clinical application; likewise, an awareness of its adverse effects is necessary, because patients may come into the office with a complaint caused by a drug effect unaware that their symptoms are because of a prescribed medication. It is only by being aware of the common and dangerous effects that the clinician can arrive at the correct diagnosis. The student is encouraged not to merely memorize the comparative adverse effect profiles of the drugs, but rather to understand the underlying mechanisms.

2. What is the likely mechanism for the clinical effect(s) and adverse effect(s)

of the medication?

As noted above, the student should strive to learn the underlying physiological, biochemical, or cellular explanation for the described drug effect. This understanding allows for the rational choice of an alternative agent, or the reasonable choice of an agent to alleviate the symptoms, or explanatory advice to the patient regarding behavioral changes to diminish any adverse affects. For example, if a 60-year-old woman who takes medications for osteoporosis complains of severe "heartburn," one may be suspicious, knowing that the bisphosphonate medication alendronate can cause esophagitis. Instruction to the patient to take the medication while sitting upright and remaining upright for at least 30 minutes would be the proper course of action, because gravity will assist in keeping the alendronate in the stomach rather than allowing regurgitation into the distal esophagus.

3. **What is the basic pharmacologic profile (absorption, elimination, volume of distribution) for medications in a certain class, and what are differences among the agents within the class**?

Understanding the pharmacological profile of medications allows for rational therapeutics. However, instead of memorizing the separate profiles for every medication, grouping the drugs together into classes allows for more efficient learning and better comprehension. An excellent starting point for the student of pharmacology would be to study how a **prototype drug** within a drug class organized by structure or mechanism of action may be used to treat a condition (such as hypertension). Then within each category of agents, the student should try to identify important subclasses or drug differences. For example, hypertensive agents can be categorized as diuretic agents, β-adrenergic-blocking agents, calcium-channel-blocking agents, and renin-angiotensin system inhibitors. Within the subclassification of renin-angiotensin system inhibitors, the angiotensin converting enzyme inhibitors can cause the side effect of a dry cough caused by the increase in bradykinin brought about by the enzyme blockade; instead, the angiotensin 1 receptor blockers do not affect the bradykinin levels and so do not cause the cough as often.

4. **Given basic pharmacological definitions such as therapeutic index (TI) or certain safety factor (TD_1/ED_{99}), or median lethal dose (LD_{50}), how do medications compare in their safety profile**?

Therapeutic Index (TI): Defined as the TD_{50}/ED_{50} (the ratio of the dose that produces a toxic effect in half the population to the dose that produces the desired effect in half the population).

Certain Safety Factor (TD_1/ED_{99}): Defined as the ratio of the dose that produces the toxic effect in 1 percent of the population to the dose that produces the desired effect in 99 percent of the population; also known as **Standard Safety Measure**.

Median Lethal Dose(LD_{50}): Defined as the median lethal dose, the dose that will kill half the population.

Based on these definitions, a desirable medication would have a high therapeutic index(toxic dose is many times that of the efficacious dose), high Certain Safety Factor, and high median lethal dose(much higher than therapeutic dose). Likewise, medications such as digoxin that have a low therapeutic index require careful monitoring of levels and vigilance for side effects.

5. **Given a particular clinical situation with described unique patient characteristics, which medication is most appropriate**?

The student must weigh various advantages and disadvantages, as well as different patient attributes. Some of those may include compliance with medications, allergies to medications, liver or renal insufficiency, age, coexisting medical disorders, and other medications. The student must be able to sift through the medication profile and identify the most dangerous adverse effects. For example, if a patient is already taking a monoamine-oxidase-inhibiting agent for depression, then adding a serotonin reuptake inhibitor would be potentially fatal, because serotonin syndrome may ensue(hyperthermia, muscle rigidity, death).

6. **What is the best treatment for the toxic effect of a medication**?

If complications of drug therapy are present, the student should know the proper treatment. This is best learned by understanding the drug mechanism of action. For example, a patient who has taken excessive opioids caused by either a heroin overdose or pain medication may develop respiratory depression, which may be fatal. The treatment of an opioid overdose includes the ABCs(airway, breathing, circulation) and the administration of naloxone, which is a competitive antagonist of opioids.

7. **What are the drug-drug interactions to be concerned with regarding a particular medication**?

Patients are often prescribed multiple medications, from either the same practitioner or different clinicians. Patients may not be aware of the drug-drug interactions; thus, the clinician must compile, as a component of good clinical practice, a current list of all medications(prescribed, over-the-counter, and herbal) taken by the patient. Thus, the student should be aware of the most common and dangerous interactions; once again, understanding the underlying mechanism allows for lifelong learning rather than short-term rote memorization of facts that are easily forgotten. For example, magnesium sulfate to stop preterm labor should not be used if the patient is taking a calciumchannel-blocking agent such as nifedipine. Magnesium sulfate acts as a competitive inhibitor of calcium, and by decreasing its intracellular availability, it slows down smooth muscle contraction such as in the uterus. Calcium-channel blockers potentiate the inhibition of calcium influx and can lead to toxic effects, such as respiratory depression.

Comprehension Questions

[I-1] Bioavailability of an agent is maximal when the drug is

A. Highly lipid soluble

B. Larger than 100 Daltons in molecular weight

C. Highly bound to plasma proteins

D. Highly ionized

[I-2] An agent is noted to have a very low calculated volume of distribution (V_d). Which of the following is the best explanation?

A. The agent is eliminated by the kidneys, and the patient has renal insufficiency.

B. The agent is extensive bound to plasma proteins.

C. The agent is extensively sequestered in tissue.

D. The agent is eliminated by zero-order kinetics.

[I-3] Which of the following describes the first-pass effect?

A. Inactivation of a drug as a result of the gastric acids.

B. Absorption of a drug through the duodenum.

C. Drug given orally is metabolized by the liver before entering the circulation.

D. Drug given intravenously accumulates quickly in the central nervous system (CNS).

[I-4] A laboratory experiment is being conducted in which a mammal is injected with a noncompetitive antagonist to the histamine receptor. Which of the following best describes this agent?

A. The drug binds to the histamine receptor and partially activates it.

B. The drug binds to the histamine receptor but does not activate it.

C. The drug binds to the receptor, but not where histamine binds, and prevents the receptor from being activated.

D. The drug irreversibly binds to the histamine receptor and renders it ineffective.

[I-5] A 25-year-old medical student is given a prescription for asthma, which the physician states has a very high therapeutic index. Which of the statements best characterizes the drug as it relates to the therapeutic index?

A. The drug's serum levels will likely need to be carefully monitored.

B. The drug is likely to cross the blood-brain barrier.

C. The drug is likely to have extensive drug-drug interactions.

D. The drug is unlikely to have any serious adverse effects.

[I-6] A drug M is injected intravenously into a laboratory subject. It is noted to have high serum protein binding. Which of the following is most likely to be increased as a result?

A. Drug interaction

B. Distribution of the drug to tissue sites

C. Renal excretion

D. Liver metabolism

[I-7] A bolus of drug K is given intravenously. The drug is noted to follow first-order kinetics. Which of the following describes the elimination of drug K?

A. The rate of elimination of drug K is constant.

B. The rate of elimination of drug K is proportional to the patient's renal function.

C. The rate of elimination of drug K is proportional to its concentration in the patient's plasma.

D. The rate of elimination of drug K is dependent on a nonlinear relationship to the plasma protein concentration.

Answers

[I-1] **A.** Transport across biological membranes and thus bioavailability is maximal with high lipid solubility.

[I-2] **B.** The volume of distribution is calculated by administering a known dose of drug (mg) intravenously and then measuring an initial plasma concentration (mg/L). The ratio of the mass of drug given (mg) divided by the initial plasma concentration (mg/L) gives the V_d. A very low V_d may indicate extensive protein binding (drug is sequestered in the bloodstream), whereas a high V_d may indicate extensive tissue binding (drug is sequestered in the tissue).

[I-3] **C.** The first pass effect refers to the process in which following oral administration, a drug is extensively metabolized as it initially passes through the liver, before it enters the general circulation. Liver enzymes may metabolize the agent to such an extent that the drug cannot be administered orally.

[I-4] **C.** A noncompetitive antagonist binds to the receptor at a site other than the agonist-binding site and renders it less effective by preventing agonist binding or preventing activation.

[I-5] **D**. An agent with a high therapeutic index means the toxic dose is very much higher than the therapeutic dose, and it is less likely to produce toxic effects at therapeutic levels.

[I-6] **A**. High protein binding means less drug to tissue, the kidney, and the liver. Drug interaction may occur if the agent binds to the same protein site as other drugs, thus displacing drugs and increasing serum levels.

[I-7] **C**. First-order kinetics means the rate of elimination of a drug is proportional to the plasma concentration.

PHARMACOLOGY PEARLS

❖ Understanding the pharmacologic mechanisms of medications allows for rational choices for therapy, fewer medication errors, and rapid recognition and reversal of toxic effects.

❖ The therapeutic index, Certain Safety Factor(TD_1/ED_{99}), and Median Lethal Dose are various methods of describing the potential toxicity of medications.

❖ There are seven key questions to stimulate the application of basic science information to the clinical arena.

REFERENCES

Braunwald E, Fauci AS, Kasper KL et al., eds. Harrison's principles of internal medicine, 16th ed. New York: McGraw-Hill, 2004.

Rosenfeld GC, Loose-Mitchell DS. Pharmacology, 3rd ed. Philadelphia: Lippincott, Williams & Wilkins, 1998: 1.

SECTION Ⅱ

Clinical Cases

❖ CASE 1

A 12-year-old girl presents to your office with a sore throat and fever. You diagnose her with pharyngitis caused by group A β-hemolytic streptococcus. She is given an IM injection of penicillin. [注1] Approximately 5 minutes later, she is found to be in respiratory distress and audibly wheezing. Her skin is mottled and cool, she is tachycardic (rapid heart rate), and her blood pressure has fallen to 70/20 mmHg. [注2] You immediately diagnose her as having an anaphylactic reaction to the penicillin and give a subcutaneous injection of epinephrine.

◆ **What effect will epinephrine have on this patient's vascular system?**

◆ **Which adrenoceptor primarily mediates the vascular response?**

◆ **What effect will epinephrine have on her respiratory system?**

◆ **Which adrenoceptor primarily mediates the respiratory system response?**

ANSWERS TO CASE 1: Autonomic Sympathetic Nervous System①

Summary: A 12-year-old girl with "strep throat" is given an injection of penicillin and develops an acute anaphylactic reaction.

- **Effect of epinephrine on vascular system**: Vasoconstriction.
- **Adrenoceptor which primarily mediates the vascular response**: Alpha-1 (α_1).
- **Effect of epinephrine on the pulmonary system**: Bronchial muscle relaxation.
- **Adrenoceptor which primarily mediates the pulmonary response**: Beta-2 (β_2).

CLINICAL CORRELATION

Anaphylaxis is an acute, immune-mediated response to an allergen characterized by bronchospasm, wheezing, tachycardia, and hypotension. Epinephrine is the drug of choice used to treat this condition because it appears, through the activation of alpha (α)-and beta(β)-adrenoceptors, to counteract the pathophysiological processes underlying anaphylaxis. As with all emergencies, the ABCs(airway, breathing, circulation) should be addressed first. Occasionally, the anaphylaxis causes laryngeal edema to the extent that the airway is compromised, and intubation(tube placed in the trachea) is impossible. In these circumstances, an emergency airway, such as a surgical cricothyroidotomy, is required.

The Autonomic Sympathetic Nervous System

Objectives

1. List the neurotransmitters of the autonomic sympathetic nervous system and describe their anatomical localization.
2. List the receptors and receptor-subtypes of the autonomic sympathetic nervous system.
3. Predict the responses to activation and inhibition of autonomic sympathetic nervous system receptors.

Definitions

Autonomic nervous system②: Subdivision of the efferent peripheral nervous system that is largely under unconscious control(the somatic subdivision of the peripheral nervous system is largely under conscious control), shown in Figure 1-1.

Sympathetic nervous system③: A division of the autonomic nervous system (the other is the parasympathetic nervous system) that originates in nuclei of the central

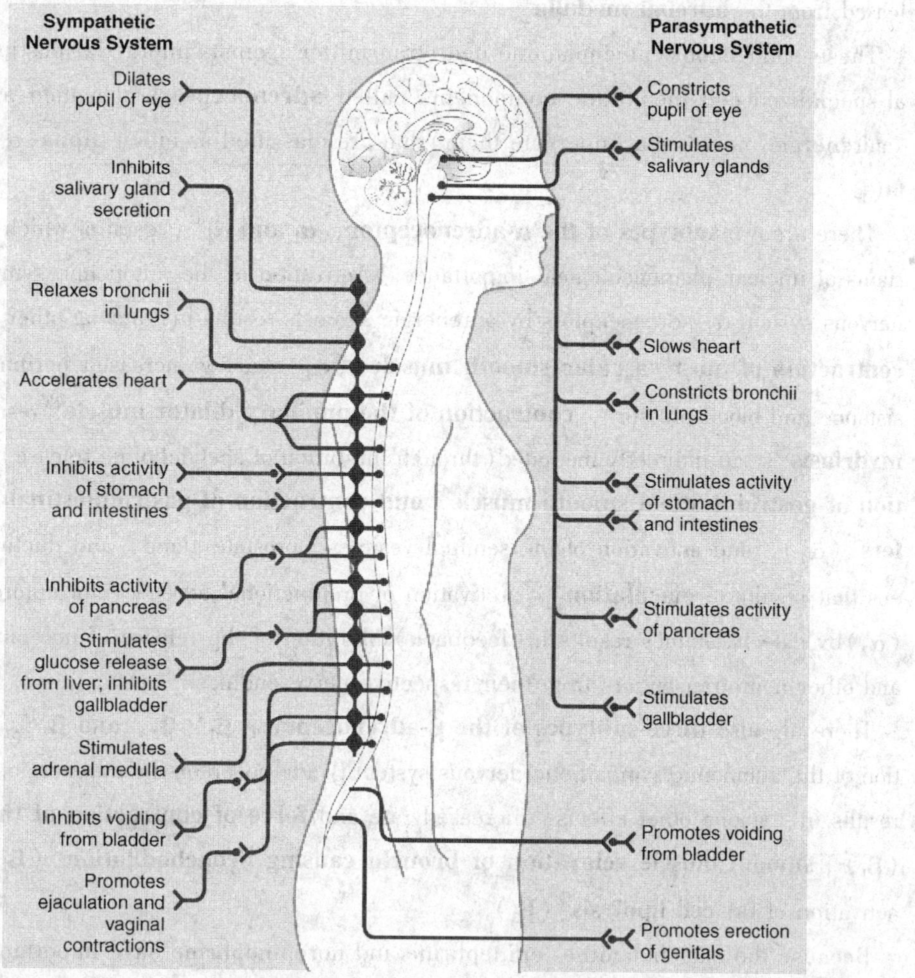

Figure 1-1. Schematic of autonomic nervous system.

nervous system. Preganglionic fibers exit through the **thoracic and lumbar spinal nerves**④ to synapse on ganglia close to the spinal cord and also on the adrenal medulla(considered a modified ganglia). Postganglionic fibers innervate a wide variety of effector organs and tissues, including arteriole and bronchial smooth muscle.

Agonist⑤: A drug that activates a receptor and results in a pharmacological response.

Antagonist⑥: A drug that binds to receptors with little or no effect of its own but that can block the action of an agonist that binds to the same receptors.

Discussion of Class

The neurotransmitter **norepinephrine**⑦ is released from the efferent nerves of the **sympathetic autonomic nervous system**⑧ at postganglionic sympathetic(also known as "adrenergic") nerve endings, whereas **epinephrine**⑨ **and some norepinephrine** are released from the **adrenal medulla**[10].

These endogenous catecholamine neurotransmitter agonists interact at postjunctional specialized cell membrane components called **adrenoceptors**[11] (named after the "adrenergic" nerves that innervate them) that are classified as either alpha(α) or beta(β).

There are two **subtypes of the α-adrenoceptor, α_1 and α_2**[12], each of which has variants of unclear pharmacological importance. Activation of the autonomic sympathetic nervous system α_1-adrenoceptors by adrenergic agonists results in, among other effects, **contraction of most vascular smooth muscle**[13] (α_1) causing increased peripheral resistance and blood pressure, **contraction of the pupillary dilator muscle**[14] resulting in **mydriasis**[15], an indirectly mediated (through inhibition of acetylcholine release) **relaxation of gastrointestinal smooth muscle**[16] **and contraction of gastrointestinal sphincters**[17] (α_1), and activation of the seminal vesicles, prostate gland, and ductus deferens that results in **ejaculation**[18]. Activation of prejunctional adrenoceptor autoreceptors (α_2) by catecholamines results in (feedback) inhibition of the release of norepinephrine and other neurotransmitters from their respective nerve endings.

There are also **three subtypes of the β-adrenoceptor, β_1, β_2, and β_3**[19]. Activation of the autonomic sympathetic nervous system β-adrenoceptors by adrenergic agonists results in, among other effects, increased rate and **force of contraction of the heart** (**β_1**), **smooth muscle relaxation of bronchi causing bronchodilation**[20] (**β_2**), and activation of **fat cell lipolysis**[21] (**β_3**).

Because the catecholamines epinephrine and norepinephrine have important physiological roles, drugs that block their actions, that is, adrenoceptor antagonists, can have important pharmacological effects, many of which are clinically useful. **α-adrenoceptor nonselective antagonists**[22] (e.g., phentolamine) are used to treat **pheochromocytoma**[23] (a tumor that secretes catecholamines) and **male erectile dysfunction**[24], whereas the more **selective α_1-adrenoceptor antagonists**[25] (e.g., prazosin, terazosin, doxazosin) are used to treat **hypertension**[26] **and benign prostatic hyperplasia**[27] (Table 1-1).

Structure

Epinephrine and norepinephrine are catecholamines, **synthesized from tyrosine**[28], that possess a catechol nucleus with an ethylamine side chain (epinephrine is the methylated side chain derivative of epinephrine). The **rate-limiting enzyme**[29] in this process is **tyrosine hydroxylase**[30].

Table 1-1

EFFECTS OF ADRENOCEPTOR ACTIVATION

ORGAN	EFFECTS (adrenoceptor subtype)
Bronchial smooth muscle	Dilates(β_2)
Heart rate and contractile force	Increases(β_1)
Eye(pupil size)	Dilates(α_1)[1]
Blood vessels	Constrict(α_1)[2,3]
Gastrointestinal tract(tone, motility, secretions)	Decrease(α_1, β_2)

[1] **Dilation(mydriasis)** results from α_1-adrenoceptor stimulation of the radial muscle.

[2] Skeletal muscle blood vessels have β_2-adrenoceptors that when activated result in **vessel constriction**.

[3] Coronary arteries have also have beta adrenoceptors that when activated the dominant effect is **vessel dilation**.

Mechanism of Action

Epinephrine binds to α_1-adrenoceptors and, through a G-protein(Gq-type GTP-binding protein[Gq])-mediated activation of phospholipase C and stimulation of polyphosphoinositide hydrolysis, results in formation of inositol 1,4,5-trisphosphate(IP_3)[31] that promotes the release of stored intracellular Ca^{2+}. Epinephrine perhaps also increases α_1-adrenoceptor mediated influx of Ca^{2+} across membrane channels. In addition to the increased formation of the "**second messenger**" **IP_3**[32], epinephrine also increases the phospholipase-mediated formation of another second messenger diacylglycerol(DAG) that activates protein kinase C that influences the activity of a number of other signaling pathways. Epinephrine also activates **β_1-and β_2-adrenoceptors to increase a G-protein-mediated stimulation of adenylyl cyclase**[33] **activity** thereby **increasing intracellular cyclic adenosine monophosphate(cAMP)**[34] **levels** and the activity of cAMP-dependent protein kinases.

Administration

Epinephrine is generally administered **parenterally**[35] (IM) for treatment of anaphylactic shock. For this and other conditions it is also available as IV, SC, ophthalmic, nasal, and aerosol preparations. Norepinephrine is only available for parenteral administration.

Pharmakocinetics

Epinephrine released from the adrenal gland is metabolized primarily by catechol-*O*-methyltransferase(COMT) and monoamine oxidase(MAO). The action of norepinephrine released from nerve endings is terminated primarily by reuptake into nerve terminals and other cells.

Comprehension Questions

[1.1] A patient with septic shock is noted to have persistent hypotension despite dopamine infusion. Epinephrine in an intravenous infusion is used. With which adrenoceptor does epinephrine act to constrict vascular smooth muscle?

A. α_1-adrenoceptors B. α_2-adrenoceptors

C. β_1-adrenoceptors D. β_2-adrenoceptors

[1.2] A 16-year-old male is having an acute asthmatic attack. Epinephrine is given subcutaneously. With which of the following adrenoceptors does epinephrine act to dilate bronchial smooth muscle?

A. α_1-adrenoceptors B. α_2-adrenoceptors

C. β_1-adrenoceptors D. β_2-adrenoceptors

[1.3] Which of the following best describes the cellular action of epinephrine?

A. Activation of adenylyl cyclase

B. Decreased activity of cAMP-dependent protein kinases

C. Increased intracellular stores of Ca^{2+}

D. Inhibition of the activity of phospholipase

[1.4] Epinephrine-mediated β_1-adrenoceptor activation results in

A. Constriction of bronchial smooth muscle

B. Decreased gastrointestinal motility

C. Dilation of the pupils

D. Increased heart rate

Answers

[1.1] **A.** α_1-adrenoceptors mediate vasoconstriction in many vascular beds. In skeletal muscle, epinephrine can act at β_2-adrenoceptors to cause vasodilation.

[1.2] **D.** Epinephrine acts on β_2-adrenoceptors to cause smooth muscle relaxation of bronchi resulting in bronchodilation. Because of adverse cardiovascular effects of epinephrine(β_1), more selective β_2-adrenoceptor agonists are now used(e.g., albuterol).

[1.3] **A.** Epinephrine activates α_1-adrenoceptors to cause a release of intracellular stored Ca^{2+} and β_1-and β_2-adrenoceptors to activate adenylyl cyclase.

[1.4] **D.** Epinephrine activation of β_1-adrenoceptors results in an increase in heart rate. Activation of α_1-adrenoceptors results in dilation of the pupil. Activation of β_2-adrenoceptors causes dilation of bronchial smooth muscle and decreased gastrointestinal(GI) motility.

PHARMACOLOGY PEARLS

- Physiologically, epinephrine acts as a hormone on distant cells after its release from the adrenal medulla.
- As one exception, sympathetic postganglionic neurons that innervate sweat glands release acetylcholine rather than norepinephrine.
- Exogenously administered epinephrine increases blood pressure through its action at β_1-adrenoceptors in the heart resulting in increased heart rate and force of contraction, and through its action at α_1-adrenoceptors in many vascular beds that results in vasoconstriction.
- In skeletal muscle, epinephrine injection can result in vasodilation(β_2) that in some cases may lead to a decreased total peripheral resistance and a decrease in diastolic pressure.
- Norepinephrine has little if any effect on β_2-adrenoceptors(norepinephrine and epinephrine have similar effects on α-and β_1-adrenoceptors), increasing both systolic and diastolic blood pressure.

REFERENCES

Goldstein S. β-blockers in hypertension and coronary heart disease. Arch Intern Med 1996; 156(12): 1267-76.

Graham RM, et al. Alpha1-adrenergic receptor subtypes. Molecular structure, function and signaling. Circ Res 1996; 78: 737-49.

Post SR, Hammond HR, Insel PA. Beta-adrenergic receptors and receptor signaling in heart failure. Ann Rev Pharmacol Toxicol 1999; 39: 343-69.

词汇

1. autonomic sympathetic nervous system[植物交感神经系统]
2. autonomic nervous system[自主神经系统]
3. Sympathetic nervous system[交感神经系统]
4. thoracic and lumbar spinal nerves[胸腰椎神经]
5. agonist[激动药]
6. antagonist[拮抗药]
7. norepinephrine[去甲肾上腺素]
8. sympathetic autonomic nervous system[交感自主神经系统]
9. epinephrine[肾上腺素]
10. adrenal medulla[肾上腺髓质]
11. adrenoceptors[肾上腺素受体]

12. subtypes of the α-adrenoceptor，α_1 and α_2［α-肾上腺素受体 α_1 和 α_2 亚型］
13. contraction of vascular smooth muscle［血管平滑肌收缩］
14. contraction of the pupillary dilator muscle［瞳孔开大肌］
15. mydrasis［瞳孔扩大］
16. relaxation of gastrointestinal smooth muscle［胃肠道平滑肌舒张］
17. contraction of gastrointestinal sphincters［胃肠道括约肌收缩］
18. ejaculation［射精］
19. subtypes of the β-adrenoceptor，β_1，β_2，β_3［β-肾上腺素受体 β_1、β_2、β_3 亚型］
20. bronchodilation［支气管扩张］
21. lipolysis［脂解作用］
22. α-adrenoceptor nonselective antagonists［非选择性 α-肾上腺素受体拮抗药］
23. pheochromocytoma［嗜络细胞瘤］
24. erectile dysfunction［勃起功能障碍］
25. selective α_1-adrenoceptor antagonist［选择性 α_1-肾上腺素受体拮抗药］
26. hypertension［高血压］
27. benign prostatic hyperplasia［良性前列腺增生］
28. tyrosine［酪氨酸］
29. rate-limiting enzyme［限速酶］
30. tyrosine hydroxylase［酪氨酸羟化酶］
31. inositol 1,4,5-trisphosphate（IP_3）［1,4,5-三磷酸肌醇］
32. second messager IP_3［第二信使 IP_3］
33. adenylyl cyclase［腺苷酸环化酶］
34. cyclic adenosine monophosphate（cAMP）［环磷酸腺苷］
35. parenterally［胃肠外］

注 1

青霉素又名苄青霉素和青霉素 G，属内酰胺类抗生素，通过抑制细菌细胞壁粘肽合成酶的活性，从而阻碍细菌细胞壁的合成而发挥抗菌作用。青霉素主要作用于革兰阳性、阴性球菌，嗜血杆菌，各种致病螺旋体和放线菌，A、B 组溶血性链球菌对其高度敏感，可用于治疗由溶血性链球菌感染引起的咽炎、扁桃体炎、丹毒、蜂窝组织炎、猩红热和产褥热等。

注 2

变态反应是药物不良的一种类型，青霉素所引起的变态反应是所有药物中较为常见且居首位的突出的不良反应，可出现药疹、药物热、哮喘发作等，甚至是过敏性休克。青霉素过敏是由于青霉素降解产物青霉噻唑蛋白、青霉烯酸等致敏原所致。过敏性休克多数发生在给药(包括皮试)后 30 分钟内，也有个别患者在持续用药 2 ~ 3 天后出现。青霉素过敏性休克如不及时救治，病人可迅速死亡。因此，为防止青霉素休克的发生，给药前必须详细询问药物过敏史，并进行青霉素皮肤过敏实验。皮试时，必须做好抢救准备，如肾上腺素注射液、氢化可的松等药物。

点评

患者肌肉注射青霉素 5 分钟之后出现青霉素过敏性休克。肾上腺素为 α、β 肾上腺素受体激动药，可通过激动较小动脉和毛细血管前括约肌上的 α 受体，明显收缩小动脉和毛细血管前括约肌，降低毛细血管的通透性，并可改善心脏功能，缓解呼吸困难，是抢救青霉素过敏性休克的首选药物。一旦发生青霉素过敏性休克，需立即停止使用青霉素，并迅速皮下或肌肉注射肾上腺素 0.5 ~ 1mg，5 ~ 10 分钟后根据病情和患者年龄等重复使用肾上腺素，用生理盐水稀释 10 倍后静脉注射。可同时应用突击量的糖皮质激素进行处理。在使用肾上腺素、激素后患者血压仍不回升，可应用血管活性药物如阿拉明等，使血压回复并维持在正常的水平。

李元建

❖ CASE 2

A 61-year-old man is noted to have increased intraocular pressure on a routine eye examination. The visual acuity is normal in both eyes. The dilated eye examination reveals no evidence of optic nerve damage. Visual field testing shows mild loss of peripheral vision. He is diagnosed with primary open-angle glaucoma and is started on pilocarpine ophthalmic drops.[注1]

◆ **What is the action of pilocarpine on the muscles of the iris and cilia?**

◆ **What receptor mediates this action?**

ANSWERS TO CASE 2: Muscarinic Cholinomimetic Agents①

Summary: A 61-year-old man with open-angle glaucoma is prescribed pilocarpine ophthalmic drops.

- **Action of pilocarpine② on muscles of the iris and cilia**: Constriction of the muscles. 注2
- **Receptor that mediates this action**: Muscarinic cholinoreceptor.

CLINICAL CORRELATION

Open-angle glaucoma is a disease caused by obstruction of the outflow of aqueous humor into the canal of Schlemm, causing an increase in intraocular pressure. The use of a direct acting muscarinic agonist, such as pilocarpine, causes contraction of the muscles of the cilia and iris. Because these are circular muscles, the pupil is constricted, which helps to relieve the outflow obstruction and lower the intraocular pressure. Although not common with the use of topical ophthalmic drops, bronchospasm and pulmonary edema has been noted with the use of pilocarpine drops. More commonly, blurred vision and myopia (near-sightedness) occur as a result of the impairment of accommodation caused by the contraction of the iris and ciliary muscles.

Muscarinic Cholinomimetic Agents

Objectives

1. Be able to list the receptors of the parasympathetic nervous system.
2. Contrast the actions and effects of direct and indirect stimulation of muscarinic cholinoreceptors.
3. List the therapeutic uses of parasympathomimetic agents.
4. List the adverse effects of parasympathomimetic agents.

Definitions

Parasympathetic Nervous System③: An anatomic division of the autonomic nervous system (the other is the sympathetic nervous system) that originates in nuclei of the central nervous system. Preganglionic fibers exit through **cranial and sacral spinal nerves④** to synapse via short postganglionic nerve fibers on ganglia, many of which are in the organs they innervate.

Cholinomimetic agents⑤: Agents that **mimic the action of acetylcholine (ACh)⑥**. These act directly or indirectly to activate **cholinoreceptors⑦**. Some directly acting agents (pilocarpine, bethanechol, carbachol) are designed to act selectively on either muscarinic or nicotinic cholinoreceptors whereas indirectly acting agents, which are acetylcholinesterase (AChE) inhibitors (such as neostigmine, physostigmine, edrophonium, demecarium) can activate both. Pilocarpine is a directly acting cholinomimetic agent that acts chiefly at muscarinic cholinoreceptors. Additional selectivity of pilocarpine and other cholinomimetics in the treatment of glaucoma is achieved by the use of an ophthalmic (topical) preparation.

Discussion of Class

The **efferent nerves of the parasympathetic autonomic nervous system**⑧ release the **neurotransmitter**⑨ **acetylcholine** at both preganglionic and post-ganglionic (aka "cholinergic") nerve endings, and also at somatic nerve endings. Nitric oxide is a cotransmitter at many of the parasympathetic post-ganglionic sites.

Acetylcholine (ACh)⑩ released from nerve endings of the parasympathetic nervous system interact at specialized cell membrane components called cholinoreceptors that are classified as either **nicotinic**⑪ **or muscarinic**⑫ after the alkaloids initially used to distinguish them.

Nicotinic cholinoreceptors⑬ are localized at **all postganglionic neurons**⑭ (the autonomic ganglia), including the adrenal medulla, and skeletal muscle endplates innervated by somatic nerves. **Muscarinic cholinoreceptors**⑮ are localized at **organs** innervated by parasympathetic postganglionic nerve endings, for example, on **cardiac atrial muscle**⑯, **sinoatrial node cells**⑰, **and atrioventricular node cells**⑱, where activation can cause a **negative chronotropic effect**⑲ and delayed atrioventricular conduction. Cholinergic stimulation of **muscarinic receptors** in the **smooth muscle**, **exocrine glands**, **and vascular endothelium**⑳ can cause, respectively, **bronchoconstriction**㉑, **increased acid secretion**, **and vasodilation**㉒ (**Table 2-1**).

Table 2-1

EFFECTS OF CHOLINORECEPTOR ACTIVATION

ORGAN	EFFECTS
Bronchial smooth muscle	Contracts
Heart rate	Decreases
Eye smooth muscles	
Pupil size	Contracts
Accommodation	Contracts
Blood vessels	Dilate[1]
Gastrointestinal tract (tone, motility, secretions)	Increase

[1] There is no parasympathetic innervation of blood vessels. However, they have cholinoreceptors that when activated result in their dilation.

There are **two subtypes of the nicotinic cholinoreceptors**: **N_N**, localized to **postganglionic neurons**, **and N_M**, localized to **the skeletal muscle endplates**[23]. There are three pharmacologically important subtypes of the **muscarinic cholinoreceptors**, **M_1, M_2, and M_3** (two additional subtypes have been identified by cloning), that alone or in combination are localized to sympathetic postganglionic neurons (and the central nervous system [CNS]), to the atrial muscle, sinoatrial (SA) cells and atrioventricular (AV) node of the heart, to smooth muscle, to exocrine glands, and to the vascular endothelium that does not receive parasympathetic innervation.

Directly and indirectly acting parasympathetic cholinomimetic agents, primarily pilocarpine and bethanechol, and neostigmine, are used most often therapeutically to treat certain diseases of the eye (acute angle-closure glaucoma), the urinary tract (urinary tract retention), the gastrointestinal tract (postoperative ileus), and the neuromuscular junction (myasthenia gravis). **Acetylcholine** is not used clinically because of its numerous actions and **very rapid hydrolysis by acetylcholinesterase (AChE)**[24] **and pseudocholinesterase**[25].

The adverse effects of direct and indirect acting cholinomimetics result from cholinergic excess and may include **diarrhea**[26], **salivation**[27], **sweating**[28], **bronchial constriction**[29], **vasodilation**, **and bradycardia**[30]. Nausea and vomiting are also common. Adverse effects of cholinesterase inhibitors (most often as a result of toxicity from pesticide exposure, e. g., **organophosphates**[31]) also may include **muscle weakness**[32], **convulsions**[33], **and respiratory failure**[34].

Structure

Acetylcholine (ACh) is a choline ester that is insoluble in lipids because of its **charged quaternary ammonium group**[35]. It **interacts with both muscarinic and nicotinic cholinoreceptors.** Choline esters similar in structure to acetylcholine that are used therapeutically include methacholine, carbachol, and bethanechol. Unlike ACh and carbachol, **methacholine**[36] **and bethanechol**[37] **are highly selective for muscarinic cholinoreceptors.** Pilocarpine is a tertiary amine alkaloid.

Mechanism of Action

Muscarinic cholinoreceptors activate **inhibitory G-proteins (G_i)**[38] to stimulate the activity of **phospholipase C**[39], which, through increased phospholipid metabolism, results in **production of inositol triphosphate (IP_3)**[40] and **diacylglycerol**[41] (**DAG**) that lead to the mobilization, respectively, of **intracellular calcium** from the endoplasmic and sarcoplasmic reticulum and, through activation of protein kinase C (PK-C), the opening of smooth muscle calcium channels with an influx of extracellular calcium. Activation of muscarinic cholinoreceptors also results in altered potassium flux that results in cell hyperpolarization, and in inhibition of adenylyl cyclase activity and cyclic adenosine monophosphate (cAMP) accumulation induced by other hormones, including the catecholamines.

The **nicotinic receptor** functions as a **cell membrane ligand-gated ion channel pore**㊷. On interaction with acetylcholine, the receptor undergoes a conformational change that results in **influx of sodium**㊸ with membrane depolarization of the nerve cell or the skeletal muscle neuromuscular endplate.

Indirectly acting parasympathetic cholinomimetic agents inhibit acetyl-cholinesterase and thereby increase acetylcholine levels at both muscarinic and nicotinic cholinoreceptors.

Administration

Directly acting muscarinic cholinomimetic agents may be administered topically as ophthalmic preparations (pilocarpine, carbachol), orally (bethanechol, pilocarpine), or parenterally (bethanechol). Depending on the agent, an indirectly acting cholinesterase inhibitor may be administered topically, orally, or parenterally.

Pharmacokinetics

Acetylcholine is synthesized from choline and acetyl-coenzyme A (acetyl-CoA) by the enzyme choline acetyltransferase and then transported into nerve ending vesicles. Like ACh, methacholine, carbachol, and bethanechol are poorly absorbed by the oral route and have limited penetration into the CNS. **Pilocarpine is more lipid soluble and can be absorbed and can penetrate the CNS.**

After release from nerve endings, acetylcholine is rapidly metabolized into choline and acetate, and its effects are terminated by the action of the enzymes AChE and pseudocholinesterase. Methacholine and particularly carbachol and bethanechol are resistant to the action of cholinesterases.

Comprehension Questions

[2.1] A 62-year-old woman is noted to have open-angle glaucoma. She inad-vertently applies excessive pilocarpine to her eyes. This may result in

A. Bronchial smooth muscle dilation
B. Decreased gastrointestinal motility
C. Dilation of blood vessels
D. Mydriasis

[2.2] Which of the following best describes the action of muscarinic cholinergic agonists?

A. Activate inhibitory G-proteins(G_i)

B. Decrease production of inositol triphosphate(IP_3)

C. Decrease release of intracellular calcium

D. Inhibit the activity of phospholipase C

[2.3] Which of the following adverse effects of choline esters like carbachol is most likely to occur?

A. Anhydrosis(dry skin)

B. Delirium

C. Salivation

D. Tachycardia(rapid heart rate)

Answers

[2.1] **C.** Excessive pilocarpine may initially result in dilation of blood vessels with a drop in blood pressure and a compensatory reflex stimulation of heart rate. Higher levels will directly inhibit the heart rate. In addition, pilocarpine stimulation of muscarinic cholinoreceptors can result in miosis, bronchial smooth muscle dilation and increased G_i motility.

[2.2] **A.** In addition to activating inhibitory G_i, muscarinic cholinergic agonists stimulate the activity of phospholipase C, increase production of IP_3 and increase release of intracellular calcium

[2.3] **C.** Diarrhea, salivation, and lacrimation may be seen. The heart rate is usually slowed. Choline esters do not cross the blood-brain barrier, and therefore delirium is not an adverse effect.

PHARMACOLOGY PEARLS

❖ Cholinoreceptors are classified as either nicotinic or muscarinic.

❖ Muscarinic cholinoreceptors are localized at organs such as the heart, causing a negative chronotropic effect.

❖ Stimulation of muscarinic receptors in the smooth muscle, exocrine glands, and vascular endothelium cause bronchoconstriction, increased acid secretion, and vasodilation.

❖ Methacholine and bethanechol are highly selective for muscarinic cholinoreceptors.

❖ Cholinomimetic agents, including anticholinesterase inhibitors, are precluded for treatment of gastrointestinal or urinary tract disease because of mechanical obstruction where therapy can result in increased pressure and possible perforation. They are also not indicated for patients with asthma.

REFERENCES

Felder C. Muscarinic acetylcholine receptors: Signal transduction through multiple effectors. FASEB J 1995; 9(8): 619-25.

Hoyng PF, van Beek LM. Pharmacological therapy for glaucoma: a review. Drugs 2000; 59(3): 411-34.

Millard CB, Broomfield CA. Anticholinesterases: medical applications of neurochemical principles. J Neurochem 1995; 64(5): 1909-18.

词汇

1. muscarinic cholinomimetic agent[毒蕈碱样拟胆碱药]
2. pilocarpine[毛果云香碱]
3. parasympathetic nervous system[副交感神经系统]
4. cranial and sacral spinal nervous[脑和脊髓骶神经]
5. cholinomimetic agent[拟胆碱药]
6. mimic the action of acetylcholine(ACh)[模拟乙酰胆碱作用]
7. cholinoreceptor[胆碱能受体]
8. efferent nerves of the parasympathetic autonomic nervous system[副交感自主神经系统传出神经]
9. neurotransmitter[神经递质]
10. acetylcholine (ACh)[乙酰胆碱]
11. nicotinic[烟碱]
12. muscarinic[毒蕈碱]
13. nicotinic cholinoreceptor[烟碱型胆碱受体,N 型胆碱受体]
14. postganglionic neurons[节后神经元]
15. muscarinic cholinoreceptor[毒蕈碱型胆碱受体,M 型胆碱受体]
16. cardiac atrial muscle[心房肌]
17. sinoatrial node cell[窦房结细胞]
18. atrioventricular node cell[房室结细胞]
19. negative chronotropic effect[负性频率作用]
20. vascular endothelium[血管内皮]
21. bronchoconstriction[支气管收缩]
22. vasodilation[血管舒张]
23. skeletal muscle endplates[骨骼肌终板]
24. acetylcholinesterase(AChE)[胆碱酯酶]
25. pseudocholinesterase[拟胆碱酯酶]
26. diarrhea[腹泻]
27. salivation[流涎]
28. sweating[出汗]
29. bronchial constriction[支气管收缩]
30. bradycardia[心动过缓]
31. organophosphates[有机磷酸]
32. muscle weakness[肌无力]
33. convulsion[抽搐惊厥]
34. respiratory failure[呼吸衰竭]
35. quaternary ammonium group[季铵基团]
36. methacholine[甲基胆碱]
37. bethanechol[氨甲酰甲胆碱]
38. inhibitory g-proteins(G_i)[抑制性 G 蛋白]
39. phospholipase C[磷脂酶 C]
40. inositol triphosphate (IP_3)[三磷酸肌醇]
41. diacylglycerol (DAG)[甘油二酯]
42. ligand-gated ion channel pore[配体门控离子通道]
43. influx of sodium[钠内流]

注 1

原发性青光眼分为闭角型青光眼和开角型青光眼（又称慢性单纯性青光眼）两种类型，其中开角型青光眼是最常见的一种青光眼。随着年龄增大，开角型青光眼的发病率增高，因此本例中的患者年龄为 61 岁。开角型青光眼患者房角虽然开放，但因小梁网及巩膜静脉窦发生变性或硬化，阻碍了房水循环，使房水不能有效的排出，引起眼内压增高。开角型青光眼早期症状轻微甚至没有，早期诊断主要依靠测定眼内压，晚期可出现视野缺损和视神经乳突凹陷。

注 2

匹罗卡品又名毛果芸香碱，为 M 胆碱受体激动药，对眼和腺体的作用最明显。可通过激动瞳孔括约肌上的 M 胆碱受体，使虹膜括约肌收缩，瞳孔缩小；通过缩瞳作用，使虹膜向中心拉紧，虹膜根部变薄，虹膜角膜角隙扩大，房水易于通过巩膜静脉窦而进入血液循环，使眼内压降低。

点评

开角型青光眼的治疗原则一般是先采用药物治疗，无效时再考虑手术治疗。治疗开角型青光眼的药物可分为五类：(1)缩瞳剂，如毛果芸香碱，通过引起睫状肌收缩，牵拉巩膜突并拉紧小梁网，以增加房水外流。(2)β-肾上腺素能受体阻滞剂，如噻吗洛尔，通过抑制睫状突上皮环腺苷酸的生成而减少房水生成。(3)α_2 肾上腺素受体激动剂，如可乐定，通过激动虹膜和睫状体的 α_2 受体，为减少房水生成，增加葡萄膜、巩膜房水外流。(4)前列腺素类药物，如拉坦前列素，通过增加葡萄膜巩膜外流而降低眼内压。(5)碳酸酐酶抑制剂，如有乙酰唑胺，通过抑制睫状上皮的碳酸酐酶的活性，从而减少房水的生成。

李元建

❖ CASE 3

A 53-year-old woman comes to see you for a consultation. She is scheduled to take a Caribbean cruise in 2 weeks but is concerned about sea sickness. She has been on boats before and is very sensitive to motion sickness. [注1] A friend mentioned to her that there is a patch that is effective for this problem. She is in good health and takes no medications regularly. Her examination is normal. You prescribe a scopolamine[①] transdermal patch for her.

◆ **What is the mechanism of action of scopolamine?**

◆ **What are the common side effects of this medication?**

◆ **What are some relative contraindications to its use?**

ANSWERS TO CASE 3: Muscarinic Cholinoreceptor[②] Antagonists

Summary: A 53-year-old woman with motion sickness is prescribed transdermal scopolamine before she takes a sea cruise.

- **Mechanism of action of scopolamine**: Competitive antagonist of muscarinic cholinoreceptors in the vestibular system and the central nervous system (CNS). [注2]
- **Common side effects**: Mydriasis, dry mouth, tachycardia, urinary retention, confusion, drowsiness.
- **Relative contraindications**[③]: Glaucoma, urinary obstruction, heart disease.

CLINICAL CORRELATION

Scopolamine, like other antimuscarinic agents, including the prototype atropine, is a selective competitive (surmountable) antagonist of acetylcholine (ACh) at muscarinic cholinoreceptors. Its actions can be overcome by increased concentrations of acetylcholine or other muscarinic cholinoreceptor agonists. **Scopolamine blocks muscarinic cholinoreceptors in the vestibular system and CNS to prevent motion sickness**[④]. It has a relatively long duration of action and can be given as a transdermal patch, making it well suited for the treatment of motion sickness.

In addition to motion sickness, muscarinic cholinoreceptor antagonists (e. g., benztropine) are used therapeutically to treat **Parkinson disease**[⑤]. Shortacting topical agents or ointments are used to facilitate ophthalmoscopic examination (e. g., cyclopentolate, tropicamide). Ipratropium bromide, a quaternary ammonium compound that does not cross the blood-brain barrier, is used to treat asthma and has efficacy in chronic obstructive pulmonary disease (COPD). Because it penetrates the CNS, a tertiary amine like atropine is used to counter the muscarinic cholinoreceptor effects of cholinergic excess resulting from organophosphate insecticide poisoning.

The **adverse effects of scopolamine and other muscarinic cholinoreceptor antagonists**[⑥] are related to inhibition of muscarinic cholinoreceptors in organ systems of the body. **Drowsiness**[⑦] **and sedation**[⑧] **are caused by actions on the CNS**. **Mydriasis**[⑨] is caused by blocking parasympathetic tone in the muscles of the cilia and iris. This could increase intraocular pressure in a person with **glaucoma**[⑩]. Cholinoreceptor blockade at the sinoatrial node results in **tachycardia**[⑪]. This could cause **arrhythmias**[⑫], especially in someone with underlying heart disease. The **urinary bladder**[⑬] **is relaxed** and the **urinary sphincter**[⑭] **constricted**, which may promote **urinary retention**[⑮]. Blockade of muscarinic cholinoreceptors in the salivary glands **reduces**

salivation[16], causing **dry mouth**[17]. Blockade of other muscarinic cholinoreceptors in the CNS can lead to **impairment of memory**[18], **confusion**[19], **restlessness**[20], **drowsiness, or hallucinations**[21].

Caution[22] **for muscarinic cholinoreceptor antagonist** drug use includes **angle-closure glaucoma**[23] (**contraindicated**), **open-angle glaucoma**[24], **urinary tract obstruction**[25] (e. g., prostatic hypertrophy), **cardiac disease, and gastrointestinal infections**[26], among others. Elderly patients are particularly sensitive to CNS effects.

Muscarinic Cholinoreceptor Antagonists

Objectives

1. Describe the mechanism of action of muscarinic cholinoreceptor antagonists.
2. Describe the physiologic effects of muscarinic cholinoreceptor antagonists.
3. List important therapeutic uses of muscarinic cholinoreceptor antagonists.
4. List the adverse effects and contraindications for muscarinic cholinoreceptor antagonists.

Discussion of Class

Cholinoreceptor antagonists are distinguished by their specificity for muscarinic and nicotinic cholinoreceptors. Muscarinic cholinoreceptor antagonists block the effects of acetylcholine at muscarinic cholinoreceptors in the parasympathetic autonomic nervous system and in the CNS. Nicotinic cholinoreceptor antagonists block the effects of acetylcholine at ganglia of the parasympathetic and sympathetic nervous system (and medulla), and at the neuromuscular junction.

Structure

Like atropine, the prototype muscarinic cholinoreceptor antagonist **scopolamine is a tertiary amine**[27]. As such, it has **ready access to the CNS** when administered parenterally, and it can be absorbed across the skin when combined with a suitable vehicle in a transdermal patch. **Quaternary amine antimuscarinic agents**[28], including **ipratropium bromide**[29], have **limited access to the CNS** and thus are used therapeutically for their peripheral effects.

Mechanism of Action

Interaction of scopolamine, atropine, or other antimuscarinic agents with muscarinic cholinoreceptors prevent the typical actions of acetylcholine such as activation of G-proteins and subsequent production of inositol triphosphate (IP_3), and diacylglycerol (DAG) that results in mobilization of calcium.

Administration

The patch formulation of scopolamine for motion sickness provides for up to 72 hours of pharmacological activity. Ipratropium bromide is administered topically to the airways as a metered-dose inhaler for asthma.

Pharmacokinetics

The duration of action of antimuscarinic agents range from less than a day (tropicamide) to 3-10 days (scopolamine, atropine).

Comprehension Questions

[3.1] A patient is prescribed a muscarinic cholinoreceptor antagonists with a quaternary amine group. Which of the following conditions is most appropriate for the patient to receive this medication?

A. A 50-year-old woman with angle-closure glaucoma
B. A 34-year-old man with gastrointestinal infectious enteritis
C. A 66-year-old man with mild dementia
D. A 56-year-old diabetic woman with urinary tract obstruction

[3.2] A 16-year-old teenager is going on his first deep sea fishing trip and is using a scopolamine patch to ward off sea sickness. Which of the following is the most likely adverse effect he will experience?

A. Bradycardia
B. Drowsiness
C. Miosis
D. Urinary urgency

[3.3] Cholinergic excess resulting from organophosphate insecticide poisoning can be treated with

A. Atropine
B. Digoxin
C. Ipratropium bromide
D. Tropicamide

Answers

[3.1] **C**. Muscarinic cholinoreceptor antagonists with quaternary amine groups do not penetrate the CNS and are therefore unlikely to impair memory. By blocking gastrointestinal motility, these agents can cause increased retention of infecting organisms.

[3.2] **B**. Scopolamine penetrates the CNS and can cause drowsiness and sedation. It also can cause mydriasis, tachycardia, and urinary retention.

[3.3] **A**. Atropine is a tertiary amine that can penetrate the CNS. In addition to its peripheral blocking actions it can also block the adverse CNS effects as a result of cholinergic excess. Tropicamide is also a tertiary amine. However, it has a very short duration of action and would be an unsuitable antidote. Ipratropium bromide is a charged quaternary ammonium compound that does not penetrate the CNS.

PHARMACOLOGY PEARLS

❖ Many antihistaminic agents, antipsychotic agents, and antidepressant agents have muscarinic cholinoreceptor antagonist (antimuscarinic) activity.

❖ Scopolamine is a tertiary amine and has ready access to the CNS when administered parenterally, whereas quaternary amine antimuscarinic agents such as ipratropium bromide have limited access to the CNS.

❖ Scopolamine can cause drowsiness and sedation, as well as mydriasis, tachycardia and urinary retention.

❖ Cholinoreceptor agonists cause symptoms of SLUD—**s**alivation, **l**acrimation, **u**rination, **d**iarrhea—whereas cholinoreceptor antagonists cause symptoms of anti-SLUD—dry mouth, dry eyes, urinary retention, constipation.

REFERENCES

Brodde O-E, Michel MC. Adrenergic and muscarinic receptors in the human heart. Pharmacol Rev 1999; 51(4): 651-90.

Eglen RM, Choppin A, Watson N. Therapeutic opportunities from muscarinic receptor research. Trends Pharmacol Sci 2001; 22(8): 409-14.

Gross NJ. Ipratropium bromide. N Engl J Med 1988; 319(8): 486-94.

词汇

1. scopolamine[东莨菪碱]
2. muscarinic cholinoreceptor[毒蕈碱型胆碱受体]
3. relative contraindications[相对禁忌证]
4. motion sickness[晕动病]
5. Parkinson disease[帕金森病]
6. muscarinic cholinoreceptor antagonists[毒蕈碱型胆碱受体拮抗药]
7. drowsiness[镇静]
8. sedation[催眠]
9. mydriasis[瞳孔散大]
10. glaucoma[青光眼]
11. tachycardia[心动过速]
12. arrhythmias[心律失常]
13. urinary bladder[膀胱]
14. urinary sphincter[尿道括约肌]
15. urinary retention[尿潴留]
16. reduce salivation[减少唾液分泌]
17. dry mouth[口干]
18. impairment of memory[记忆力受损]
19. confusion[意识错乱]
20. restlessness[坐立不安]

21. hallucinations［幻觉］
22. caution［慎用］
23. angle-closure glaucoma［闭角型青光眼］
24. open-angle glaucoma［开角型青光眼］
25. urinary tract obstruction［尿路梗阻］
26. gastrointestinal infections［胃肠道感染］
27. tertiary amine［叔胺］
28. quaternary amine antimuscarinic agents［季胺抗毒蕈碱剂］
29. ipratropium bromide［异丙托溴铵］

注 1

晕动病（motion sickness）即晕车病、晕船病、晕机病和由于各种原因引起的摇摆、颠簸、旋转、加速运动等所致疾病的统称，多发生于儿童和妇女，主要与影响前庭功能有关。本例的患者为53岁的妇女。前庭器内的囊斑或毛细胞受到一定量的不正常运动刺激所引起的神经冲动，可通过前庭神经传至前庭神经核，再传至小脑和下丘脑，引起一系列以眩晕为主要症状的临床表现如恶心、呕吐、血压下降和眼球震颤等。

注 2

东莨菪碱属阿托品类生物碱，为 M 胆碱受体竞争性拮抗药，对前庭和中枢神经系统 M 胆碱受体的选择性较高。本品小剂量可引起镇静，较大剂量有催眠作用，可用于晕动病和帕金森病的治疗以及麻醉前给药。此外，本品也可以阻断外周 M 胆碱受体，其抑制腺体分泌的作用强于阿托品，对心血管的系统的作用较阿托品弱，将其制成贴片经皮肤吸收可避免其外周作用而引起的口干、便秘、瞳孔散大和视力模糊等不良反应。

点评

晕动病发病时患者宜闭目仰卧；坐位时头部紧靠在固定椅背或物体上，避免较大幅度的摇摆；环境要安静，通风要良好。其药物治疗可以选用抗胆碱药物和抗组胺药物。前者如东莨菪碱，主要通过降低迷路 M 胆碱受体的应激性并抑制前庭小脑通路的传导而起到防晕止吐的作用；后者如苯海拉明，其止吐和防晕作用与阻断中枢 H_1 受体以及中枢抗胆碱作用有关。在旅行前 1.5～1 小时服用上述药物一次，可减轻症状或避免发病。

李元建

❖ CASE 4

A healthy 25-year-old man is undergoing a brief surgical procedure requiring general anesthesia. 注1 He underwent an unremarkable intubation and induction of anesthesia using IV succinylcholine and inhaled halothane. During the surgery the patient develops muscle rigidity and tachycardia, and his temperature rapidly rises.

◆ **What is the mechanism of action of succinylcholine?**

◆ **What reaction is occurring in the patient?**

◆ **What drug should immediately be given to the patient, and what is its mechanism of action?**

ANSWERS TO CASE 4: Skeletal Muscle Relaxants[注2]

Summary: A 25-year-old man develops muscle rigidity, tachycardia, and high fever during surgery.

- **Mechanism of action of succinylcholine**: Nicotinic receptor agonist at the motor endplate of the neuromuscular junction, which causes persistent stimulation and depolarization of muscle cells.
- **Reaction that is occurring**: Malignant hyperthermia.
- **Drug given for treatment and its mechanism of action**: Dantrolene, which acts by interfering with calcium release from the sarcoplasmic reticulum.

CLINICAL CORRELATION

Succinylcholine is the only depolarizing neuromuscular agent in wide clinical use. It is used for the rapid induction of a brief flaccid paralysis. It works as an agonist of the nicotinic receptor at the motor endplate of the neuromuscular junction. This causes a persistent stimulation and depolarization of the muscle, preventing stimulation of contraction by acetylcholine (ACh). It has a rapid onset and short duration of action because it is quickly hydrolyzed by plasma and liver cholinesterase. **Malignant hyperthermia**①, a rare but significant cause of anesthetic morbidity and mortality, is an inherited **autosomal dominant disorder**② that causes **tachycardia**③, **muscle rigidity, and high body temperatures** in response to the use of certain **inhaled anesthetics**④ in combination with **muscle relaxants**⑤, **usually succinylcholine**⑥. It is caused by a **release of calcium ions from the sarcoplasmic reticulum**⑦ **in muscle cells. Dantrolene**⑧ interferes with this release and is therefore the treatment of choice for this condition.

Pharmacology of Skeletal Muscle Relaxants

Objectives

1. Contrast the mechanism of action of depolarizing and nondepolarizing neuromuscular junction blocking agents.
2. List the therapeutic uses and adverse effects of skeletal muscle relaxants.

Discussion of Class

Neuromuscular blocking agents⑨ are classified as either **depolarizing**⑩ or **nondepolarizing** (**Table 4-1**) and are used mostly as adjuncts with general anesthetics to block motor endplate activity of acetylcholine at the neuromuscular junction. **Succinylcholine** is the prototype for **depolarizing agents** and used for **brief paralysis**[11] for surgery and for intubation. **Tubocurarine**[12], the prototype, and other **nondepolarizing agents**(e. g., cisatracurium, vecuronium, rocuronium) are used for **longer-term paralysis** for surgery.

Table 4-1

SELECTED SKELETAL MUSCLE RELAXANTS

TYPE OF AGENT	MECHANISM OF ACTION	SELECTED ADVERSE EFFECTS
Depolarizing agents (succinylcholine)	Persistent endplate depolarization and desensitization	Malignant hyperthermia, hyperkalemia, myalgia
Nondepolarizing agents (tubocurarine, cisatracurium vecuronium, rocuronium)	Reversible competitive antagonists that block the action of ACh at nicotinic cholinoreceptor	Hypotension, tachycardia

In addition to malignant hyperthermia, succinylcholine administration may result in **hyperkalemia**[13], particularly in patients with **burn and trauma**[14], which could result in **cardiac arrest**[15]. Myalgia is also commonly reported.

Certain **nondepolarizing agents** may produce **hypotension**[16], as a result of histamine release and some ganglionic blocking activity, and tachycardia as a result of vagolytic activity.

Numerous drug interactions between neuromuscular blocking agents and other drugs have been reported that lead to increased neuromuscular blockade, particularly with certain antibiotics and inhaled anesthetics.

Structure

The **neuromuscular blocking agents resemble acetylcholine**[17] (succinylcholine contains two linked acetylcholine molecules) and contain **one or two quaternary nitrogens**[18] that **limit entry into the central nervous system(CNS)**[19].

Mechanism of Action

After a single dose, **succinylcholine occupies the nicotinic receptor**[20] to produce a **persistent endplate depolarization**[21] (phase I block) that results in flaccid paralysis because the muscles become unresponsive to endogenously released acetylcholine. The initial depolarization is accompanied by muscle fasciculations. **Continued exposure of endplates to succinylcholine results in their repolarization**. However, through an unclear mechanism, they become relatively insensitive to subsequent depolarization (so-called desensitization, or phase Ⅱ block).

Nondepolarizing blocking agents act as reversible competitive antagonists that block the action of acetylcholine at nicotinic cholinoreceptors in muscle endplates and autonomic ganglia.

Cholinesterase inhibitors[②] (e.g., neostigmine, pyridostigmine) can effectively **antagonize and reverse the neuromuscular blocking action of nondepolarizing agents and succinylcholine during phase Ⅱ**. However, they will augment the action of succinylcholine during phase Ⅰ.

Administration

The neuromuscular blocking agents are **highly polar** and therefore must be administered parenterally.

Pharmacokinetics

Neuromuscular blocking agents are **highly ionized** and therefore have limited volume of distribution and **limited access to the CNS**.

Comprehension Questions

[4.1] Succinylcholine action when used as an adjunct to general anesthetics during surgery is based on its ability to

A. Block the action acetylcholine at the motor endplate.

B. Increase release of acetylcholine from autonomic ganglia.

C. Increase release of histamine from mast cells.

D. Inhibit cholinesterase.

[4.2] Continued exposure of muscle endplates to succinylcholine results in the

A. Development of diabetes mellitus

B. Enhanced sensitivity of muscle endplates to acetylcholine

C. Regeneration of muscle endplate acetylcholine receptors

D. Repolarization of muscle endplates

[4.3] Cholinesterase inhibitors can reverse the action of

A. Cisatracurium only B. Succinylcholine only

C. Both A and B D. Neither A or B

[4.4] A 35-year-old man undergoes surgery for a hernia repair. After the surgery, he complains of diffuse muscle aches, which the anesthesiologist states is likely caused by the skeletal muscle relaxant. He has a temperature of 37.8℃ (100℉). Which of the following is the most accurate statement?

A. The agent also commonly causes hypokalemia.

B. The agent blocks acetylcholine at the nicotinic receptor.

C. The agent causes persistent endplate depolarization and desensitization.

D. The patient likely has malignant hyperthermia.

Answers

[4.1] **A.** Succinylcholine acts like acetylcholine to cause depolarization of the muscle endplate. However, unlike acetylcholine, succinylcholine is not metabolized at the synapse. Therefore, the endplate remains depolarized and unresponsive to endogenous acetylcholine, resulting in muscle paralysis.

[4.2] **D.** Continued exposure of the muscle endplate to succinylcholine results in desensitization (phase Ⅱ block), where the endplate repolarizes but cannot readily be depolarized.

[4.3] **C.** Cholinesterase inhibitors like neostigmine can effectively antagonize and reverse the neuromuscular blocking action of nondepolarizing agents and succinylcholine during phase Ⅱ. However, they will augment the action of succinylcholine during phase Ⅰ.

[4.4] **C.** Myalgia (muscle aches) is a common adverse reaction of depolarizing agents such as succinylcholine; these agents also may induce hyperkalemia and malignant hyperthermia.

PHARMACOLOGY PEARLS

❖ Malignant hyperthermia is a rare autosomal dominant disorder characterized by tachycardia, muscle rigidity, and high body temperatures that occurs when the patient is exposed to inhaled anesthetics in combination with muscle relaxants, usually succinylcholine.

❖ Dantrolene interferes with the release of intracellular calcium and is therefore the treatment of choice for the muscle rigidity and hyperthermia associated with malignant hyperthermia.

❖ The neuromuscular blocking agents are highly polar and highly ionized and therefore, must be administered parenterally and have limited volume of distribution and limited access to the CNS.

❖ A small number of patients (1:10,000) with atypical cholinesterase experience long lasting apnea of 1-4 hours following succinylcholine. Mechanical ventilation is used to manage the apnea even though prescreening could detect this rare condition.

REFERENCES

Bevan DR. Reversal of neuromuscular blockade. Anesthesiology 1992; 77(4): 785-805.

Lee C. Structure, conformation, and action of neuromuscular blocking drugs. Br J Anaesth 2001; 87(5): 755-69.

Sparr HJ, Beaufort TM, Fuchs-Buder T. Newer neuromuscular blocking agents. How do they compare with established drugs? Drugs 2001; 61(7): 919-42.

词汇

1. malignant hyperthermia[恶性高热]
2. autosomal dominant disorder[常染色体显性疾病]
3. tachycardia 心动过速
4. inhaled anesthetics[吸入性麻醉剂]
5. muscle relaxants[肌松药]
6. succinylcholine[琥珀胆碱]
7. sarcoplasmic reticulum[肌浆网]
8. dantrolene[丹曲洛林]
9. neuromuscular blocking agents[神经肌肉阻断剂]
10. depolarizing[除极化]
11. brief paralysis[短暂麻痹]
12. tubocurarine[氯筒箭毒碱]
13. hyperkalemia[高钾血症]
14. burn and trauma[烧伤和损伤]
15. cardiac arrest[心脏停搏]
16. hypotension[低血压]
17. acetylcholine[乙酰胆碱]
18. nitrogen[氮]
19. central nervous system[中枢神经系统]
20. nicotinic receptor[烟碱性受体]
21. persistent endplate depolarization[持续性终板除极化]
22. cholinesterase inhibitor[胆碱酯酶抑制药]

注 1

全身麻醉药是一类能抑制中枢神经系统功能的药物。全身麻醉药作用于中枢神经系统(脑和脊髓),使其被抑制,从而使意识、感觉和反射暂时消失,骨骼肌松弛,主要用于外科手术麻醉。全身麻醉药可分为吸入麻醉药和静脉麻醉药。吸入麻醉药经呼吸道吸入而达到全身麻醉,为挥发性液体或气体,前者如乙醚、氟烷、异氟烷、恩氟烷等,后者如氧化亚氮;静脉麻醉药经静脉或肌肉注射而引起全身麻醉,常用的静脉麻醉药有硫喷妥钠、氯胺铜等。目前,吸入性全身麻醉药中最古老的氧化亚氮仍在临床广泛使用,乙醚、甲氧氟烷等现已基本不用,由恩氟烷、异氟烷、七氟烷、脱氟烷等替代。静脉全身麻醉药除硫喷妥钠外,尚有氯胺酮、依托咪酯、异丙酚等作用更好的新药相继补充。此外,各种新型肌肉松弛剂也替代了箭毒。

注 2

骨骼肌松弛药又称神经肌肉接头阻滞药,简称肌松药,主要作用于接头后膜处的乙酰胆碱 N_2 受体,能暂时干扰神经肌肉接头的兴奋(冲动)传导,产生一过性骨骼肌松弛。肌松药用于临床麻醉后改变了靠加深全麻获得肌肉松弛满足手术的要求。因此，肌松药已成为全麻时重要的辅助用药。此外，肌松药可用于机械通气病人。肌松药也可不同程度地作用在位于神经节细胞的 N_1 乙酰胆碱受体和 M(毒蕈碱样)乙酰胆碱受体，通过兴奋或抑制周围自主神经系统产生心血管效应。某些肌松药还具有组胺释放作用。这些肌松药的不良反应可导致血流动力学改变。

点评

恶性高热这种紊乱来自于并用去极化肌松药(通常为琥珀胆碱)和强的挥发性全身麻醉药(最常见为氟烷,还有异氟烷和七氟烷)引起的高代谢反应，出现威胁生命的体温升高，这种合并应用产生的效应类似于某些患有肌肉营养不良或肌强直病人的反应。受恶性高热影响的病人约为 1:20000，对这种疾患的易感性是由常染色体显性的病人经遗传而获得的。编码在斯里兰卡肉桂碱受体(钙释放通道)的基因变异可能引起这种疾患，这种机制看来和氟烷引起骨骼肌肌浆网中钙活性增强有关。敏感病人骨骼肌组织对钙呈现高反应性，其结果是，钙引起的生化反应加速了，引起了剧烈的肌肉收缩和代谢率加快。恶性高热可以发生在麻醉期和手术后的早期。临床表现不一，依所用的药物以及病人的敏感性而异。如发生恶性高热应立即停止吸入麻醉药及司可林的使用，大流量纯氧过度通气，准备治疗药物。更换回路及 CO_2 吸收罐，或高流量氧气冲洗回路。降温及纠正酸中毒。同时给予特效药物丹曲林(Dantrolene)，初剂量 2.5mg/kg，最大可达 10mg/kg，根据病情可用到更大，因为丹曲林的出现，如抢救处理及时，从理论上讲恶性高热的死亡率可降到零。

李 清

❖ CASE 5

A 65-year-old woman is admitted to the intensive care unit (ICU) of the hospital with sepsis caused by a urinary tract infection. [注1] She is hypotensive, with a blood pressure of 80/40 mmHg and has an elevated heart rate (tachycardia) and decreased urine output (oliguria). Along with the institution of appropriate antibiotic therapy and IV fluids, a decision is made to start her on an intravenous infusion of dopamine to attempt to raise her blood pressure.

◆ **What effects can be expected with low-dose dopamine?**

◆ **Which receptors mediate these effects?**

◆ **What effects occur with higher dose dopamine and which receptors mediate these?**

ANSWERS TO CASE 5: Sympathomimetic Agents

Summary: A 65-year-old woman in septic shock has persistent hypotension and oliguria requiring intravenous dopamine.

- **Effects of low-dose dopamine**: Reduces arterial resistance and increases blood flow in renal, coronary, and splanchnic systems; positive inotropic effect [注2]
- **Receptors involved**: β_1-receptors and specific dopamine receptors
- **Effects of higher dose dopamine and receptors involved**: Vasoconstriction mediated by α-receptors

CLINICAL CORRELATION

Dopamine is frequently used to treat cardiogenic or septic shock. The β_1-adrenoceptor mediated effects in the heart result in an increase in cardiac output with minimal peripheral vasoconstriction. This contributes to dopamine's ability to raise systolic blood pressure with no effect or only a slight effect on diastolic pressure. Specific dopamine receptors in the vasculature of the renal, coronary, and splanchnic systems allow for reduced arterial resistance and increased blood flow. At higher doses there is a peripheral α-adrenoceptor effect that overrides dopamine receptor-mediated vasodilation and results in vasoconstriction. The combination of renal blood-flow preservation, while supporting the blood pressure, is desirable in conditions of shock. This also contributes to increasing blood pressure. Prolonged high doses of dopamine can result in peripheral tissue necrosis because of the α-adrenoceptor-mediated vasoconstriction that reduces blood flow to the extremities, particularly in the digits.

Pharmacology of Autonomic Sympathetic Agents

Objectives

1. Outline the effects of sympathomimetic agents on peripheral organ systems.
2. List the major sympathomimetic agonists and their routes of administration.
3. Describe the therapeutic and adverse effects of the major sympathomimetic drugs.

Definitions

Sympathomimetic agents: Drugs that either directly or indirectly mimic all or some of the effects of epinephrine or norepinephrine.

Receptor Selectivity: Preferential binding (greater affinity) of a drug to a specific receptor group or receptor subtype at concentrations below which there is little if any interaction with another receptor group or subtype.

Discussion of Class

Sympathomimetic agents[1] act **directly** (e. g., epinephrine[2], norepinephrine, dopamine, dobutamine[3], phenylephrine, metaraminol[4], methoxamine[5], albuterol[6], terbutaline[7]) or indirectly (amphetamine[8], ephedrine[9]) to activate **α- and β-adrenoceptors**[10] (**Table 5-1**). Sympathomimetic agent adrenoceptor selectivity varies. Some are **nonselective** (e. g., ephedrine), whereas some have greater affinity for α-adrenoceptors (e. g., phenylephrine, metaraminol, methoxamine) or β_1-adrenoceptor (e. g., dobutamine, metaproterenol[11]) or β_2-adrenoceptor (e. g., terbutaline, albuterol) subgroups. However, selectivity is often lost as the dose of a sympathomimetic agent is increased. Compared to nonselective betareceptor agonists (isoproterenol[12]), **β_1-selective sympathomimetic agents may increase cardiac output**[13] **with minimal reflex tachycardia**[14]. **α_2-selective agents**, which **decrease blood pressure** by a prejunctional action in the central nervous system (CNS) (clonidine[15], methyldopa[16]), are used to treat hypertension. Fenoldopam is a potent D_1 agonist with a short half-life, useful in severe hypertension; its effects include decreasing systemic vascular resistance.

Dopamine interacts with specific subtypes of **dopamine receptors**[17] in the **periphery**[18] (**D_1 and D_2**). Stimulation of the D_1 receptor on the vasculature is principally vasodilation[19], and on the renal proximal tubules leads to natriuresis and diuresis; stimulation of the D_2 receptor on the presynaptic sympathetic nerve endings inhibits norepinephrine release. It also has direct and indirect sympathomimetic activity where, at lower doses, it has greater affinity for β-adrenoceptors than it does for α-adrenoceptors.

The clinical utility of a particular sympathomimetic agent depends on, among other factors, the specific organ system and receptor subtypes that are involved. In the **cardiovascular**[20] system, a reduction in blood flow by relatively selective α-adrenoceptor sympathomimetic agents is used to achieve surgical hemostasis, reduced diffusion of local anesthetics, and a reduction of mucous membrane congestion in hay fever and for the common cold. An increase in blood flow or blood pressure by α-adrenoceptor sympathomimetic agents is beneficial for the management of hypotensive emergencies (e. g., phenylephrine, methoxamine, norepinephrine) and chronic orthostatic hypotension (oral ephedrine). Sympathomimetic agents such as isoproterenol (and epinephrine) are also used for emergency short-term treatment of complete heart block and cardiac arrest.

Treatment of **bronchial asthma**[21] represents a major use of **β_2-selective sympathomimetic agents** (e. g., terbutaline, albuterol). Its effect is bronchodilation and relaxation of the smooth muscles of the bronchioles.

Ophthalmic examination[22] is facilitated with the use of the **directly acting α-adre-**

noceptor sympathomimetic agonist, phenylephrine. Phenylephrine (and the indirectly acting sympathomimetic agent, cocaine) is also used to localize the lesion in Horner's syndrome. In addition to β-adrenoceptor blocking agents, α-selective agents (e. g., apraclonidine) are used to lower intraocular pressure in glaucoma.

Table 5-1

AUTONOMIC NERVOUS SYSTEM EFFECTS[1]

ORGAN	ADRENERGIC RECEPTOR/ACTION	MUSCARINIC CHOLINERGIC RECEPTOR/ACTION
Heart	β_1—increased heart rate and contractility	Decreased heart rate and contractility
Blood vessels[2]	α_1—constriction β_2—dilation	Dilation
Bronchi	β_2—bronchial smooth muscle relaxation	Bronchial smooth muscle contraction
GI tract	α_1—sphincter contraction β_2—relaxation	Overall contraction Relaxation of spincter
Kidney	β_1—renin release	No effect
Urinary bladder	α_1—sphincter contraction β_2—wall relaxation	Wall contraction Spincter relaxation
Adipose tissue	β_1—increased lipolysis	No effect
Eye	α_1—radial muscle contraction with pupil dilation	Sphincter muscle contraction with pupil constriction Ciliary muscle contraction

[1] Also see Figure 1-1.

[2] No direct parasympathetic innervation

The peripheral adverse effects of the sympathomimetic agents are generally an extension of their pharmacological effects. These are most often cardiovascular in nature, particularly when they are administered parenterally, and may include increased blood pressure, arrhythmias, and cardiac failure.

Structure

Sympathomimetic agents, as well as norepinephrine and epinephrine, are **derived from phenylethylamine**[23]. Substitutions on the amino group, the benzene ring or the alpha or beta carbon markedly alter the selectivity, activity and metabolism of the sympathomimetic agents. For example, alkyl substitutions on the amino group tends to markedly increased β-adrenoceptor selectivity.

Mechanism of Action

Directly acting sympathomimetic agents bind to and activate adrenoceptors to mimic the actions of epinephrine or norepinephrine. Indirectly acting sympathomimetic agents mimic the actions of norepinephrine by either displacing or inhibiting its reuptake from adrenergic nerve endings.

Administration

Sympathomimetic agents are available for administration by **topical**, **nasal**, **oral**, **ophthalmic**, **and parenteral routes** depending on the drug and condition being treated.

Pharmacokinetics

Like the catecholamines norepinephrine and epinephrine, direct and indirect sympathomimetic agent may be subject to **metabolism and inactivation** by **catechol-*O*-methyltransferase(COMT)**[24] **and monoamine oxidase(MAO)**[25]. Phenylephrine is not metabolized by COMT, whereas metaraminol and methoxamine are not substrates for either COMT or MAO. Their durations of action, therefore, are relatively long(20-60 minutes).

Comprehension Questions

[5.1] A 25-year-old man is noted to be in septic shock. A low-dose dopamine infusion is administered, and will likely

A. Decrease cardiac output.

B. Decrease systolic blood pressure.

C. Increase renal blood flow.

D. Produce significant peripheral vasoconstriction.

[5.2] In contrast to norepinephrine, metaraminol, and methoxamine are metabolized by

A. COMT B. MAO C. Both D. Neither

[5.3] Which of the following is the most accurate statement?

A. α-adrenoceptor sympathomimetic agonists are used to reduce mucous membrane congestion.

B. α-adrenoceptor agonists are used to treat bronchospasm.

C. β-adrenoceptor agonists are used to reduce surgical bleeding.

D. β_2-adrenoceptor agonist agents are used to prolong local anesthesia.

Answers

[5.1] **C.** Dopamine binding to specific dopamine receptors in the vasculature in the kidney increases renal blood flow. Cardiac output is increased by dopamine action on β_1-adrenoceptors. Dopamine causes minimal peripheral vasoconstriction.

[5.2] **D.** Metaraminol and methoxamine are not substrates for either COMT or MAO and have a longer duration of action than norepinephrine, which is a substrate for both.

[5.3] **A.** α-adrenoceptor sympathomimetic agents will cause vasoconstriction and thereby reduce mucous membrane congestion.

PHARMACOLOGY PEARLS

❖ β_1-selective sympathomimetic agents may increase cardiac output with minimal reflex tachycardia.

❖ α_2-selective agents decrease blood pressure by a prejunctional action in the CNS.

❖ Terbutaline and albuterol are preferred over ephedrine for relieving the bronchoconstriction of asthma, and other bronchial conditions, because of their greater bronchiolar selectivity.

❖ Dopamine binding to specific dopamine receptors in the vasculature in the kidney increases renal blood flow. Cardiac output is increased by dopamine action on β_1-adrenoceptors. Low-dose dopamine causes minimal peripheral vasoconstriction.

REFERENCES

Graham RM, et al. Alpha$_1$-adrenergic receptor subtypes. Molecular structure, function and signaling. Circ Res 1996; 78(5): 737-49.

Insel PA, Feldman RD. β-adrenergic receptors in health and disease. Boca Raton, FL: CRC 1994.

Limbird E, ed. The alpha$_2$-adrenergic receptors. Clifton, NJ: Humana, 1988.

Missale C, et al. Dopamine receptors: from structure to function. Physiol Rev 1998; 78(1): 189-225.

词汇

1. sympathomimetic agents[拟交感神经药]
2. epinephrine[肾上腺素]
3. dobutamine[多巴酚丁胺]
4. metaraminol[间羟胺]
5. methoxamine[甲氧明]
6. albuterol[沙丁胺醇]
7. terbutaline[特布他林]
8. amphetamine[安非他命]
9. ephedrine[麻黄碱]
10. α-and β-adrenoceptor[α-和 β-肾上腺素受体]
11. metaproterenol[奥西那林]
12. isoproterenol[异丙肾上腺素]
13. cardiac output[心输出量]
14. reflex tachycardia[反射性心动过速]
15. clonidine[可乐定]
16. methyldopa[甲基多巴]
17. dopamine receptor[多巴胺受体]
18. periphery[外周]
19. vasodilation[血管舒张]
20. cardiovascular[心血管的]
21. bronchial asthma[支气管哮喘]
22. hypoglycemic examination[眼科检查]
23. phenylethylamine[苯乙胺]
24. catechol-*O*-methyltransferase(COMT)[儿茶酚-邻-甲基转移酶]
25. monoamine oxidase(MAO)[单胺氧化酶]

注 1

在尿路感染的治疗中，急性膀胱炎症状轻的可给予口服氧氟沙星或环丙沙星、头孢拉定、阿莫西林、复方新诺明等，选其中一种即可。疗程 2～3 天，甚至有的抗生素单剂量也行。对于症状较重的可肌注 3 天庆大霉素或丁胺卡那霉素，必要时加用阿托品或黄酮哌酯片。急性肾盂肾炎在药敏试验结果未弄清楚之前，可凭经验选择抗生素。一般可用庆大霉素或丁胺卡那霉素肌注，或氨苄青霉素静脉给药。如症状减轻可继续治疗 1 周，然后改用适当的抗生素口服 2 周。

注 2

多巴胺为体内合成肾上腺素的前体，具有 β 受体激动作用，也有一定的受体激动作用。能增强心肌收缩力，增加排血量，加快心率作用较轻微(不如异丙肾上腺素明显)；对周围血管有轻度收缩作用，升高动脉压，对内脏血管(肾、肠系膜、冠状动脉)则使之扩张，增加血流量；使肾血流量及肾小球滤过率均增加，从而促使尿量及钠排泄量增多。用于各种类型休克，包括中毒性休克、出血性休克、中枢性休克、特别对伴有肾功能不全、心排出量降低、周围血管阻力增高而已补足血容量的病人更有意义。

点评

激动交感神经系统肾上腺素受体和位于肾、肠系膜、冠状动脉、脑动脉的多巴胺受体其效应为剂量依赖性。(1)小剂量的多巴胺：即用量2~5微克/(公斤·分)。主要是通过激动多巴胺受体起作用。多巴胺受体除存在于中枢神经系统外，还存在于肾、肠系膜、脑和冠状血管。外源性多巴胺不能透过血脑屏障。多巴胺受体被激动的结果是使血管扩张，肾血流量增加尤其明显，肾小球滤过率增加，从而产生强大的利尿作用，并使尿钠增加。小剂量的多巴胺还能使总血管外周阻力降低，血压下降。(2)中等剂量的多巴胺：即用量6~10微克/(公斤·分)。可直接兴奋心脏的β受体，使心肌收缩力增强，心输出量增加，对心率影响不明显；能扩张冠状动脉；还能作用于交感神经末梢，使之释放去甲肾上腺素。(3)大剂量的多巴胺：即用量>10微克/(公斤·分)。主要兴奋血管α受体，对全身血管(除冠状动脉外)均产生强烈收缩反应，使血压升高，总外周血管阻力增高。通过兴奋β_1受体，使心肌收缩力增强，心率增快心肌耗氧量明显增加。大剂量时，由于它对肾血管的强烈收缩作用，使肾血流量减少。总之，小剂量多巴胺主要有扩张血管作用，使总外周阻力降低，对心脏前、后负荷均有降低。大剂量多巴胺以兴奋α、β受体为主，使心率加快，心肌收缩力增强，血管总外周阻力高，心肌耗氧量增加。

李 清

❖ CASE 6

A 70-year-old man is seen in follow-up at your office after he has been hospitalized for a myocardial infarction (MI). He underwent successful angioplasty and is currently asymptomatic. Prior to his MI, he was on no medications. He is not a smoker and is not diabetic. During his hospitalization, he was noted to have persistently elevated blood pressure readings. He had asthma as a child, but has not had any recent wheezing episodes. While in the hospital, he was started on oral metoprolol.

◆ **Metoprolol is selective for which adrenoceptor?**

◆ **What effects do agents such as metoprolol have on the cardiovascular system?**

◆ **In which organ is metoprolol primarily metabolized?**

◆ **Why must β-adrenergic antagonists be used with caution in asthmatics?**

ANSWERS TO CASE 6: Adrenoceptor Antagonists

Summary: A 70-year-old hypertensive man with a childhood history of asthma had a recent myocardial infarction and is prescribed metoprolol.

- **Adrenoceptor selectively antagonized by metoprolol**: β_1
- **Effect of β-adrenoceptor antagonists on the cardiovascular system**: Reduction of sympathetic-stimulated increases in heart rate, contractility and cardiac output; lower blood pressure as a result of effects on the heart, renin-angiotensin system, and central nervous system (CNS); increased atrioventricular (AV) conduction time and refractoriness.
- **Organ in which metoprolol is metabolized**: Liver.
- **Reason for caution in use in asthmatics**: Blockade of β_2-adrenoceptor in bronchial smooth muscle may cause increased airway resistance and bronchospasm.

CLINICAL CORRELATION

β-adrenergic receptor antagonists are widely used in medicine, primarily for their beneficial effects on the cardiovascular system and for lowering intraocular pressure in patients with glaucoma. Both the nonselective β-adrenoreceptor antagonists and the relatively β_1-adrenoceptor selective antagonists are used to treat hypertension. The mechanism of their action is multifactorial, probably including reduction in cardiac output, reduction in renin release and some CNS effect. They are also beneficial for treating coronary artery disease and postmyocardial infarction patients as they reduce sympathetic-stimulated increases in heart rate and contractility. This helps to reduce myocardial oxygen demand, providing prophylaxis for angina. **β-adrenoceptor antagonists**① **have a proven benefit in prolonging survival after heart attacks**②. They lengthen AV conduction time and refractoriness and suppress automaticity. This helps to prevent both supraventricular and ventricular arrhythmias. Caution must be used when giving β-blockers to patients with asthma, chronic obstructive pulmonary disease and diabetes. All β-adrenoceptor blockers, including those that are β_1-adrenoceptor selective, have some β_2-adrenoceptor antagonist activity and **may cause bronchospasm**③ by their effects on bronchial smooth muscle. They **can also mask the symptoms of hypoglycemia**④ in a diabetic by blocking the adrenergic stimulated symptoms of tremor, tachycardia, and nervousness that would normally occur.

Pharmacology of Adrenoceptor Agonists

Objectives

1. Describe the therapeutic uses and adverse effects of α-adrenoceptor antagonists.
2. Describe the therapeutic uses and adverse effects of α-adrenoceptor antagonists.
3. Contrast the differences between the nonselective and relatively β_1-selective adrenoceptor antagonists.

Definitions

Pheochromocytoma⑤: A tumor of the adrenal medulla that releases excess levels of epinephrine and norepinephrine that can result in hypertension, cardiac anomalies, and severe headache.

Myocardial Infarction⑥: Death of cardiac muscle as a result of ischemia.

Discussion of Class

There are two classes of clinically important α-adrenoceptor antagonists: nonselective antagonists and selective α_1-antagonists. **Phentolamine**⑦, **a nonselective**, **competitive α-adrenoceptor antagonist**, and **phenoxybenzamine**⑧, a **nonselective**, **noncompetitive α-adrenoceptor antagonist** are used for the preoperative management of the marked catecholamine-induced **vasoconstriction**⑨ associated with **pheochromocytoma**. **Prazosin**⑩ and other **α_1-adrenoceptor selective antagonists** (doxazosin, terazosin) are used to manage **chronic mild to moderate hypertension**⑪ and **benign prostatic hypertrophy**⑫.

In addition to the nonselective β-adrenoceptor antagonists, there are two classes of clinically important selective β-adrenoceptor antagonists, β_1 and β_2 (Table 6-1). The

Table 6-1

BETA-ADRENOCEPTOR ANTAGONIST SELECTIVITY

Nonselective β-Adrenoceptor Antagonists
Propranol[注1]
Nadolol
Timolol
Selective β_1-Adrenoceptor Antagonists
Atenolol
Metoprolol
Esmolol
Non-selective β- and α_1-Adrenoceptor Antagonists
Labetalol
Carvedilol

major clinical uses for β-adrenoceptor antagonists include ischemic heart disease, cardiac arrhythmias, hypertension, hyperthyroidism, and glaucoma. Ischemic heart disease is managed with nonselective β-adrenoceptor antagonists, propranolol, timolol, and nadolol, as well as β_1-adrenoceptor selective antagonists, metoprolol, atenolol, and esmolol. **Cardiac arrhythmias**⑬ are managed, depending on the arrhythmia, with **propranolol**⑭ **and esmolol**⑮. **Hypertension** is managed with a wide variety of **nonselective and β_1-adrenoceptor selective antagonists**, except esmolol. **Timolol**⑯ and other β-adrenoceptor antagonists are used to manage **glaucoma**⑰ by decreasing aqueous humor production and thereby reducing intraocular pressure.

Labetalol⑱ (and several other agents, including carvedilol), **blocks both β-and α-adrenoceptors in a 3:1 ratio**. Labetalol **lowers blood pressure** by **decreasing systemic vascular resistance** without any major effect on heart rate or cardiac output. It is used to treat hypertensive emergencies and hyper-tension from **pheochromocytoma**. Table 6-2 has a listing of selected sympa-thomimetic agents.

Table 6-2

SELECTED DRUGS AND THEIR EFFECTS ON THE AUTONOMIC NERVOUS SYSTEM

DRUG	ADRENOCEPTOR ACTIVITY	MECHANISM OF ACTION	CLINICAL USE
Epinephrine	Nonselective α- and β-adrenoceptor agonist	Bronchial smooth muscle dilation	Asthma and other allergic diseases to relax airways and reduce swelling
Phenylephrine	α_1-adrenoreceptor stimulation	Vasoconstriction	Rhinitis and colds as decongestant
Propranolol	Nonselective β-adrenoceptor agonist	Decreases heart rate, cardiac contractility	Hypertension, coronary heart disease
Albuterol	β_2-adrenoceptor agonist	Bronchial smooth muscle dilation	Asthma
Phentolamine	Nonselective competitive α-adrenoceptor antagonist	Vasodilation	Preoperative management of the marked catecholamine-induced vasoconstriction associatedwith pheochromocytoma
Prazosin	α_1-adrenoreceptor selective anatagonists	Vasodilation	Chronic mild to moderate hypertension and benign prostatic hypertrophy

The **major adverse effects**[19] **of nonselective β-adrenoceptor antagonists** are **cardiac stimulation**, primarily **tachycardia**[20] because of baroreflex mediated sympathetic discharge, and **postural hypotension**[21]. Additional cardiac stimulation by phentolamine may be caused by antagonist activity at prejunctional α_2-adrenoceptors that results in increased norepinephrine release. (Prazosin and other selective α_1-adrenoceptor selective antagonists are less likely to cause reflex tachycardia). A β-adrenoceptor antagonist may be required to counter the cardiac effects.

The **major adverse effects of nonselective β-adrenoceptor antagonists** are related to their effects on **bronchial smooth muscle**[22] **and on carbohydrate**[23] **metabolism. Blockade of β_2-receptors in smooth muscle may increase airway resistance in patients with asthma**[24] **or other airway obstruction diseases**. Although the clinical use of a selective β_1-adrenoceptor antagonist may offer some protection in patients with asthma, the selectivity of these agents is not great, and therefore they should be used judiciously, if at all. In patients with **insulin-dependent diabetes**[25], **nonselective β-adrenoceptor antagonists** increase the incidence and severity of **hypoglycemic episodes**[26]. The use of selective β_1-adrenoceptor antagonists in patients with this condition offers some potential benefit.

Mechanism of Action

α-adrenoceptor antagonists and β-adrenoceptor antagonists interact directly, and either competitively or irreversibly with, respectively, α-adrenoceptors and β-adrenoceptors to block actions of the endogenous catecholamines, norepinephrine and epinephrine, and exogenously administered sympathomimetic agents.

Administration

α-and β-adrenoceptor antagonists are administered orally or parenterally. β-adrenoceptor antagonists are also available for ophthalmic application.

Pharmacokinetics

Metoprolol and propranolol[注2] undergo extensive and variable interindividual first-pass hepatic metabolism resulting in relatively low bioavailability. Oral sustained-release preparations of these agents are available. Drugs that inhibit cytochrome P_{450} 2D6 may decrease the metabolism of carvedilol. Esmolol is ultra-short-acting as a result of its ester linkage that is rapidly metabolized by plasma esterases.

Comprehension Questions

[6.1] Which of the following actions of epinephrine are blocked by prazosin?

A. Bronchial dilation B. Increased cardiac stroke volume
C. Increased heart rate D. Mydriasis

[6.2] A 34-year-old man is prescribed labetalol for hypertension. The effect on the cardiovascular system is a result of its action as an antagonist at

A. α-adrenoceptors only B. β-adrenoceptors only
C. Both α-and β-adrenoceptors D. Muscarinic cholinoreceptors

[6.3] Which of the following is the least likely clinical use for β-adrenoceptor antagonists?

A. Benign prostatic hypertrophy B. Cardiac arrhythmias
C. Hypertension D. Ischemic heart disease

Answers

[6.1] **D.** Prazosin is an α-adrenoceptor antagonist that will block epinephrine mediated contraction of the radial smooth muscle of the eye that results in mydriasis. All the other actions listed are mediated by β-adrenoceptors, which would be blocked by β-adrenoceptor antagonists like propranolol.

[6.2] **C.** Labetalol blocks both β- and α-adrenoceptors. It lowers blood pressure by decreasing systemic vascular resistance (α-adrenoceptor antagonist activity), without any major effect on heart rate or cardiac output (β-adrenoceptor antagonist activity).

[6.3] **A.** β-adrenoceptor antagonists are used therapeutically to manage ischemic heart disease, cardiac arrhythmias, and hypertension. α_1-adrenoceptor selective antagonists are used to manage benign prostatic hypertrophy.

PHARMACOLOGY PEARLS

❖ α_1-adrenoceptor selective antagonists such as doxazosin and terazosin are used for mild chronic hypertension and benign prostatic hypertrophy.

❖ The major clinical uses for β-adrenoceptor antagonists include ischemic heart disease, cardiac arrhythmias, hypertension, hyperthyroidism, and glaucoma.

❖ The **major adverse effects of nonselective β-adrenoceptor antag-onists** are related to their effects on **bronchial smooth muscle** (increased airway resistance in asthmatics) and on **carbohydrate metabolism** (hypoglycemia in **insulin-dependent diabetics**).

REFERENCES

Cruickshank JM, Prichard BNC. Beta-blockers in clinical practice, 2nd ed. London: Churchill Livingstone, 1994.

Piascik MT, Perez DM. Alpha 1-adrenergic receptors: New insights and directions. J Pharmacol Exp Ther 2001; 293(2): 403-10.

词汇

1. β-adrenoceptor antagonist[β-肾上腺素受体拮抗剂]
2. heart attack[心脏病发作]
3. bronchospasm[支气管痉挛]
4. hypoglycemia[低血糖]
5. pheochromocytoma[嗜铬细胞瘤]
6. myocardial infarction[心肌梗死]
7. phentolamine[酚妥拉明]
8. phenoxybenzamine[酚苄明]
9. vasoconstriction[血管收缩]
10. prazosin[哌唑嗪]
11. hypertension[高血压]
12. prostatic hypertrophy[前列腺肥大]
13. cardiac arrhythmias[心律失常]
14. propranolol[普萘洛尔]
15. esmolol[艾司洛尔]
16. timolol[噻吗洛尔]
17. glaucoma[青光眼]
18. labetalol[拉贝洛尔]
19. adverse effect[副作用]
20. tachycardia[心动过速]
21. postural hypotension[直立性低血压]
22. bronchial smooth muscle[支气管平滑肌]
23. carbohydrate[碳水化合物,糖类]
24. asthma[哮喘]
25. insulin-dependent diabetes[胰岛素依赖性糖尿病]
26. hypoglycemic episode[低血糖发作]

注 1

普萘洛尔为β肾上腺素受体阻断药(β阻滞剂)，阻断心肌的β受体，减慢心率，抑制心脏收缩力与房室传导，循环血流量减少，心肌氧耗量降低。它可抑制肾素的释放，故血浆肾素的浓度下降。临床上用于治疗多种原因所致的心律失常，如房性及室性早搏(效果较好)、窦性及室上性心动过速，心房颤动等，但室性心动过速宜慎用。锑剂中毒引起的心律失常，当其他药物无效时，可试用本品。

此外，也可用于心绞痛、高血压、嗜铬细胞瘤(手术前准备)等。治心绞痛时，常与硝酸酯类合用，可增高疗效，并互相抵消其副作用。对高血压有一定疗效，不易引起直立性低血压为其特点。

注 2

美托洛尔属于心脏选择性β受体阻断药，它对β_1受体有选择性阻断作用，无PAA(部分激动活性)，无膜稳定作用。其阻断β受体的作用约与普萘洛尔(PP)相等，对β_1-受体的选择性稍逊于阿替洛尔。美托洛尔对心脏的作用如减慢心率、抑制心收缩力、降低自律性和延缓房室传导时间等与普萘洛尔、阿替洛尔（AT）相似，其降低运动试验时升高的血压和心率的作用也与PP、AT相似。其对血管和支气管平滑肌的收缩作用较PP为弱，因此对呼吸道的影响也较小，但仍强于AT。美托洛尔用于治疗高血压、心绞痛、心肌梗死、肥厚型心肌病、主动脉夹层、心律失常、甲状腺功能亢进、心脏神经官能症等。近年来尚用于心力衰竭的治疗，此时应在有经验的医师指导下使用。

点评

肾上腺素受体阻断药能阻断肾上腺素受体从而拮抗去甲肾上腺素能神经递质或肾上腺素受体激动药的作用。对于整体动物，它们的作用强度取决于机体的去甲肾上腺素能神经张力。这类药物按对α和β肾上腺素受体选择性的不同，分为α肾上腺素受体阻断药（简称α受体阻断药）和β肾上腺素受体阻断药（β受体阻断药）二大类。α受体阻断药能选择性地与α肾上腺素受体结合，其本身不激动或较少激动肾上腺素受体，却能妨碍去甲肾上腺素能神经递质及肾上腺素受体激动药与α受体结合，从而产生抗肾上腺素作用。它们能将肾上腺素的升压作用翻转为降压，这个现象称为“肾上腺素作用的翻转”。这可解释为α受体阻断药选择性地阻断了与血管收缩有关的α受体，留下与血管舒张有关的β受体；所以能激动α受体和β受体的肾上腺素的血管收缩作用被取消，而血管舒张作用得以充分地表现出来。对于主要作用于血管α受体的去甲肾上腺素，它们只能取消或减弱其升压效应而无“翻转作用”。对于主要作用于β受体的异丙肾上腺素的降压作用则无影响。

李　清

❖ CASE 7

A 64-year-old woman with a history of two previous myocardial infarctions[1] (MIs) comes to the emergency room with shortness of breath. In the previous 2 weeks, she has developed dyspnea[2] with exertion and swelling of her legs. She sleeps on three pillows[3] because she coughs and gets short of breath if she tries to lie flat. In the emergency department, she is sitting upright, appears to be in moderate respiratory distress[4], and is tachycardic[5] and hypertensive. She has jugular venous distension[6] to the angle of her jaw. On auscultation[7] of her lungs, wet rales[8] are heard bilaterally[9]. She has pitting edema[10] of both lower legs up to her knees. A chest x-ray confirms the diagnosis of pulmonary edema. She is placed on oxygen and immediately given an IV injection of furosemide.

◆ **What is the mechanism of action of furosemide?**

◆ **What electrolyte abnormalities can be caused by furosemide?**

ANSWERS TO CASE 7: Diuretics

Summary: A 64-year-old woman with pulmonary edema is prescribed furosemide.

- **Mechanism of action of furosemide**: Inhibit active NaCl reabsorption in the ascending limb of the loop of Henle, increasing water and electrolyte excretion.
- **Potential electrolyte abnormalities**[11]: Hypokalemia[12], hypomagnesemia[13], and metabolic alkalosis[14] because of enhanced H^+ excretion.

CLINICAL CORRELATION

Loop diuretics given intravenously promote diuresis within minutes, making them ideal for the treatment of acute pulmonary edema. Furosemide is the prototype and most widely used drug in this class. Loop diuretics inhibit NaCl reabsorption in the ascending limb of the loop of Henle. This causes a marked *increase* in the excretion of both water and electrolytes. **The excretion of potassium**[15], **magnesium, and calcium ions are all increased**, which may cause clinically significant adverse effects. A metabolic alkalosis may also occur as a result of the excretion of hydrogen ions[16]. However, the ability to cause excretion of these electrolytes may also provide a clinical benefit in certain situations. **Forced diuresis by giving IV saline and furosemide is a primary method of treatment of hypercalcemia.**

Pharmacology of the Loop Diuretics

Objectives

1. Know the site and mechanism of action of diuretic agents.
2. Know the electrolyte effects of the various diuretic agents.
3. Know the therapeutic uses, adverse effects, and contraindications to diuretic use.

Definitions

Diuretic: An agent that increases the production of urine. The most common are natriuretic diuretics, agents that increase urine production by interfering with sodium reabsorption in the kidney.

Edema: Accumulation of water in interstitial spaces. Causes include elevated blood pressure, a decrease in plasma oncotic pressure[17] caused by a reduction in hepatic protein synthesis, or an increase in the oncotic pressure within the interstitial space[18].

Discussion of Class

Natriuretic diuretics all act within the kidney to reduce the reabsorption of Na^+ and Cl^-. There are **four sites within the kidney** where various diuretics act; these correspond to four anatomic regions of the nephron. The **proximal tubule** (**site 1**) is the site of about 60 percent Na^+ reabsorption, but diuretics acting here are relatively ineffective because of the sodium-reabsorbing capacity in more distal regions of the nephron. The **ascending loop of Henle**⑲ (**site 2**) has active reabsorption of about 35 percent of the filtered Na^+. This is mediated by a cotransporter termed NKCC2 that transports 1 Na^+, 1 K^+, and 2 Cl^-, and this is the molecular target of **furosemide** and other loop or "high-ceiling" diuretics. The **distal convoluted tubule** ⑳ (**site 3**) is responsible for transport of about 15 percent of filtered sodium. **Thiazide** diuretics act in this segment of the nephron by interfering with another cotransporter, NCC, that co-transports Na^+ and Cl^-. **Site 4 diuretics** act in the **collecting tubule** by interfering with Na^+ reabsorption through a specific channel, epithelial sodium channel (ENaC), also called the amiloride-sensitive sodium channel (Fig. 7-1). [注1]

Loop diuretics—furosemide, ethacrynic acid, bumetanide, and torsemide—are **highly acidic drugs** that act on the **luminal side of the tubule**. They reach this site by being secreted into the tubule by anion secretion in the proximal tubule. Compared with other diuretics, loop diuretics cause the greatest diuresis because the $Na^+K^-2Cl^-$ transporter is responsible for a large fraction of Na^+ reabsorption, and regions distal to the ascending limb have more limited capacity for sodium transport. Loop diuretics are useful for the treatment of peripheral and pulmonary edema, which may occur secondarily as a consequence of cardiac failure, liver failure, or renal failure. Loop diuretics increase the excretion of Na^+, Cl^-, K^+, Mg^{2+}, Ca^{2+} and decrease the excretion of Li^+. The increased excretion of Ca^{2+} is clinically relevant, and loop diuretics can be used to treat hypercalcemia. Some of the diuretic actions of furosemide are mediated via prostaglandins because inhibitors of prostaglandin biosynthesis diminish the increase in diuresis produced by the drug. In addition, furosemide has actions on the vascular system that occur prior to diuresis and may in part be mediated by prostaglandins. These effects include changes in renal blood flow and a reduction in left ventricular filling pressure. Loop diuretics increase urine production and decrease plasma K^+ in patients with acute renal failure.

Major adverse effects of loop diuretics are electrolyte imbalances. Increased delivery of Na^+ to the collecting duct increases K^+ and H^+ excretion. Loop diuretics therefore cause **hypokalemic, hypochloridemic, and metabolic alkalosis. Hyperuricemia** may be caused by the volume contraction and enhanced uric acid reabsorption by the proximal tubule. Loop diuretics can produce dose-dependent **ototoxicity**㉑.

Structure

Most loop diuretics are **sulfonamide derivatives**; the exceptions are ethacrynic acid, which is a phenoxyacetic acid derivative㉒, and torsemide, which is a sulfonylurea㉓.

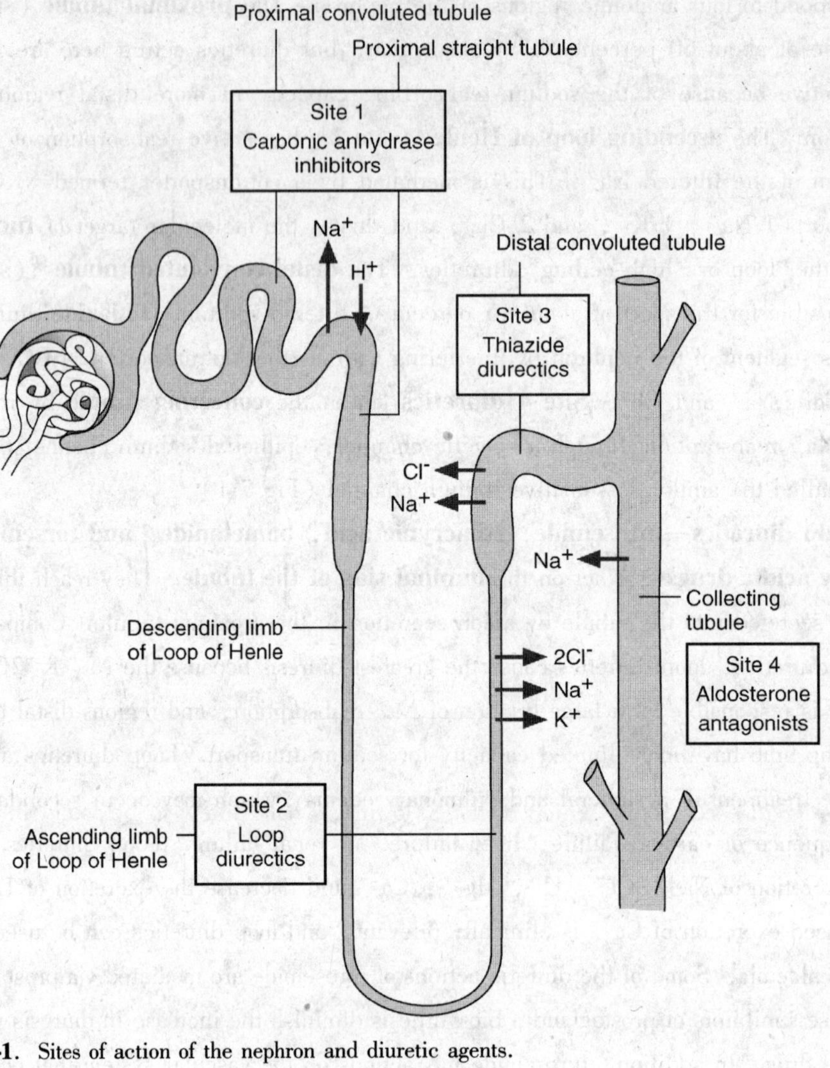

Figure 7-1. Sites of action of the nephron and diuretic agents.

Mechanism of Action

The molecular target of furosemide and other loop or high-ceiling diuretics is the sodium-potassium-2 chloride cotransporter (NKCC2), which transports 1 Na^+, 1 K^+, and 2 Cl^-. The activity of this transporter is blocked by loop diuretics.

Administration

All loop diuretics can be administered orally, and their onset of action is about 1 hour (torsemide) to 2 hours (furosemide). Loop diuretics can also be administered IV, and for furosemide, this produces vasodilation in as little as 5 minutes and diuresis in 20 minutes.

Pharmacokinetics

All loop diuretics are extensively bound to plasma proteins. Half-lives vary from 45 minutes (bumetanide) to 3.5 hours (torsemide). About 65 percent of a dose of furosemide is eliminated by the kidney, and the remainder is metabolized. Only 20 percent of torsemide is eliminated by the kidney, and 80 percent is metabolized.

Comprehension Questions

[7.1] Furosemide acts to inhibit Na^+ reabsorption in the

A. Ascending limb of the loop of Henle
B. Collecting duct
C. Descending limb of the loop of Henle
D. Distal convoluted tubule

[7.2] A patient arrives in the emergency room in a coma and has a serum Ca^{2+} of 4.5 mM. You start a saline infusion and which of the following drugs:

A. Calcitonin B. Ethacrynic acid
C. Hydrochlorothiazide D. Spironolactone

[7.3] A 55-year-old man with congestive heart failure is noted to be taking furosemide each day. Which of the following is most likely to be found in the serum?

A. Decreased potassium level B. Decreased uric acid level
C. Elevated magnesium level D. Low bicarbonate level

Answers

[7.1] **A.** Furosemide acts specifically on a $Na^+ K^+ 2Cl^-$ transporter in the ascending limb of the loop of Henle.

[7.2] **B.** Loop diuretics such as ethacrynic acid increase the excretion of Ca^{2+}.

[7.3] **A.** Furosemide leads to hypokalemia, hypomagnesemia, and metabolic alkylosis (elevated bicarbonate level).

PHARMACOLOGY PEARLS

❖ Furosemide, which acts on the loop of Henle, is the most efficacious diuretic.

❖ Hypokalemia is a frequent adverse effect encountered with loop diuretics, and this can be managed with the concomitant use of potassium-sparing diuretics such as triamterene or spironolactone.

❖ Loop diuretics can produce dose-dependent ototoxicity.

REFERENCES

Paul RV. Rational diuretic management in congestive heart failure: a case-based review. Crit Care Nurs Clin North Am 2003; 15(4): 453-60.

Plant L. Clinical Use of Diuretics. Clin Med 2003 Nov-Dec; 3(6): 517-20.

词汇

1. myocardial infraction[心肌梗死]
2. dyspnea[呼吸困难]
3. pillow[枕头]
4. respiratory distress[呼吸性窘迫]
5. tachycardic[心搏过速的]
6. jugular venous distension[颈静脉怒张]
7. auscultation[听诊]
8. wet rales[湿啰音]
9. bilaterally[双侧的]
10. pitting edema[凹陷性水肿]
11. electrolyte abnormality[电解质紊乱]
12. hypokalemia[低钾血症]
13. hypomagnesemia[低镁血症]
14. metabolic alkalosis[代谢性碱中毒]
15. potassium[钾]
16. hydrogen ion[氢离子]
17. oncotic pressure[胶体渗透压]
18. interstitial space[间质间隙]
19. ascending loop of Henle[亨利(氏)袢升支]
20. distal convoluted tubule[远曲小管]
21. ototoxicity[耳毒性]
22. phenoxyacetic acid derivative[苯氧(基)乙酸衍生物]
23. sulfonylurea[磺酰脲类]

注 1

NaCl 重吸收依赖于肾小管髓袢升支粗段管腔膜上的 Na^+-K^+-$2Cl^-$ 共转运子(NKCC2)，吸收的 Na^+ 主动转运至细胞间质，细胞内聚集的 K^+ 扩散回官腔维持管腔内正电位，驱动 Ca^+ 和 Mg^+ 的重吸收。呋塞米等袢利尿剂可选择性阻断 NKCC2，导致 NaCl 排出增加，减轻水钠潴留；但同时也可能抑制 K^+ 和 Mg^+ 的重吸收，使之排出增加，可能导致临床上明显的低钾血症和低镁血症。

点评

病人为 64 岁老人，有两次心肌梗死病史，2 周前发展为呼吸困难和下肢水肿，不能平卧(需垫三个枕头)，并伴有心动过速、颈静脉怒张和肺部双侧湿啰音，为典型心衰引起的肺水肿征兆(经 x 光胸片确诊)。故立即给予吸氧和呋塞米静注对症治疗。利尿药是心衰传统治疗药之一。能促进 Na^+、水排泄，减少体液量，减轻容量超负荷，降低心脏前、后负荷，消除或缓解静脉充血及其所引起的肺淤血、肺水肿和外周水肿。也能降低房室舒张压，从而降低室壁肌张力，并改善心内膜下灌流，阻止左室功能的恶性进展而改善左室功能。低、中、高效能的利尿药均可用于心衰的治疗，对轻度心衰单独应用利尿药效果良好，对心衰有容量负荷征象如水肿或有明显充血和淤血者尤为适用。静注呋塞米 20～40mg，于 2min 内推完，利尿作用于 5min 内开始，30min 达高峰，持续约 2h。呋塞米可迅速扩张容量血管，使回心血量减少，降低左心室充盈压，在利尿作用发生前即可缓解肺水肿；其利尿作用亦可降低循环血容量，降低前负荷而改善心功能。

张　伟

❖ CASE 8

Following his third episode of gouty arthritis①, a 50-year-old man sees you in the clinic. Each case was successfully treated acutely; however, your patient is interested in trying to prevent future episodes. He is on no medications regularly and has a normal physical examination today. Blood work reveals an elevated serum uric acid② level and otherwise normal renal function and electrolytes③. A 24-hour urine collection for uric acid reveals that he is underexcreting④ uric acid. Suspecting that this is the cause of his recurrent gout, you place him on probenecid⑤.

◆ **What is the mechanism of action of probenecid?**

◆ **Which drugs could have their excretion inhibited by probenecid?**

ANSWERS TO CASE 8: Nondiuretic Inhibitors of Tubular Transport

Summary: A 50-year-old man with recurrent gout is prescribed probenecid.

- **Mechanism of action of probenecid**: Inhibits secretion of organic acids and decreases reabsorption of uric acid, causing a net increase in secretion.
- **Other drugs whose secretion could be inhibited**: Penicillin, indomethacin, and methotrexate.

CLINICAL CORRELATION

Gout is a disease in which uric acid crystals deposit in joints, causing an extremely painful acute inflammatory arthritis. Persons with recurrent gout often have chronically elevated levels of uric acid in their blood. [注1]This hyperuricemia[⑥] is frequently caused by either overproduction of uric acid or underexcretion of uric acid by the kidneys. Probenecid (and other uricosuric drugs[⑦]) promotes the excretion of uric acid. It works by inhibiting the secretion of organic acids from the plasma into the tubular lumen and blocking the reuptake of uric acid. The net result of this is an **increase in the secretion of uric acid**. The benefit of this is the prevention of recurrent gout attacks in chronic underexcreters of uric acid. In those individuals who overproduce uric acid, allopurinol[⑧] is used. This inhibits xanthine oxidase[⑨], a key enzyme in the production of uric acid.

Pharmacology of Uricosuric Agents

Objectives

1. Understand the mechanism of action of uricosuric agents.
2. Know the therapeutic uses, adverse effects, and contraindications to uricosurics.
3. Know the mechanism of action and use of allopurinol.

Definitions

Uricosuric agents: Increase the mass of uric acid that is excreted in the urine.
Renal secretion: Moves solutes such as urate from the plasma into the urine.
Renal reabsorption: Moves solutes from the urine back into the plasma.

Discussion of Class

Urate[⑩] is both secreted and reabsorbed by at least three independent molecular transporters located in the proximal tubule. Urate is nearly completely secreted into the lumen of the nephron[⑪] against an electrochemical gradient by the action of **organic acid transporter-1 (OAT-1) and transporter-3 (OAT-3)**. [注2] These cotransporters exchange α-ketoglutarate[12] and urate (or other organic anions) and move urate from the plasma into the tubular cell. The protein UAT is an electrically neutral channel that permits uric acid to leave tubular cells and enter either the lumen or the plasma. URAT1, located on the apical membrane of tubular cells, is thought to be responsible for most of the reabsorption of urate from the filtrate. URAT1 is a transporter that is capable of exchanging a variety of anions with urate in an electrically neural manner. Interaction of uricosuric agents such as probenecid with URAT1 diminishes the reabsorption of urate and increases urate excretion. All of these transporters or channels are relatively nonselective with respect to the organic acid transported. OAT-1 and OAT-3 are capable of secreting most organic acids including penicillin, aspirin, furosemide, and hydrochlorothiazide[13].

In patients with **gout**, **probenecid can be used prophylactically**[14]; **uricosuric drugs will not diminish the severity of an acute attack**. An **acute gouty attack** may be **precipitated** by the **initiation of probenecid treatment** as uric acid is mobilized out of joints. **Adequate hydration**[15] should be ensured, because probenecid predisposes patients to the formation of **uric acid kidney stones**.

The alternate therapeutic approach to the treatment of gout is to reduce the **production of uric acid with allopurinol**[16]. The enzyme **xanthine oxidase** produces uric acid in a two-step reaction from the purine hypoxanthine. Allopurinol is metabolized to alloxanthine by xanthine oxidase, and this metabolite is a long-lasting inhibitor of the enzyme.

Probenecid is also useful for decreasing the excretion of penicillin, because **penicillin is eliminated** primarily by renal secretion mediated by **OAT-1** and **OAT-3**. Probenecid competes for this secretion and thereby reduces the rate of elimination and **increases both the biological half-life of penicillin and increases the plasma concentration** of the antibiotic more than twofold. This adjunct use of probenecid is particularly useful in singledose regimens for the treatment of gonococcal infections with long-acting penicillins such as penicillin G.

Secretion of organic acids is quite nonspecific, and most acidic drugs are secreted by the same transporters OAT-1 and OAT-3. This implies that nearly any combination of acidic drugs will compete for elimination at the level of the transporters, and the effects on elimination of each individual drug must be considered. For example, the half-life of diuretics such as furosemide will be increased by probenecid, and this may require dosage adjustment. **Aspirin**, another acidic drug, **will compete with probenecid for secretion**. This reduces the action of probenecid to increase uric acid excretion and thus increases plasma urate. Therefore **aspirin is contraindicated in patients with gout who are taking probenecid**.

The most common adverse effect of probenecid is gastrointestinal (GI) upset[17], and about 2 percent of patients experience a hypersensitivity reaction usually manifest as a skin rash[18]. The incidence of hypersensitivity is lower with sulfinpyrazone[19], but the incidence of GI upset is higher.

Structure

Probenecid is a lipid-soluble benzoic acid derivative. Sulfinpyrazone is a pyrazolone derivative similar to the antiinflammatory agent phenylbutazone. Both are strong acids (pKa 3.4 and 2.8, respectively).

Mechanism of Action

Both probenecid and sulfinpyrazone are secreted into the lumen of the nephron via OAT-1 and OAT-3 where the drugs can diminish the ability of URAT1 to reabsorb urate.

Administration

Both drugs are active orally, and both are nearly completely absorbed.

Pharmacokinetics

The half-life of probenecid is 5-8 hours; sulfinpyrazone is about 3 hours, but its uricosuric actions can last as long as 10 hours. Increased excretion of uric acid occurs promptly after oral administration. Both agents are eliminated in the urine.

Comprehension Questions

[8.1] Probenecid is effective in treating gout because it decreases

A. Inflammation in affected joints

B. Production of uric acid

C. Reabsorption of uric acid

D. Secretion of uric acid

[8.2] Which of the following describes the action of allopurinol?

A. Inhibits metabolism of purines to uric acid

B. Inhibits prostaglandin biosynthesis

C. Inhibits uric acid reabsorption

D. Interferes with cytokine production

[8.3] An 18-year-old man who is known to have non-penicillinase-producing gonococcal urethritis is given an injection of penicillin and probenecid. What is the mechanism used by probenecid that makes penicillin more efficacious?

A. Decreases the bacterial resistance by inhibiting penicillinase production

B. Increases the half-life and serum level by decreasing the renal excretion of penicillin

C. Prolongs the duration of action by affecting the liver metabolism of penicillin

D. Promotes entry of the penicillin into the bacteria

Answers

[8.1] **C.** Probenecid does inhibit renal tubular secretion of urate, but at therapeutic doses it inhibits reabsorption to a greater degree, thereby increasing net excretion urate.

[8.2] **A.** Allopurinol interferes with the metabolism of purines by inhibiting the enzyme xanthine oxidase.

[8.3] **B.** Probenecid decreases the renal excretion of penicillin, thereby increasing both the half-life and the serum level.

PHARMACOLOGY PEARLS

❖ At low doses, probenecid inhibition of urate secretion predominates, and this paradoxically increases plasma urate.

❖ At higher doses, inhibition of reabsorption predominates, leading to the therapeutically useful increased excretion of urate.

❖ An acute gouty attack may be precipitated by the initiation of probenecid treatment as uric acid is mobilized out of joints.

❖ Probenecid is also useful for decreasing the excretion of penicillin.

❖ Patients are typically begun on a high loading dose to ensure the action on reabsorption is achieved.

REFERENCES

Dantzler WH. Regulation of renal proximal and distal tubule transport: sodium, chloride and organic ions. Comp Biochem Physiol Part A 2003; 136: 453-78.

Rafey MA, Lipkowitz MS, Leal-Pinto E, et al. Uric acid transport. Curr Opin Nephrol Hyperten 2000; 12: 511-5.

词汇

1. gouty arthritis[痛风性关节炎]
2. uric acid[尿酸]
3. electrolyte[电解质]
4. under-excreting[排泄障碍]

5. probenecid［丙磺舒］
6. hyperuricemia［高尿酸血症］
7. uricosuric drugs［尿酸排泄剂］
8. allopurinol［别嘌醇］
9. xanthine oxidase［黄嘌呤氧化酶］
10. urate［尿酸盐］
11. nephron［肾单位］
12. α-ketoglutarate［α-酮戊二酸］
13. hydrochlorothiazide［氢氯噻嗪］
14. prophylactically［预防地］
15. hydration［水合(作用)］
16. alloxanthine［别黄嘌呤］
17. gastrointestinal(GI) upset［胃肠不适］
18. skin rash［皮疹］
19. sulfinpyrazone［磺吡酮］

注 1

痛风为嘌呤代谢紊乱所致的疾病，因血中尿酸过高，尿酸盐在关节、肾脏及结缔组织中结晶沉积而导致关节炎及粒细胞浸润；如未及时治疗则可发展成慢性痛风性关节炎或肾病变。痛风可通过抑制尿酸的生成或促进尿酸的排泄，降低血中尿酸水平。原发性痛风好发于中老年男性，要确诊此类疾病除血尿酸增高外，还需以下几条：(1)关节腔穿刺取滑囊液进行旋光检查，发现白细胞内有针形尿酸盐结晶；(2)痛风石活检证实为尿酸盐结晶；(3)受累关节 X 线检查。

注 2

由于尿酸的排泄几乎完全依靠有机酸转运蛋白(OAT-1 和 OAT-3)，水杨酸类、青霉素等药物可通过竞争有机酸转运蛋白而影响丙磺舒作用。

点评

丙磺舒口服液吸收完全，大部分通过肾近曲小管主动分泌排出，脂溶性高，易被肾小管再吸收。此时可竞争性抑制尿酸的再吸收，增加尿酸排泄而降低血中尿酸浓度，适用于本病例(该病人肾功能正常,日尿排出)。少数病人可有胃肠道反应、皮疹、发热等，用时还应注意大量饮水及碱化尿液。治疗初期可使痛风发作加重，这是由于尿酸盐由关节移出所致。加服碳酸氢钠并大量饮水可防止尿酸在泌尿到沉积，促进其排出。如病人尿酸生成过多，对排尿酸药过敏或无效，则需要考虑使用抑制尿酸合成药，如别嘌醇。

张 伟

❖ CASE 9

A 72-year-old man presents to the office for routine followup[①]. He is under treatment for hypertension and congestive heart failure with enalapril and a diuretic. His blood pressure is under acceptable control and he has no symptoms of heart failure at present. He does complain that he has been coughing frequently in the past few months. History and exam reveal no other cause of a chronic cough, so you decide to discontinue his enalapril and start him on losartan.

◆ **What is the mechanism of action of enalapril?**

◆ **By what mechanism does enalapril convert to its active form enalaprilat?**

◆ **What is the likely cause of the cough?**

◆ **What is the mechanism of action of losartan?**

ANSWERS TO CASE 9: Drugs Active on the Renin-Angiotensin System

Summary: A 72-year-old man with hypertension and congestive heart failure presents with an ACE inhibitor-induced cough, and is switched to losartan.

- **Mechanism of action of enalapril**: Inhibit the conversion of angiotensin I to angiotensin II, this also inhibits the angiotensin II-stimulated release of aldosterone[2]. Angiotensin-converting enzyme (ACE) inhibitors also impair the inactivation of bradykinin[3].
- **Mechanism of converting enalapril to enalaprilat**: Deesterification[4] in the liver.
- **Mechanism of ACE inhibitor induced cough**: Secondary to the increased bradykinin levels, which is caused by reduction in the inactivation of bradykinin.
- **Mechanism of action of angiotensin receptor blockers**: Antagonists of angiotensin-1 (AT-1), receptors which mediate the pressor effects[5] of angiotensin II.

CLINICAL CORRELATION

Angiotensin-converting enzyme inhibitors have gained wide-scale use in medicine for their effectiveness in hypertension, congestive heart failure, coronary artery disease, and renal protection in diabetics. They inhibit the conversion of angiotensin I to angiotensin II. Angiotensin II is a *potent* vasoconstrictor and stimulates the release of aldosterone, which promotes sodium retention. *Inhibition of the production of angiotensin II* reduces vascular resistance and sodium and water retention. Another effect of ACE inhibitors is to reduce the inactivation of bradykinin. Active bradykinin is a vasodilator, providing an additive effect in lowering blood pressure. However, raising bradykinin levels contributes to one of the ACE inhibitors most bothersome side effects, chronic dry cough. Angiotensin-converting enzyme inhibitors in general are well tolerated, but along with cough, can cause hyperkalemia and should be used with caution with potassium-sparing diuretics or in persons with impaired renal function. Angiotensin receptor blockers (ARBs) are antagonists of the angiotensin I receptor, which mediates the direct vasoconstrictor effect of angiotensin II. This also blocks the release of aldosterone. Angiotensin receptor blockers extra do not affect the bradykinin system and therefore do not cause a cough. They are also well tolerated but, like ACE inhibitors, can cause hyperkalemia.

Pharmacology of the Renin-Angiotensin System

Objectives

1. Know the mechanism of action of angiotensin converting enzyme inhibitors.
2. Know the therapeutic uses, side effects and contraindications to ACE inhibitor use.
3. Know the mechanism of action of angiotensin receptor blockers.
4. Know the therapeutic uses, side effects and contraindications to ARB use.

Definitions

Hypertension: From the Seventh Report, Joint National Committee on Detection, Evaluation, and Treatment of High Blood Pressure, normal blood pressure is 120/80 mm Hg.[注]

Bradykinin: a member of a class of peptides, the kinins, that have a variety of effects on the cardiovascular system, including vasodilatation, and inflammation.

ARB: Angiotensin receptor blocker, more precisely angiotensin AT-1 receptor blockers.

Discussion of Class

The **renin-angiotensin-aldosterone system provides a humoral system**[⑥] **for controlling blood pressure and electrolyte levels**. The "sensors" in this **system monitor Na^+, K^+, vascular volume, and blood pressure**. A reduction in blood pressure, detected by intrarenal stretch receptors, or a fall in the delivery of Na^+ to the distal portions of the nephron results in release of renin from the juxtaglomerular apparatus[⑦] (JGA). Renin secretion can also be increased through the baroreceptor[⑧] reflex mediated by increased central nervous system (CNS) outflow and β_1-adrenergic receptors on the JGA. Renin is an aspartyl protease[⑨] that cleaves angiotensinogen, a 56 Kd polypeptide produced in the liver, to the decapeptide[⑩] angiotensin I (Figure 9-1, "classic" pathway).

Angiotensin I is biologically inactive and is **rapidly converted to the octapeptide**[⑪] **angiotensin II** by the action of ACE, a dipeptidyl peptidase[⑫]. Angiotensin II is further metabolized within the brain and in the plasma by aminopeptidase A[⑬], which removes the N-terminal aspartic acid[⑭] to produce angiotensin III, which may itself be further metabolized by aminopeptidase N, which removes the N-terminal arginine yielding angiotensin IV. The latter two metabolites may play a critical role in regulating blood pressure in the brain. Distinct from this classic intravascular pathway for the formation of angiotensins, evidence has accumulated indicating that angiotensins can also be produced within various tissues by a local conversion to angiotensins II, III, and IV (see Fig. 9-1).

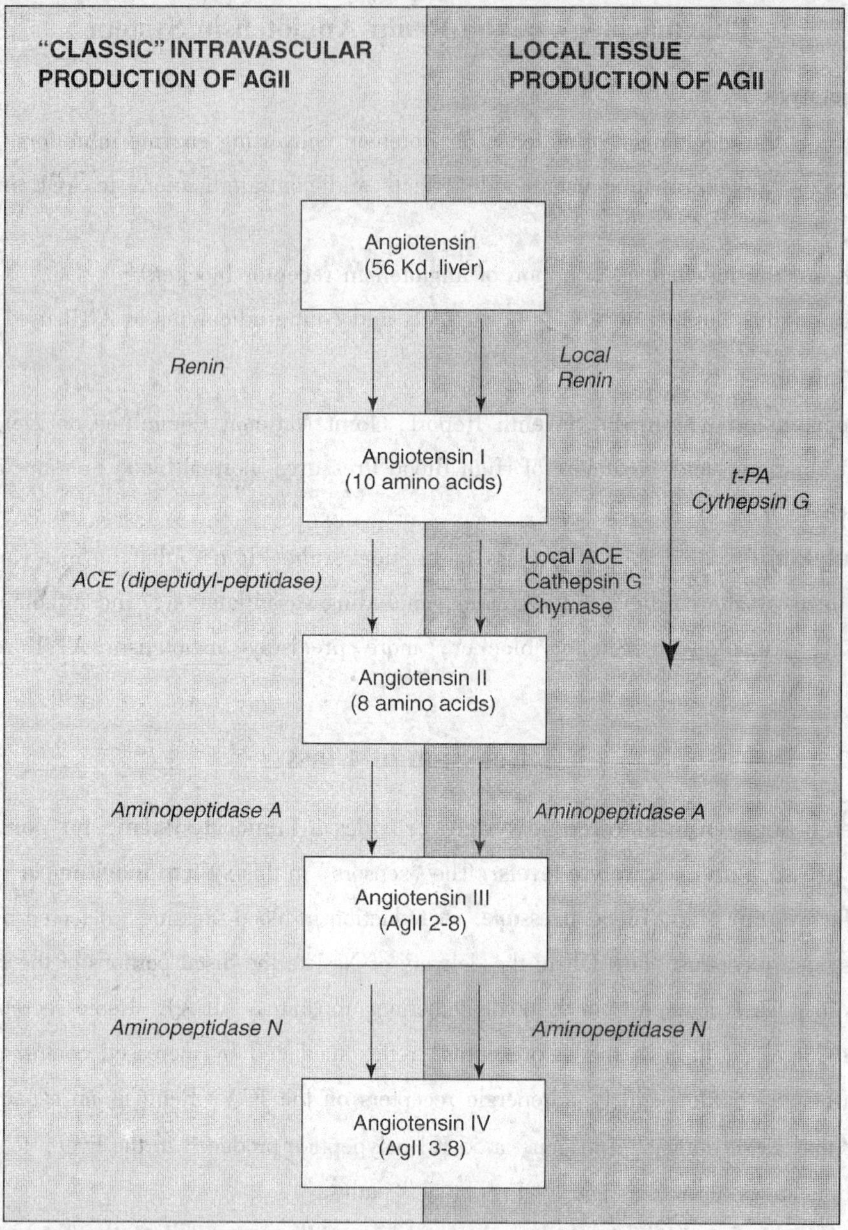

Figure 9-1. Schematic of angiotensin pathway.

Angiotensin II has multiple actions that act in concert to increase blood pressure and alter electrolyte levels. **Angiotensin II is a potent vasoconstrictor**, 10-40 times more potent than epinephrine[15], an effect **mediated by receptor-coupled Ca^{2+} channels** in **vascular smooth muscle cells**, as described below. **Angiotensin II enhances the release of catecholamines** from both the adrenal medulla[16] and at peripheral nerve endings. Within the adrenal gland, angiotensin II increases the biosynthesis of aldosterone, which leads to an increase in Na^+ and water reabsorption in the kidneys and volume expansion. Angiotensin II has several actions within the CNS including altering vagal tone[17] to increase blood pressure, increasing thirst and increasing the release of antidiuretic hormone.

Angiotensin II also has effects on the heart and the vasculature that do not directly affect blood pressure. **Angiotensin II induces cardiac hypertrophy**[18], is proproliferative, and enhances matrix remodeling and the deposition of matrix proteins, which leads to **increased myocardial stiffness**. Within vessel walls, angiotensin II is proinflammatory[19] and can stimulate the release of several chemokines.

Three angiotensin receptors mediate these actions. The AT-1 and angiotensin-2 (AT-2) receptors have been described in various tissues. Both are seven-transmembrane receptors that appear to couple to various signaling pathways. AT-1 receptors bind angiotensin II, angiotensin III, and angiotensin IV. This receptor mediates most of the cardiovascular and central responses to angiotensin II, including vasoconstriction of vascular smooth muscle and aldosterone biosynthesis in the adrenal medulla. AT-1 receptors also mediate the cardiac hypertrophic and proproliferative responses to angiotensin II. AT-2 receptors also bind angiotensin II and play a role in the development of the cardiovascular system. In general, activation of AT-2 receptors is physiologically antagonistic to the action of AT-1 receptors. Activation of AT-2 receptors is hypotensive and antiproliferative and is coupled to distinctly different signaling pathways compared to AT-1 receptors. Angiotensin-4 (AT-4) receptors appear to be identical to transmembrane aminopeptidase insulin-regulated aminopeptidase (IRAP) and has a single transmembrane domain. AT-4 receptors are expressed in the numerous tissues and bind angiotensin IV. Activation of these receptors has been reported to regulate cerebral blood flow, and to stimulate endothelial cell expression of plasminogen activator inhibitor, and has effects on both memory and learning.

Inhibition of the renin angiotension system (RAS) is accomplished pharmacologically two ways: inhibition of the production of angiotensin II or a blockade of AT-1 receptors. **Angiotensin-converting enzyme inhibitors** (ACE inhibitors), or peptidyl dipeptidase (PDP) inhibitors, include **enalapril**, **lisinopril**, **fosinopril**, **captopril**, and seven others. These drugs differ in their chemistry and pharmacokinetic properties, but all are orally active, have the same range of activities, and are equally effective clinically. **ACE is the enzyme responsible for both *activation* of angiotensin I (metabolism to angiotensin II) and *inactivation* of bradykinin**. The decreased metabolism of bradykinin is partly responsible for the hypotensive action of ACE inhibitors, and the decreased metabolism of **bradykinin** is also responsible for enhancing the irritability of airways that leads to the **dry cough** associated with ACE inhibitors.

ARBs block the action of angiotensin II by acting as antagonists at AT-1

receptors. These nonpeptide antagonists include **losartan**[20], **valsartan**[21], **candesartan**[22], and others. ARBs bind with high affinity to AT-1 receptors without interfering with AT-2 or AT-4 receptors.

The **ACE inhibitors and ARBs are equally effective in reducing blood pressure**. More clinical experience exists with the ACE inhibitors and it has been well established that this class of drugs reduces the risk of second events in patients who have had a myocardial infarction and in reducing renal damage in patients with diabetic nephropathy. **Hypotension and hyperkalemia are adverse effects seen with both classes of RAS inhibitors**. **Cough and angioedema**, **caused by increased bradykinin** levels, are more frequently seen with the **ACE inhibitors**.

Structure

Although the various ACE inhibitors have different chemical structures, they are mostly based on extensive modifications of L-proline. The ARBs are also quite distinct chemically: Valsartan is an L-valine derivative, and losartan is an imidazole derivative.

Mechanism of Action

ACE inhibitors are all competitive inhibitors of angiotensin converting enzyme. ARBs are competitive antagonists of the angiotensin II type 1 receptor (AT-1)

Administration

All ACE inhibitors are available for oral administration. Enalaprilat, the active metabolite of enalapril, is available for intravenous infusion.

Pharmacokinetics

Most of the current ACE inhibitors are prodrugs and require conversion to the active metabolite in the liver. For example, enalapril is converted to enalaprilat, fosinopril is converted into fosinoprilat. Captopril and lisinopril are active drugs that do not require metabolism. The onset of action of ACE inhibitors is 0.5-2 hours, and the duration of action is typically 24 hours (captopril is 6 hours). Most are eliminated in the urine.

Comprehension Questions

[9.1] Losartan acts to

A. Decrease AT-1 receptor activity

B. Decrease bradykinin production

C. Decrease production of angiotensin II

D. Decrease renin production

[9.2] A limiting adverse effect of ACE inhibitors is

A. Acidosis
B. Hyperkalemia
C. Hypernatremia
D. Hypokalemia
E. Hyponatremia

[9.3] Which of the following is an advantage of losartan over enalapril?

A. Better efficacy in lower blood pressure
B. Better prevention of secondary myocardial events
C. Less cost
D. Less incidence of angioedema

Answers

[9.1] **A**. Losartan is a prototypical angiotensin AT-1 receptor antagonist.

[9.2] **B**. By reducing aldosterone levels, ACE inhibitors decrease K^+ excretion in the distal nephron.

[9.3] **D**. Losartan does not lead to elevated bradykinin levels; thus, there is less of an incidence of angioedema and dry cough. The effects on blood pressure are equal. The track record for prevention of secondary cardiovascular events is well established for ACE inhibitors, although the same is speculated for ARBs.

PHARMACOLOGY PEARLS

- Elevation of the bradykinin levels is thought to be the etiology of the dry cough and angioedema of ACE inhibitors.
- ACE inhibitors improve outcome in patients with cardiovascular disease and have been recommended as therapy in several guidelines.
- Clinical experience suggest that inhibitors of the renin angiotensin system are somewhat less effective in African Americans.
- ARBs block the action of angiotensin II by acting as antagonists at AT-1 receptors.

REFERENCES

Yusuf S, Sleight P, Pogue J, et al. Effects of an angiotensin-converting-enzyme inhibitor, ramipril, on cardiovascular events in high-risk patients: the heart outcomes prevention evaluation study investigators. N Engl J Med 2000; 342: 145-53.

词汇

1. followup[随访]
2. aldosterone[醛固酮]
3. bradykinin[缓激肽]
4. deesterification[脱脂作用]
5. pressor effect[加压效应]
6. humoral system[体液系统]
7. juxtaglomerular apparatus[球旁器]
8. baroreceptor[压力感受器]
9. aspartyl protease[天冬氨酰蛋白酶]
10. decapeptide[十肽菌素]
11. octapeptide[辛肽]
12. dipeptidyl peptidase[二肽基肽酶]
13. aminopeptidase A[氨基肽酶 A]
14. aspartic acid[门冬氨酸]
15. epinephrine[肾上腺素]
16. medulla[髓质]
17. vagal tone[迷走神经张力]
18. cardiac hypertrophy[心脏肥厚]
19. proinflammatory[促炎症反应]
20. losartan[氯沙坦]
21. valsartan[缬沙坦]
22. candesartan[坎地沙坦]

注

高血压的诊断标准已多次修改，目前世界高血压联盟的新标准为：理想血压，收缩压<120mmHg、舒张压<80mmHg；正常血压，收缩压<130mmHg、舒张压<85mmHg，其中收缩压变动范围为130~139mmHg，舒张压变动范围为85~89mmHg。

点评

病例为高血压伴充血性心力衰竭患者，一直用利尿药和ACEI类药物(依那普利)治疗。依那普利为不含巯基的长效、高效血管紧张素转化酶抑制药。降压作用强而持久。依那普利为前体药，在体内被肝脏酯酶水解转化为生物活性更强的依那普利拉，后者能与血管紧张素转化酶持久结合而发挥抑制作用。降压机制与卡托普利相似，但抑制血管紧张素转化酶的作用较卡托普利强10倍。高血压病人口服2.5~40mg后血压下降，口服吸收率39%~64%，吸收不受饮食影响，0.5~1h血药浓度达峰值。可每日给药一次。其不良反应、药物相互作用与卡托普利相似，但因为不含巯基，故无典型的青霉胺样反应(皮疹、嗜酸细胞增多等)，因作用强，引起咳嗽较多，合并有心力衰竭或利尿药时应减小剂量至每日口服2.5mg。

由于病史和检查均未发现其他引起慢性干咳的原因，所以考虑干咳为依那普利副作用所致。几乎所有的ACEI都可引起咳嗽，表现为刺激性、持续性干咳，停药后易恢复，其原因是因缓激肽降解受阻而作用于呼吸道引起，与ACEI的剂型无关。血管紧张素II受体阻断药主要与AT1受体选择性地结合，并间接激活AT2受体，对抗血管紧张素II的缩血管作用，使血压降低。也能拮抗血管紧张素II的促细胞生长作用，逆转心肌肥厚。因此血管紧张素II受体阻断药较血管紧张素转化酶抑制药可以更强地阻断血管紧张素II已知的所有作用，且不良反应少于血管紧张素转化酶抑制药，是ACEI药物引起干咳时很好的替代药物。

张 伟

❖ CASE 10

A 69-year-old man sees you in the office for follow-up of his chronic congestive heart failure[1]. He has a marked reduction in his ejection fraction following a series of myocardial infarctions (MIs)[2]. He also has hypertension and type II diabetes mellitus. His symptoms include dyspnea[3] on exertion, orthopnea[4], paroxysmal nocturnal dyspnea[5], and peripheral edema[6]. He has normal renal function. He is on appropriate treatment of his diabetes, along with an angiotensinconverting enzyme (ACE) inhibitor and a loop diuretic. You decide to add digoxin to his regimen.

- **What is the effect of digoxin on the normal heart?**
- **What is the effect of digoxin on the failing heart?**
- **What neural effects does digoxin have?**
- **What are the side effects and toxicities of digoxin?**

ANSWERS TO CASE 10: Agents Used to Treat Congestive Heart Failure

Summary: A 69-year-old man with congestive heart failure, hypertension, and diabetes mellitus has a markedly low ejection fraction and is prescribed digoxin.

- **Effect on a normal heart**:[注1] Increased systemic vascular resistance and constriction of smooth muscle in veins, which may decrease cardiac output.
- **Effect on a failing heart**: Increased stroke volume and increased cardiac output.
- **Neural effects**: Decrease sympathetic tone and increased vagal[7] activity, resulting in inhibition of sinoatrial (SA) node[8] and delayed conduction through atrioventricular (AV) node[9].
- **Side effects and toxicities**: Induction of arrhythmias[10], anorexia[11], nausea[12], vomiting, diarrhea[13], disorientation[14], and visual disturbance[15].

CLINICAL CORRELATION

Digoxin can be useful in improving some of the symptoms of congestive heart failure, but its use must be closely monitored. Digoxin works by inhibiting the sodium-potassium adenosine triphosphatase (ATPase)[16], primarily in cardiac muscle cells. This causes increased intracellular sodium and decreased intracellular potassium.[注2] The increased sodium reduces the exchange of intracellular calcium for extracellular sodium, causing an increased intracellular calcium level. The overall effect of this is to allow for a greater release of calcium with each action potential. This has a positive inotropic effect. In a failing heart, stroke volume[17] and cardiac output[18] are increased. End-diastolic volume, venous pressure, and blood volume are decreased. These circulatory improvements also result in a reduction of sympathetic tone. This further improves circulation by lowering systemic vascular resistance. **Digoxin also has the effect of increasing vagal activity**, which inhibits the SA node and slows conduction through the AV node. This is beneficial in patients with atrial tachyarrhythmias[19] such as atrial fibrillation[20], atrial flutter[21], and atrial tachycardias. **Digoxin has a narrow therapeutic index**, and its **level in the blood must be closely monitored**. The **dose must be adjusted for renal impairment**, because it is cleared by the kidney. Toxic digoxin levels may produce many types of **arrhythmias**, with **AV blocks and bradycardia** being common. Mental status changes and gastrointestinal symptoms are common as well. Asymptomatic elevations in digoxin levels are usually treated by discontinuing or reducing the drug's dosage. Symptomatic toxicity, particularly arrhythmias, is **most often trea-**

ted by the IV infusion of digoxin-binding antibodies. [注3]

Pharmacology of the Cardiac Glycosides

Objectives

1. Know the mechanism of action of the cardiac glycosides.
2. Know the therapeutic uses, adverse effects, and toxicities of cardiac glycosides.
3. Know the other agents used frequently in the treatment of congestive heart failure.

Definitions

Cardiac Glycosides[22]: The cardenolides include digitalis, digoxin, digitoxin, and ouabain.

Inotropic: Affecting myocardial contractility[23].

Chronotropic: Affecting heart rate.

Congestive heart failure: A syndrome with multiple causes that may affect either systole or diastole. Left heart failure leads to pulmonary congestion and reduced cardiac output and appears in patients with myocardial infarction, aortic[24], and mitral valve[25] disease and hypertension. Right heart failure leads to peripheral edema and ascites and appears in patients with tricuspid valve[26] disease, cor pulmonale[27], and prolonged left heart failure. The New York Heart Association classification of congestive heart failure includes class I (mild disease) to class IV (severe disease).

Discussion of Class

The medicinal actions of the cardiac glycosides, digitalis, have been used successfully for over 200 years, and they have both positive inotropic and antiarrhythmic properties. **Digoxin is the most commonly used cardiac glycoside. Cardiac glycosides act to indirectly increase intracellular calcium** (Fig. 10-1). **Digitalis binds to a specific site on the outside of the Na^+-K^+-ATPase** and this reduces the activity of the enzyme. All cells express Na^+/K^+-ATPase but different isoforms of the enzyme; the isoforms expressed by **cardiac myocytes and vagal neurons are the most susceptible to digitalis**. Inhibition of the enzyme by digitalis causes an increase in intracellular Na^+ and decreases the Na^+ concentration gradient across the plasma membrane. It is this Na^+ concentration that provides the driving force for the Na^+-Ca^{2+} antiporter. The rate of transport of Ca^{2+} out of the cell is reduced, and this leads to an increase in intracellular Ca^{2+}, greater activation of contractile elements, and an increase in the force of contraction of the heart. The **electrical characteristics of myocardial cells** are also **altered** by the **cardiac glycosides**. The most important effect is a **shortening of the**

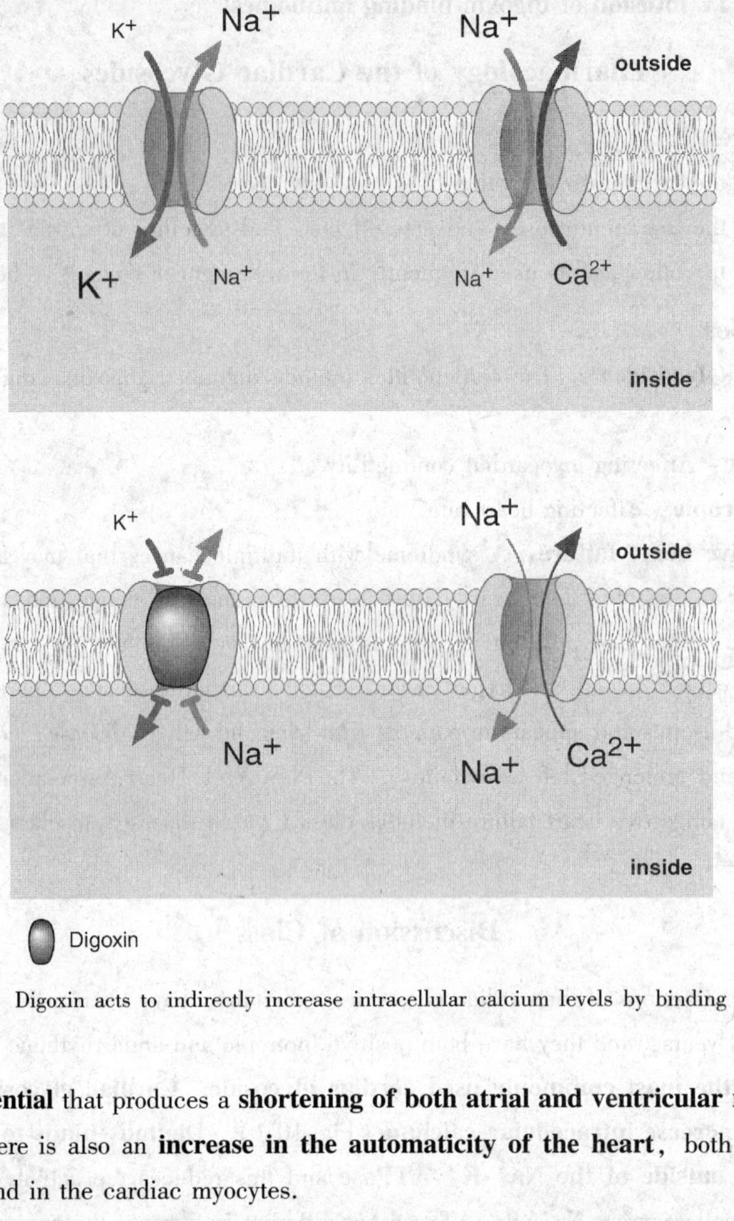

Figure 10-1. Digoxin acts to indirectly increase intracellular calcium levels by binding to the Na^+-K^+-ATPase.

action potential that produces a **shortening of both atrial and ventricular refractoriness**㉘. There is also an **increase in the automaticity of the heart**, both within the AV node and in the cardiac myocytes.

Within the nervous system cardiac glycosides affect both the sympathetic and parasympathetic systems, and parasympatheticomimetic effects predominate at therapeutic doses. **Increased vagal activity inhibits the SA node and delays conduction through the AV node.**

In **acute heart failure, digitalis clearly improves contractility**. Ejection fraction and cardiac output is increased and symptoms are decreased. **In congestive heart failure, digitalis is used primarily in patients who are symptomatic after optimal therapy with diuretics, ACE inhibitors, and beta blockers**. In this setting, digitalis decreases symptoms and increases exercise tolerance. However, in patients with **normal sinus rhythm**㉙, there is **no decline in overall mortality** because of deaths associated with digitalis toxicity.

Because of its action in **increasing vagal tone**, **cardiac glycosides** are useful in the treatment of **several supraventricular arrhythmias** including **atrial flutter** and **atrial fibrillation**. **Digitalis can control paroxysmal atrial and atrioventricular nodal tachycardia**. Its use is **contraindicated in Wolff-Parkinson-White syndrome**, where it can induce arrhythmias in the alternate pathway.

Cardiac glycosides have a **narrow therapeutic index. Toxic levels of cardiac glycosides leads to depletion of intracellular K^+ and accumulation of Na^+** (because of inhibition of Na^+/K^+-ATPase). This leads to partial depolarization of the cell and increased excitability, both of which can lead to arrhythmias including supraventricular and ventricular tachyarrhythmias. Bradycardia[30] and heart block are also manifestations of digitalis toxicity in the heart. **Adverse effects of digitalis on the gastrointestinal (GI) tract** are common including **anorexia**, **vomiting**, **pain**, and **diarrhea**. Central nervous system effects include **yellowed and blurred vision**[31], **dizziness**[32], **fatigue**[33], **and delirium**[34]. At very high toxic ranges digitalis inhibits Na^+/K^+ ATPase in skeletal muscle, resulting in hyperkalemia[35].

K^+ competes with digitalis for binding to the Na^+/K^+ ATPase; **hypokalemia increases the effectiveness of digitalis and increases toxicity**. Hypercalcemia can also increase the action of digitalis and increase toxicity.

Dopamine and dobutamine[36] **are positive inotropic agents**[37] that can be used on a **short-term basis in congestive heart failure**. **Dobutamine stimu-lates β_1 and β_2-adrenergic receptors**. The action on **β_1-adrenoreceptors** is responsible for **most of the beneficial actions of dobutamine**. It is useful in patients with acute left ventricular failure or to prevent pulmonary edema[38] in heart failure. At sufficient doses, **dopamine** interacts with **β-1 receptors** and **increases myocardial contractility**. It is useful in the treatment of **cardiogenic and septic shock**[39].

Structure

These compounds share two structural features: an aglycone steroid nucleus with a lactone at carbon 17 in the D ring, which confers the cardiotonic properties, and polymeric sugar moieties attached to carbon 3 of the A ring. Both features are necessary for pharmacologic activity; the sugar groups are largely responsible for the pharmacokinetic properties of these drugs.

Mechanism of Action

Inhibition of the activity the Na^+-K^+-ATPase; this indirectly increases intracellu-

lar Ca^{2+}.

Administration

Digoxin can be administered IV or orally. Oral bioavailability is approximately 75 percent. Digitoxin is available only as an oral agent and its bioavailability is greater than 90 percent. Ouabain has limited bioavailability and is not used clinically.

Pharmacokinetics

Digoxin is excreted by the kidney and is not metabolized. Patients with com-promised renal function must be monitored carefully for digoxin toxicity. Digitoxin is metabolized in the liver and renal impairment does not affect the half-life of the drug.

Comprehension Questions

[10.1] Digoxin increases cardiac contractility by directly

A. Activating L-type Ca^{2+} channels

B. Inhibiting cardiac phosphodiesterase

C. Inhibiting myocardial Na^{+}/Ca^{2+} ATPase

D. Inhibiting myocardial Na^{+}/K^{+} ATPase

[10.2] Which of the following drugs may be used to increase cardiac output in a patient with pulmonary edema secondary to myocardial infarction?

A. Captopril B. Dobutamine

C. Metoprolol D. Verapamil

[10.3] Which of the following is the most accurate statement regarding digoxin?

A. Decreased mortality in patients with congestive heart failure with normal sinus rhythm

B. Increases vagal tone and decreases AV nodal conduction

C. Lengthens the action potential and increases the refractoriness of the heart

D. Useful in the treatment of Wolff-Parkinson-White Syndrome

Answers

[10.1] **D**. While digoxin reduces the amount of Na^{+}-Ca^{2+} exchange, this effect is indirect and mediated by the inhibition of the Na^{+}/K^{+} ATPase.

[10.2] **B**. Dobutamine is useful in this setting, the other choices would not increase cardiac output.

[10.3] **B**. Cardiac glycosides increase vagal tone and decrease AV node conduction. The action potential is decreased and the refractoriness of the heart is decreased. Mortality is not decreased in patients with normal sinus rhythm because of digoxin toxicity. Digoxin is contraindicated in WPW.

PHARMACOLOGY PEARLS

- ❖ Cardiac glycosides inhibit the activity the Na^+-K^+-ATPase; this indirectly increases intracellular Ca^{2+}.
- ❖ While several studies have found that digitalis does not improve mortality, it is still useful in reducing symptoms in congestive heart failure.
- ❖ The increased effectiveness of digitalis as serum K^+ falls is significant because most patients with congestive heart failure are also frequently treated with diuretics that cause potassium loss.
- ❖ Hypokalemia exacerbates digoxin toxicity.

REFERENCES

Hood W Jr, Dans A, Guyatt G, et al. Digitalis for treatment of congestive heart failure in patients in sinus rhythm. Cochrane Database Syst Rev 2004; 2: CD002901.

词汇

1. congestive heart failure[充血性心力衰竭]
2. myocardial infarctions(MIS)[心肌梗死]
3. dyspnea[呼吸困难]
4. orthopnea[端坐呼吸]
5. paroxysmal nocturnal dyspnea[阵发性夜间呼吸困难]
6. peripheral edema[外周水肿]
7. vagal[迷走神经]
8. sinoatrial(SA) node[窦房结]
9. atrioventricular(AV) node[房室结]
10. arrhythmias[心律失常]
11. anorexia[厌食症]
12. nausea[恶心]
13. diarrhea[腹泻]
14. disorientation[定向力消失]
15. visual disturbance[视觉障碍]
16. sodium-potassium adenosine triphosphatase (ATPase)[Na^+-K^+-ATP 酶]
17. stroke volume[每搏输出量]
18. cardiac output[心输出量]
19. atrial tachyarrhythmias[快速性心律失常]
20. atrial fibrillation[心房纤颤]
21. atrial flutter[心房扑动]
22. cardiac glycosides[强心苷(洋地黄类药物)]
23. myocardial contractility[心肌收缩力]
24. aortic[主动脉的]
25. mitral valve[二尖瓣]
26. tricuspid valve[三尖瓣]
27. cor pulmonale[心肺]
28. refractoriness[失效]
29. normal sinus rhythm[正常窦性节律]
30. bradycardia[心动过缓]
31. blurred vision[视力模糊]

32. dizziness[头晕]
33. fatigue[疲劳]
34. delirium[妄想]
35. hyperkalemia[高钾血症]
36. dobutamine[多巴酚丁胺]
37. inotropic agents[收缩性物质]
38. pulmonary edema[肺水肿]
39. septic shock[败血性休克]

注 1

强心苷对正常人和CHF患者心脏都有正性肌力作用，但是它只增加患者心搏出量而不增加正常心搏出量。因为强心苷对正常人还有收缩血管提高外周阻力的作用，由此限制了心搏出量的增加。但是在CHF患者中，通过反射作用，强心苷同时也降低了交感神经活性，因此这一收缩血管的作用难以发挥，使搏出量得以增加。

注 2

强心苷可加强心肌的收缩力。一方面，强心苷与心肌细胞膜上的强心苷受体 Na^+-K^+-ATP 酶结合并抑制其活性，使细胞内 Na^+ 量增加，而 K^+ 减少。胞内 Na^+ 量增加后，又通过 Na^+-Ca^{2+} 双向交换机制或使 Na^+ 内流减少，Ca^{2+} 外流减少或使 Na^+ 外流增加，Ca^{2+} 内流增加，最终导致细胞内 Na^+ 减少，Ca^{2+} 增加，肌浆网摄取 Ca^{2+} 也增加，储存 Ca^{2+} 增多。另有研究证实，细胞内 Ca^{2+} 增加时，还可增加钙离子流，使动作电位2相内流的 Ca^{2+} 增多，此又能促使肌浆网释放出 Ca^{2+}，即“以钙释钙”的过程。这样，在强心苷的作用下，心肌细胞内可利用的 Ca^{2+} 增加，心肌的收缩加强。

注 3

地高辛抗体Fab片断对强心苷有强大选择性亲和力，能使强心苷自 Na^+-K^+-ATP 酶的结合中解离出来，对严重中毒有明显效果。它与地高辛的结合物可经肾排泄。

点评

地高辛治疗心力衰竭(心衰)已有200多年的历史，已成为治疗心衰的主要药物之一，但因个体差异大，影响因素多，是临床治疗药物中最主要的监测药品之一。影响地高辛药代动力学参数的因素主要包括个体因素、制剂因素以及药物相互作用影响。个体因素包括年龄，心肌病变的程度，疾病状态等等。地高辛在体内仅有5%～10%经肝脏代谢，由于肝功能下降导致血浆蛋白较少，血中游离药物浓度提高而易被代谢，故在肝病严重者地高辛的消除反而加快。地高辛主要以原形经肾排除，肾功能对总清除率起决定性作用。另外，胃肠道疾病者，地高辛吸收减少，血药浓度降低。甲状腺功能也直接影响地高辛的清除，甲状腺功能亢进者地高辛清除率增加，需要增加用量；甲状腺功能减退者对地高辛敏感性提高，可使地高辛的清除率不变或微降。另外，不同厂家生产的制剂其口服利用度也有很大的差异，患者服用相同剂量不同厂家生产的地高辛片，达到稳态血药浓度的时间有显著的差异，并可发生意外的地高辛中毒。因此在治疗过程中病人最好使用同一厂家生产的制剂。在使用地高辛治疗心衰时，临床医生与药师需根据血药浓度监测结果，结合病人的病理、生理情况制定合理的给药方案，使给药方案由常规化、经验化转向个体化、科学化。

周宏灏

❖ CASE 11

A 62-year-old man is being managed in the intensive care unit following a large anterior wall myocardial infarction (MI). He has been appropriately managed with oxygen, aspirin, nitrates, and β-adrenergic receptor blockers but has developed recurrent episodes of ventricular tachycardia. During these episodes he remains conscious but feels dizzy, and he becomes diaphoretic and hypotensive. He is given an IV bolus of lidocaine and started on an IV lidocaine infusion.

◆ **To what class of antiarrhythmic does lidocaine belong?**

◆ **What is lidocaine's mechanism of action?**

ANSWERS TO CASE 11: Antiarrhythmic Drugs

Summary: A 62-year-old man develops symptomatic ventricular tachycardia after a myocardial infarction. He is begun on IV lidocaine.

- **Class of antiarrhythmic to which lidocaine belongs**: IB.
- **Mechanism of action**: Specific Na^+ channel blocker, reducing the rate of phase 0 depolarization, primarily in damaged tissue.

CLINICAL CORRELATION

Lidocaine is a common treatment for ventricular tachycardia in a patient who is symptomatic and remains conscious. It works by blocking Na^+ channels and is highly selective for damaged tissue. This makes it useful for the treatment of ventricular ectopy associated with an MI. It is administered as an IV bolus followed by a continuous drip infusion. It is metabolized in the liver and undergoes a large first-pass effect. It has many neurological① side effects, including agitation, confusion, and tremors, and can precipitate seizures.

Pharmacology of the Antiarrhythmics

Objectives

1. Know the classes of antiarrhythmic agents and their mechanisms of action.
2. Know the indications for the use of antiarrhythmic agents.
3. Know the adverse effects and toxicities of the antiarrhythmic agents.

Definitions

Paroxysmal atrial tachycardias (PAT)②: Arrhythmia③ caused by reentry through the atrioventricular④ (AV) node.

Heart block: Failure of normal conduction from atria⑤ to ventricles.

WPW: Wolff-Parkinson-White syndrome.

Discussion of Class

Arrhythmias arise as a result of improper impulse generation or improper impulse conduction. The abnormal action potentials cause disturbances in the rate of contraction or in the coordination of myocardial contraction. The molecular target of antiarrhythmics are ion channels in the myocardium or conduction pathways; these may be direct or indirect effects. **There are four ion channels of pharmacologic importance in the heart**[注1]:

Voltage-activated Na^+ channel—SCN5A

Voltage-activated Ca^{2+} channel—L-type

Voltage-activated K^+ channel—IKr

Voltage-activated K^+ channel—IKs

Most antiarrhythmic drugs either bind directly to sites within the pore of a channel or indirectly alter channel activity.

There are about 20 antiarrhythmics approved for use today. They are classified according to which of the ion channels⑥ they affect and their mechanism of action (Table 11-1). The major arrhythmias of clinical concern are ventricular arrhythmias, atrial arrhythmias, bradycardias⑦, and heart blocks. There is also the pharmacologic need to convert an abnormal rhythm to normal sinus rhythm (cardioconversion). The class of antiarrhythmic used for any particular arrhythmia depends on the clinical circumstances. The treatment of acute, life-threatening disease, in contrast with the long-term management of chronic disease, requires a different selection of antiarrhythmics.

Table 11-1

SELECTED ANTIARRHYTHMIC AGENTS

CLASS	PROTOTYPE DRUG	Na^+	K^+	Ca^{2+}	EFFECT
Ia	Quinidine	X	X		Increases refractory period, slows conduction
Ib	Lidocaine	X			Shortens duration of refractory period
Ic	Flecadine	X	X		Slows conduction
II	Propranolol			X[1]	Blocks β_1-adrenergic receptors
III	Amiodarone	X		X	Increases refractory period
IV	Verapamil			X	Increases refractory period AV node
Other					
	Adenosine		X	X[1]	Decreases AV node conduction
	Moricizine	X[3]			
	Atropine				Decreases vagal tone
	Digoxin				Increases vagal tone
	Sotalol		X[2]		Also nonselective beta blocker

[1] Indirect effect mediated by decreasing cAMP.

[2] Solotol has α- and β-adrenergic antagonist properties and also inhibits K^+ channels.

[3] Moricizine blocks Na^+ channels and is usually considered a class 1 antiarrythtmic, but is hasproperties of Ia, IIb, and Ic drugs.

Class I Antiarrhythmics

Class I antiarrhythmics bind to Na^+ channels and prevent their activation. This increases their effective refractory[8] period and decreases conduction velocity. Class I antiarrhythmics have a greater effect on damaged tissue compared to normal tissue. This may be because of several factors:

Depolarization[9]. Damaged tissues tend to be depolarized because of K^+ leakage—many class I antiarrhythmics preferentially bind to depolarized tissues.

pH. Ischemic[10] tissues are more acidic, and many Class I antiarrhythmics preferentially bind to membranes at low pH.

Inactivation frequency. During arrhythmias, Na^+ channels undergo more rapid cycles of activation/inactivation. At any given time there will be an increase in the number of inactive channels compared to normal tissues in a normal rhythm. Class I antiarrhythmics generally bind preferentially to Na^+ channels in the inactive state.

The subclasses, a, b, and c of class I antiarrhythmics are distinguished based on their ability to inhibit K^+ channels.

Class 1a. Procainamide[11] is a prototype class 1a antiarrhythmic that suppresses the activity of Na^+ and also suppresses K^+ channel activity. **Administered IV**, it is used for the acute suppression of supraventricular and ventricular arrhythmias and for suppressing episodes of atrial flutter and atrial fibrillation. **It may be administered orally for the long-term suppression of both supraventricular and ventricular arrhythmia, but toxicity limits this application. Procainamide can suppress sinoatrial (SA) and AV nodal activity, especially in patients with nodal disease, and cause heart block. Prolonged use of procainamide is associated with increased risk of ventricular tachycardias[12]. Procainamide has some ganglionic[13] blocking activity and can cause hypotension and decreased myocardial contractility[14].** A limiting adverse effect of procainamide is the development of lupus-like syndrome characterized by skin rash, arthritis, and serositis[15]. **All patients on procainamide will develop antinuclear antibodies within 2 years.** Procainamide is metabolized to N-acetyl procainamide (NAPA), **which has K^+-channel blocking effects. NAPA is excreted by the kidney, and plasma levels of procainamide and** NAPA should both be moni-tored especially in patients with renal disease.

Class 1b. Lidocaine is very specific for the Na^+ channel and it blocks both activated and inactivated states of the channel. **It must be administered parenterally. Lidocaine has been used extensively to suppress ventricular arrhythmias associated with acute MI** or cardiac damage (surgery). **It has been used prophylacti-**

cally to prevent arrhythmias in patients with MI, but there is controversy as to the overall benefit in decreasing mortality. Lidocaine is metabolized in the liver and has relatively short half-life (60 minutes). This limits its adverse effects which generally are mild and rapidly reversible. Overdose can produce sedation, hallucinations[16], and convulsions[17].[注2]

Class 1c. Flecainide[18] inhibits both Na^+ and K^+ channels but shows no preference for inactivated Na^+ channels. It delays conduction and increases refractoriness. **It is effective for the control of atrial arrhythmias and it is very effective in suppressing supraventricular arrhythmias.** A recent large clinical trial with patients with **ischemic heart disease**, demonstrated that flecainide is **associated with increased mortality. Currently its use is restricted to patients with atrial arrhythmias without underlying ischemic heart disease.**

Class II Agents

Endogenous catecholamines[19] increase myocardial excitability and can trigger ventricular arrhythmias. β-adrenergic receptor blockade indirectly suppresses L-type Ca^{2+} channel activity. **This slows phase 3 repolarization and lengthens the refractory period. Reduction in sympathetic tone depresses automaticity, decreases AV conduction, and decreases heart rate and contractility. Beta blockers are useful for the long-term suppression of ventricular arrhythmias particularly in patients at risk for sudden cardiac arrest. Beta blockers are most effective in patients with increased adrenergic activity**:

Surgical or anesthetic stress
Anginal pain[20] and myocardial infarction
Congestive heart failure and ischemic heart disease
Hyperthyroidism

Beta blockers have been shown to reduce mortality and second cardiovascular events by 25% to 40% in patients with postmyocardial infarction.

There are a large number of beta blockers approved for use as antiarrhythmics. Two of particular interest are

1. **d, l-sotalol**, which is particularly effective as an antiarrhythmic because it combines inhibition of K^+ channels with betablocker activity.
2. Metoprolol, a specific β_1 antagonist, which reduces the risk of pulmonary complications.

d, l-sotalol is a racemic mixture; l-sotalol is an effective, **nonselective β-adrenergic antagonist**; and d-sotalol is a class III antiarrhythmic that inhibits K^+ channels. It is an oral agent with a long half-life (20 h) that can maintain therapeutic blood levels with once a day dosing. d, l-sotalol is useful for the long-term suppression of ventricular arrhythmias, especially in patients at risk of sudden death. It is also used to suppress atrial flutter and fibrillation and paroxysmal atrial tachycardia. It is a valuable adjunct in the use of implantable cardiac defibrillators㉑, decreasing the number of events that require defibrillation. At low doses, the β-adrenergic blocking activity, and associated adverse effects, predominate. At higher doses, the K^+-channel inhibitory effects predominate with the risk of developing ventricular tachycardia.

Class III Antiarrhythmics

Drugs in this class **include bretylium**㉒, **dofetilide**㉓, **and amiodarone**㉔. These agents act predominantly to **inhibit cardiac K^+ channels (IKr)**. This lengthens the time to repolarize and prolongs the refractory period. Amiodarone is also a potent inhibitor of Na^+ channels and has α- and β-adrenergic antagonist activity.

Amiodarone has an unusual structure related to thyroxine. It can be administered IV or orally, but its actions differ depending on route of admin-istration. IV-administered amiodarone has acute effects to inhibit K^+-channel activity, slowing repolarization and increasing the refractory period of all myocardial cell types. Administered orally in a more chronic setting leads to long-term alterations in membrane properties with a reduction in both Na^+ and K^+ channel activity and decreases in adrenergic receptor activity. **Amiodarone is used extensively for ventricular and atrial arrhythmias and has little myocardial depressant activity**, allowing it to be used in patients with diminished cardiac function. Administered IV amiodarone is effective in treating ventricular tachycardia and to prevent recurrent ventricular tachycardia, and to suppress atrial fibrillation. Oral amiodarone is useful for arrhythmias that have not responded to other drugs (such as adenosine) and for long-term suppression of arrhythmias in patients at risk of sudden cardiac death.

Amiodarone has little myocardial toxicity, does not impair contractility, and rarely induces arrhythmias. Most of the adverse effects of amiodarone result from its **long half-life** (13-103 days) and **poor solubility**. **Amiodarone deposits in the lung** and can cause **irreversible pulmonary damage**. Similarly, **amiodarone can be deposited in the cornea causing visual disturbances or in the skin where it can cause a bluish tinge**.

Class IV Antiarrhythmics

The class IV antiarrhythmics act by directly blocking the activity of L-type Ca^{2+} channels. **Verapamil**㉕ and **diltiazem**㉖ are the major members of this class, and they have a similar pharmacology. **Verapamil blocks both active and inactive Ca^{2+} channels** and has effects that are equipotent in cardiac and peripheral tissues. The

dihydropyridines such as **nifedipine** have **little effect on Ca^{2+} channels in the myocardium. Verapamil** has marked effects on both **SA and AV nodes** because these tissues are highly dependent on Ca^{2+} currents. AV nodal conduction and refractory period are prolonged and the SA node is slowed. **Verapamil and diltiazem are useful for reentrant supraventricular tachycardias** and can also be used to reduce the ventricular rate in atrial flutter or fibrillation. The **major adverse effect of verapamil** is related to its **inhibition of myocardial contractility**. It can cause heart block at high doses.

Other Antiarrhythmics

Adenosine is a **very short-acting drug (approximately 10 seconds)** used specifically to **block paroxysmal atrial tachycardias (PAT). Adenosine binds to purinergic A1 receptors**. Activation of these receptors leads to increased potassium conductance and a decrease in calcium influx. This results in hyperpolarization and a decrease in Ca^{2+} dependent action potentials. The effect in the AV node is marked with a decrease in conduction and an increase in nodal refractory period. Effects on the SA node are smaller. Adenosine is nearly 100 percent effective in converting PAT to sinus rhythm. Adenosine must be given IV, and because of its short half-life, it has few adverse effects. Flushing and chest pain are frequent but typically resolve quickly.

Digoxin (see Case 10) blocks Na^+ K^+ ATPase and indirectly increases intracellular Ca^{2+}. In the myocardium this causes an increase in contractility; in nerve tissue the predominant effect is to increase neurotransmitter release; and the parasympathetic system (vagus) is affected more than the sympathetic system. The increased vagal tone results in increased stimulation of muscarinic acetylcholine receptors that slow conduction in the AV node. **Digoxin is very effective controlling the ventricular response rate in patients with atrial fibrillation or flutter**. Digoxin can be administered IV to acutely treat atrial arrhythmias or orally for long-term suppression of abnormal atrial rhythms. Digitalis is less effective than adenosine in PAT and **should not be used in WPW**.

Atropine[27] **is a muscarinic antagonist that can be used in some bradycardias and heart blocks. It can be administered to reverse heart block caused by increased vagal tone such as a myocardial infarction or digitalis toxicity. Atropine is administered IV, and it exerts its effect within minutes.**

Comprehension Questions

[11.1] The most effective agent for converting paroxysmal atrial tachycardia to normal sinus rhythm is

A. Adenosine B. Atropine

C. Digoxin D. Lidocaine

[11.2] Which of the following best describes a pharmacologic property of amiodarone?

A. α-adrenergic agonist B. β-adrenergic agonist

C. activation of Ca^{2+} channels D. inhibition of K^+ channels

[11.3] A 45-year-old man is noted to have dilated cardiomyopathy with atrial fibrillation and a rapid ventricular rate. An agent is used to control the ventricular rate, but the cardiac contractility is also affected, placing him in pulmonary edema. Which of the following agents was most likely used?

A. Amiodarone B. Digoxin

C. Nifedipine D. Verapamil

Answers

[11.1] **A.** Adenosine is nearly 100 percent effective in converting PAT. Digoxin could be used but is less effective.

[11.2] **D.** Amiodarone blocks both Na^+ and K^+ channels and has α- and β-adrenoreceptor **antagonist** activities. The latter would indirectly decrease Ca^{2+} channel activity.

[11.3] **D.** Verapamil is a calcium channel-blocking agent that slows conduction in the AV node, but it also has a negative inotropic effect on the heart.

PHARMACOLOGY PEARLS

- Amiodarone is typically the first choice in acute ventricular arrhythmias.
- Adenosine is the best choice to convert PAT to sinus rhythm.
- Long-term benefit of using class I antiarrhythmics is uncertain, but mortality is not decreased.
- Beta blockers have been shown to reduce mortality and second cardiovascular events by 25-40% in patients postmyocardial infarction.

REFERENCES

Kowey PR, Yan GX, Dimino TL, et al. Overview of the management of atrial fibrillation: What is the current state of the art? J Cardiovasc Electrophysiol 2003 Dec; 14(suppl 12): S275-80.

Cooper HA, Bloomfield DA, Bush DE, et al. Relation between achieved heart rate and outcomes in patients with atrial fibrillation (from the atrial fibrillation follow-up investigation of rhythm management [AFFIRM] study): AFFIRM Investigators. Am J Cardiol 2004 May 15; 93(10): 1247-53.

词汇

1. neurological[神经学的]
2. paroxysmal atrial tachycardia(PAT)[阵发性前房心跳加快]
3. arrhythmia[心律失常]
4. atrioventricular[房室的]
5. atria[心房]
6. ion channel[离子通道]
7. bradycardia[心动过缓]
8. refractory[抗感染的]
9. depolarization[去极化]
10. ischemic[局部缺血]
11. procainamide[普鲁卡因胺]
12. tachycardia[心动过速]
13. ganglionic[神经节的]
14. myocardial contractility[心肌收缩力]
15. serositis[浆膜炎]
16. hallucination[幻觉]
17. convulsion[抽搐,惊厥]
18. flecainide[氟卡尼]
19. catecholamines[儿茶酚胺]
20. anginal pain[心绞痛]
21. defibrillator[除颤器]
22. bretylium[溴苄胺]
23. dofetilide[多非利特]
24. amiodarone[胺碘酮]
25. verapamil[维拉帕米]
26. diltiazem[地尔硫草]
27. atropine[阿托品]

注 1

钙通道阻滞剂或称钙拮抗剂是在通道水平上选择性的阻滞钙离子经细胞膜上的钙离子通道内流，减少细胞内钙离子浓度的药物。它们是20世纪70年代发展起来的，临床上主要用于治疗高血压、心绞痛、心律失常、脑血管痉挛、心肌缺血等疾病的一类心脑血管药物。钙离子是心肌和血管平滑肌兴奋-收缩偶联中的关键物质，钙离子进入血管平滑肌细胞后，可直接收缩平滑肌，是冠脉痉挛，阻力增大，耗氧增加。钙通道阻滞剂通过抑制细胞外钙离子内流，使心肌和血管平滑肌细胞内缺乏足够的钙离子，结果导致心肌收缩力减弱，心率减慢，同时松弛血管，血压下降，从而减少心肌耗氧量。

注 2

利多卡因是目前防治急性心肌梗死及各种心脏病并发快速室性心律失常的药物。该药只能通过静脉途径给药，毒性发生率低。特别适用于危急病例。利多卡因也是一种常用的局部麻醉药，其穿透力较其他局部麻醉药强，且作用快而持久，毒性小、无刺激性，可有效地阻断病灶周围神经末梢反射，减轻药物对局部血管神经的不良刺激，止痛效果好。剂量过大时可引起惊厥及心跳骤停。严重房室传导阻滞、室内传导阻滞者禁用。与奎尼丁、普鲁卡因胺、普萘洛尔、美西律或妥卡胺合用时，本品的毒性增加，甚至引起窦性停搏。

点评

依据药物的电生理作用，可将抗心律失常药物分为四类：

Ⅰ类：药物的主要作用是阻断快速流出钠通道。根据阻滞钠通道特性和程度的不同，对 K^+ 通道和 APD 影响的差异又将其分为ⅠA、ⅠB 和ⅠC，对传导速度的作用强度依次为ⅠC > ⅠA > ⅠB。

ⅠA 类：中度减慢动作电 0 期上升速率 Vmax，减慢传导，延长动作电位时程。代表药有奎尼丁、普鲁卡因胺等。

ⅠB 类：轻度减慢，稍减慢传导，缩短动作电位。代表药有利多卡因、美西律等。IC 类：明显减慢，显著减慢传导，轻微延长动作电位时程。代表药有氟卡胺、英卡胺、普罗帕酮。

Ⅱ类：阻断肾上腺素能受体，减慢动作电位上升速率，抑制 4 相除极。代表药有普萘洛尔等。

Ⅲ类：延长动作电位时程。代表药有胺碘酮、溴苄胺、索托洛尔等。

Ⅳ类：阻断钙通道。代表药有维拉帕米、地尔硫䓬等。

其他抗心律失常药物还有地高辛，用于治疗心房颤动和阵发性室上性心动过速；腺苷用于治疗室上性心动过速等。

李 清

❖ CASE 12

A 50-year-old man presents for follow-up of his hypertension. He is maintaining a low-sodium diet, exercising regularly, and taking metoprolol at maximum dosage. [注1] He is on no other medications. His blood pressure remains elevated at 150/100 mmHg. His examination is otherwise unremarkable. You decide to add a thiazide diuretic to his regimen. [注2]

◆ **What is the mechanism of action of metoprolol?**

◆ **What is the mechanism of action of thiazide diuretics?**

◆ **What electrolyte abnormalities commonly occur with thiazide diuretics?**

ANSWERS TO CASE 12: Antihypertensive Agents

Summary: A 50-year-old man with inadequately controlled hypertension is prescribed a thiazide diuretic.

- **Mechanism of action of metoprolol**: β_1-selective adrenoreceptor antagonist.
- **Mechanism of action of thiazide diuretics**: Inhibit active reabsorption of NaCl in the distal convoluted tubule by interfering with a specific Na^+/Cl^- cotransporter.
- **Electrolyte abnormalities seen with thiazide diuretics**: Hypokalemia, hyponatremia, hypochloremia.

CLINICAL CORRELATION

Thiazide diuretics and beta blockers are the recommended first-line agents for most people with hypertension. They are frequently used in combination with each other and with other classes of antihypertensives. Thiazides inhibit the active reabsorption of NaCl. This causes an increase in the excretion of Na^+, Cl^-, and K^+. They also reduce the excretion of Ca^{2+} by increasing its absorption. The excretion of sodium and water reduces intravascular volume and contributes to their antihypertensive effect. Thiazides are used as single agents primarily in mild to moderate hypertension. They are often added as second agents when other drugs alone cannot control a patient's hypertension. The electrolyte abnormalities caused by thiazides can be clinically important. Hypokalemia occurs frequently, especially when higher doses of thiazides are used. Patients need to be instructed to follow a high potassium diet and frequently require potassium supplementation. Thiazides can also elevate serum uric acid levels, which can precipitate gout in susceptible individuals.

Pharmacology of Antihypertensive Agents

Objectives

1. Know the classes of antihypertensive medications and their mechanisms of action.
2. Know the common side effects of the antihypertensive agents.

Definitions

Hypertension: Blood pressure continuously elevated to levels greater than 120/80 mmHg. Pressures of 130/90 mmHg are considered prehypertensive.

Essential hypertension: Hypertension of unknown etiology makes up about 90 percent of hypertensive patients.

Discussion of Class

There are 10 major classes of drugs that are used as oral antihypertensive drugs, and these include drugs that act centrally and those that work in the periphery. Antihypertensive drugs may cause vascular smooth-muscle relaxation, vascular volume reduction, or a decrease in cardiac output. This is accomplished by decreasing Ca^{2+} in vascular smooth muscle cells or by reducing Na^+ reabsorption on the kidney. Table 12-1 lists these major classes. **Lifestyle modifications include smoking cessation, weight management①, and commencement of an exercise program.**

The Joint National Commission(JNC) also emphasized the need to recognize and treat **systolic hypertension②**, which is associated with a **higher degree of risk of myocardial infarction(MI)③** in patients **older than 45years.** Systolic hypertension is more difficult to treat than diastolic hypertension and frequently requires multiple drugs acting via different mechanisms.

The JNC recommendation for treatment of hypertension recommends **diuretics or** beta blockers **as first choices for monotherapy④(Table 12-2)**. This conservative approach is based on the fact that data support that these **agents decrease morbidity and mortality⑤** in clinical trials. The other agents that should be considered for initial monotherapy include the reninangiotensin system inhibititors (either angiotensin-converting enzyme [ACE] inhibitors or angiotensin receptor blockers[ARBs]), α-adrenoreceptor antagonists, calcium-channel antagonists, and arterial vasodilators. All have been shown to reduce blood pressure by 10-15 mmHg.

Diuretics

Diuretics cause an initial reduction in blood pressure by **facilitating loss of Na^+ and water**. This leads to a decrease in cardiac output and blood pressure. However, after 8 weeks, cardiac output returns to normal while blood pressure remains reduced. This is thought to be caused by a **reduction in the vasoconstrictive activities⑥ of Na^+ on vascular smooth muscles** that include **elevation of intracellular Ca^{2+} via the Ca^{2+}/Na^+ antiporter⑦. Thiazide** diuretics, which reduce the activity of a specific Na^+Cl^- cotransporter(NCC2) in the **distal convoluted tubule⑧**, are the class of diuretics most often used for hypertension. In refractory cases or in patients with concomitant edema, loop diuretics can be used with caution. Loop diuretics reduce Na^+ reabsorption in the ascending limb of the loop of Henle by reducing the activity of another Na^+-K^+-$2Cl^-$ cotransporter (NKCC) and can produce a profound loss of Na^+ and K^+. **Both thiazides and loop diuretics⑨ can cause hypokalemia and hyponatremia**. A common complaint associated with diuretic use is the increased **frequency of urination⑩**.

Table 12-1
SELECTIVE CLASSES OF ANTIHYPERTENSIVE AGENTS

CLASS	PROTOTYPE DRUG	MOA	COMMON ADVERSE EFFECT
beta blocker	Propranolol	Adrenergic β-receptor antagonist	Fatigue, reduction on libido
α_1-antagonist	Prazosin	Adrenergic receptor antagonist	Orthostatic hypotension
ACE inhibitor	Enalapril	Reduces production of angiotensin II	Hyperkalemia
ARB (angiotenson receptor blocker)	Losartan	AT-1 receptor antagonist	Hyperkalemia
Diueretic—loop	Furosemide	Reduces Na^+ reabsorption in loop of Henle	Hypokalemia
Diuretic—distal tubule	Hydrochlorothiazide	Reduces Na^+ reabsorption at site 3	Hypokalemia
Ca^{2+} channel blocker	Nifedipine	Blocks Ca^{2+} entry in vascular smooth muscle cells	Hypotension arrhythmias
Arterial vasodilators	Minoxidil	Hyperpolarizes VSMC	Orthostatic hypotension
Central acting Vasodilator	Clonidine	α_2-adrenergic Agonist, I_2 receptor agonist	Sedation, depression
Adrenergic neuron blockers	Guanethidine	Inhibits release of norepinephrine	Postural hypotension
Neuronal uptake inhibitor	Reserpine	Depletes neurons of neurotransmitters	Sedation

Table 12-2

THE JOINT NATIONAL COMMITTEE ON HYPERTENSION HAS DEFINED 4 CATEGORIES OF HYPERTENSION

STAGE	BLOOD PRESSURE SYSTOLIC (mmHg)	BLOOD PRESSURE DIASTOLIC (mmHg)	RECOMMENDED TREATMENT
Normal	< 120	and < 80	—
Pre-hypertensive	120-139	Or 80-89	Lifestyle modification
Hypertensive stage 1	140-159	Or 90-99	Lifestyle modification, R_x
Hypertensive stage 2	≥160	Or ≥100	Lifestyle modification, R_x

Beta (β)-blockers

Use of β-adrenoreceptor blockers for hypertension relies on **decreasing cardiac output and decreasing peripheral vascular resistance**⑪. The various drugs in this class vary in their potency on β_2 receptors; **metoprolol**⑫ is more than 1000 times more potent in blocking β_2 compared to β_1 receptors, giving this drug a relative **cardioselectivity**⑬. Blockade of β_1-adrenoreceptors in the juxtaglomerular apparatus of the kidney reduces renin secretion, and this reduces the production of angiotensin II. Nonselective beta blockers such as propanolol cause a number of predictable adverse effects including bronchoconstriction (contraindicating use in asthmatics); a decrease in the production of insulin (contraindicating use in diabetics); and central nervous system (CNS) effects including depression, insomnia, and a decline in male potency. In addition, the nonselective agents increase both triglycerides and low-density lipoprotein (LDL). These effects are reduced but not eliminated with the more β_1 selective agents.

α_1-Blockers

Prazosin⑭, **doxazosin**⑮, **and terazosin**⑯ reduce blood pressure by **antagonizing α_1-adrenoreceptors in vascular smooth muscle**. Blockade of this receptor reduces intracellular **cyclic adenosine monophosphate** (cAMP)⑰ and leads to a reduction in intracellular Ca^{2+}. **Orthostatic hypotension**⑱ is common on initiation of therapy but diminishes. Dizziness and headache are also adverse effects. α_1-blockers appear to reduce LDL cholesterol.

Ca^{2+}-Channel Blockers

Calcium channel blockers are useful antihypertensives and can reduce blood pressure by 10-15 mmHg. These agents exert their antihypertensive effect by **blocking L-type (voltage-sensitive) calcium channels**. By blocking the entry of Ca^{2+} into the cell, less is available to activate the contractile apparatus, and within vascular smooth muscle, this produces a reduction in vascular tone. Three distinct chemical classes comprise the Ca^{2+}-channel antagonists, **dihydropyridines**⑲ include nifedipine, diphenylalkylamines include verapamil, and **benzothiazepines**⑳ include diltiazem. All are approved for treating hypertension. Nifedipine and the other dihydropyridines have less of an effect on the heart than verapamil and diltiazem. **Verapamil has the greatest effect on the heart and can significantly reduce contractility**. Because of its effect on the heart, verapamil can be used to treat supraventricular arrhythmias as well as variant angina. Depression of cardiac function is the greatest adverse effect of the Ca^{2+} channel blockers, and this is markedly diminished with the dihydropyridines. However, clinical trials with short-acting nifedipine suggested that there was an increase in the risk of MI in patients treated for hypertension, and these agents should not be used to treat the disease.

Renin-Angiotensin System Inhibitors

Inhibitors of the renin-angiotensin system, both **angiotensin-converting enzyme (ACE)**㉑ **inhibitors and angiotensin receptor blockers (ARBs)** are effective for hypertension monotherapy. ACE inhibitors block the conversion of the inactive angiotensin I to the potent angiotensin II. Angiotensin II acts to increase blood pressure in several ways. In vascular smooth muscle it increases intracellular Ca^{2+} and produces pronounced vasoconstriction. At peripheral nerve endings and in the adrenal medulla it increases the amount of catecholamines released on stimulation. In the zona glomerulosa of the adrenal cortex it acts to stimulate the biosynthesis of aldosterone, which increases renal Na^{+} and water retention. Adverse effects include hypotension, dizziness, and fatigue; rarely, hyperkalemia may occur. A dry cough and angioedema may occur as a result of the reduction in degradation of bradykinin that is brought about by these drugs.

Angiotensin II acts through AT-1 and AT-2 receptors, which in turn couple to numerous signal transduction pathways. The hypertensive actions of angiotensin II are mediated by AT-1 receptors. Losartan, valsartan, and other AT-1 receptor blockers are also effective in reducing blood pressure by 10-15 mmHg. The adverse effect profile is similar to the ACE inhibitors but without the cough or angioedema.

Direct Arterial Vasodilators

Arterial vasodilators㉒ **act by increasing the efflux of potassium from the cell.** This causes **hyperpolarization**㉓ across the plasma membrane that diminishes the activity of the voltage-regulated L-type calcium channel. In vascular smooth muscle cells this produces a reduction in vascular tone. **Minoxidil**[24] **and hydralazine**[25] are the two most commonly used oral vasodilators used to treat hypertension. Both have pronounced effects on the resistance vessels and little effect on veins. Because of their predominant effect on arterioles, these agents provoke the **baroreceptor reflex**[26] **that includes tachycardia, vasoconstriction, and the release of renin**. For this reason, these agents are usually combined with a beta blocker and a diuretic.

Centrally Acting Agents

Central acting vasodilators such as clonidine[27] **and methyldopa**[28] act as **α_2-adrenergic receptor agonists**[29] **in the vasomotor center within the medulla**[30]. These agents decrease sympathetic outflow and thereby decrease vascular tone and cardiac output. The use of these agents as antihypertensives has been overshadowed by the introduction of ACE inhibitors and ARBs and calcium channel blockers. This is largely a result of the adverse effects, which are mostly in the CNS and include sedation, depression, and dry mouth. However, they are still used in cases of refractory hypertension.

Peripheral Sympathetic Inhibitors

Peripheral sympatholytic agents used for hypertension include guanethidine and reserpine. Guanethidine enters sympathetic nerve terminals by transport and replaces norepinephrine in transmitter vesicles. Release of norepinephrine is thereby diminished. Reserpine blocks the uptake and storage of biogenic amines, and this diminishes the amount of transmitter released on stimulation. Because of much higher rates of adverse effects, these agents are rarely used to treat simple hypertension but may be combined in the treatment of refractory hypertension.

Comprehension Questions

[12.1] The inclusion of spironolactone with a thiazide diuretic in a regimen to treat hypertension is done to

A. Reduce hyperuricemia
B. Reduce Mg^+ loss
C. Decrease the loss of Na^+
D. Reduce K^+ loss

[12.2] Which of the following drugs would be the best to treat moderate hypertension in a diabetic patient with mild proteinuria?

A. Enalapril
B. Propranolol
C. Hydrochlorothiazide
D. Nifedipine

[12.3] A 33-year-old man is diagnosed with essential hypertension. He is started on a blood pressure medication, and after 6 weeks, he notes fatigue, rash over his face, joint aches, and effusions. A serum antinuclear antibody (ANA) test is positive. Which of the following is the most likely agent?

A. Hydralazine
B. Propranolol
C. Thiazide diuretic
D. Nifedipine
E. Enalapril

Answers

[12.1] **D**. Spironolactone is a "potassium-sparing" diuretic that reduces K^+ excretion in the collecting duct. It diminishes the K^+-wasting effects of thiazide diuretics.

[12.2] **A**. ACE inhibitors such as enalapril have been shown to reduce the progressive loss of renal function that is often seen is diabetic patients. The nonselective beta blocker propranolol would worsen the diabetes.

[12.3] **A**. Hydralazine is associated with a lupus-like presentation, with photosensitivity, malar rash, joint pain, and sometimes pericardial effusion or pleural effusion.

PHARMACOLOGY PEARLS

❖ The ALLHAT clinical trial (Antihypertensive and Lipid-Lowering Treatment to Prevent Heart Attack) compared amlodipine, a dihydropyridine Ca^{2+} channel blocker, lisinopril, an ACE inhibitor, doxazosin, an α_1-adrenergic antagonist with chlorthalidone, a thiazide diuretic.

❖ Thiazide diuretics and beta blockers are the preferred initial therapy for hypertension.

❖ Beta-blocking agents can cause depression, insomnia, male impotency, bronchoconstriction, and decreased production of insulin.

REFERENCES

Tatti P, Pahor M, Byington RP, et al. Outcome results of the fosinopril versus amlodipine cardiovascular events randomized trial (FACET) in patients with hypertension and NIDDM. Diabetes Care 1998 Apr; 21(4): 597-603.

ALLHAT Officers and Coordinators for the ALLHAT Collaborative Research Group. Major outcomes in moderately hypercholesterolemic, hypertensive patients randomized to pravastatin vs usual care: the antihypertensive and lipidlowering treatment to prevent heart attack trial (ALLHAT-LLT). The antihypertensive and lipid-lowering treatment to prevent heart attack trial. JAMA 2002 Dec 18; 288(23): 2998-3007.

词汇

1. weight management[保持体重]
2. systolic hypertension[收缩期高血压]
3. myocardial infarction(MI)[心肌梗死]
4. monotherapy[单一疗法]
5. morbidity and mortality[发病率和死亡率]
6. vasoconstrictive activities[血管收缩反应]
7. Ca^{2+}/Na^{+} antiporter[Ca^{2+}/Na^{+}反向转运体]
8. distal convoluted tubule[远曲小管]
9. loop diuretics[髓袢利尿剂]
10. increased frequency of urination[尿频]
11. peripheral vascular resistance[外周血管阻力的下降]
12. metoprolol[美托洛尔]
13. cardioselectivity[心选择性]
14. prazosin[哌唑嗪]
15. doxazosin[喹唑嗪]
16. terazosin[特拉唑嗪]
17. cyclic adenosine monophosphate(cAMP)[环磷腺苷]
18. orthostatic hypotension[直立性低血压]
19. dihydropyridines[二氢吡啶类]
20. benzothiazepine[苯并噻氮䓬类]
21. angiotensin-converting enzyme(ACE)[血管紧张素转化酶]
22. arterial vasodilators[血管扩张剂]
23. hyperpolarization[超极化]
24. minoxidil[米诺地尔 周围血管扩张剂]
25. hydralazine[肼屈嗪 周围血管扩张剂]
26. baroreceptor reflex[压力感受器反射]
27. clonidine[可乐定 降血压药]
28. methyldopa[甲基多巴 降血压药]
29. α_2-adrenergic receptor agonist[α_2 肾上腺素受体激动剂]
30. medulla[髓质]

注 1

近年来，世界卫生组织(WHO)推出了高血压患者的“阶梯用药法”，亦叫分级治疗。所谓“阶梯用药法”，就是在一般治疗的基础上，首先选用一种作用缓和且副作用小、经济方便的降压药，适当的降压，以后则根据疗效、副作用等情况而逐级增加药物联合应用，是相加性疗法。具体方法是：第一级可以在利尿剂或β-阻滞剂普萘洛尔任选一种，大多数病人以单用利尿剂为合适，用药7～10天。若无效要加用第二阶段药物。第二级在第一级治疗用药无效的基础上加用另一类药物，常采用利尿剂加β-阻滞剂或甲基多巴或肼苯达嗪或硝苯地平。第三级在第二级用药无效的基础上，加用第三类药物，如利尿剂、普萘洛尔加利血平或哌唑嗪或肼苯达嗪或甲巯丙脯酸。

注 2

噻嗪(类)利尿剂：噻嗪类利尿药是广泛用于临床的口服利尿药，对各种原因引起的水肿、以心源性水肿为佳。对高血压者有降压作用、与其他抗高血压药物合用，可增强降压作用。对尿崩症有一定疗效。严重肝病患者应慎用，以防诱发肝昏迷。严重肾功能不良者禁用。最近发表的试验研究结果显示，小剂量噻嗪类利尿剂对所有的预后终点事件(冠心病、充血性心力衰竭 CHF、脑卒中、心血管疾病事件、心血管病死亡率)的改善都显著优于安慰剂。对上述任何一项预后终点，其他抗高血压药物(β受体阻断剂、ACEI、ARB、CCB和α受体阻断剂都不优于噻嗪类利尿剂。

点评

临床上常联合应用几种降压药物治疗高血压，其优点是：药物的协同作用可提高疗效；几种药物共同发挥作用，可减少各药的单剂量；减少每种药物的副作用，或使一些副作用互相抵消；使血压下降较为平稳。最常用的联合是利尿剂和其他降压药合用，利尿剂既可增强多种降压药疗效，又可减轻引起水肿的副作用；利血平和肼屈嗪，β受体阻滞剂和米诺地尔合用时，各自减慢和增快心率的副作用互相抵消。近年来多选用钙离子拮抗剂作为首选药，尤其对伴有冠心病心绞痛者尤为适宜，对有传导阻滞、心动过缓者亦甚安全；亦可选用酶抑制剂，对伴有心功能欠佳者更好，对血压过高上述两药可同时应用；对有心动过速者可选用β受体阻滞剂，尤其对心肌梗死后伴有高血压、心动过速或过早搏动可能有预防猝死的作用；对持久血压不易下降者有时需上述三药同时应用，但应从小剂量开始，并经常随访血压。近年研究证明，硝苯地平与卡托普利有逆转高血压引起的左心室肥厚的作用，故特别适合高血压合并心脏病患者。不同个体对高血压药物治疗的反应存在差异，CYP2C9、CYP2C19、CYP2D6、受体和血管紧张素Ⅱ受体基因多态性是已知的抗高血压药物疗效和不良反应个体差异产生的主要原因。

李 清

❖ CASE 13

A 60-year-old man with hypertension and type II diabetes comes in to the office for a follow-up visit. Along with making appropriate diet and lifestyle changes, he is taking an angiotensin-converting enzyme(ACE) inhibitor-thiazide diuretic combination for his hypertension and metformin for his diabetes. His blood pressure and diabetes arc under acceptable control. Routine blood work revealed normal electrolytes, renal function, and liver enzymes. He is noted to have elevated total cholesterol and low-density lipoprotein(LDL) levels, which have remained high in spite of his lifestyle changes. In an effort to reduce his risk of developing coronary artery disease, you start him on a 3-hydroxy-3-methylglutaryl-coenzyme A(HMG-CoA) reductase inhibitor.

◆ **What is the mechanism of action of HMG-CoA reductase inhibitors?**

◆ **What effect do they have on total and LDL cholesterol levels?**

◆ **What are the common adverse effects of HMG-CoA reductase inhibitors?**

ANSWERS TO CASE 13: Lipid-Lowering Agents

Summary: A 60-year-old man has hypertension, diabetes, and hyperlipidemia and is started on an HMG-CoA reductase inhibitor.

- **Mechanism of action of HMG-CoA reductase inhibitors**: Competitive inhibition of the rate limiting enzyme in cholesterol biosynthesis, results in compensatory increase in plasma cholesterol uptake in the liver mediated by an increase in the number of LDL receptors.
- **Effect on total cholesterol**: Up to 30 percent reduction.
- **Effect on LDL cholesterol**: Up to 50 percent reduction.
- **Common adverse events**: Elevated liver enzymes and hepatotoxicity, myalgia and myositis, irritability, sleep disturbance, anxiety.

CLINICAL CORRELATION

HMG-CoA reductase inhibitors are in wide clinical use with proven benefit in lowering cholesterol levels and reducing the risk of coronary artery disease in susceptible individuals. **They competitively antagonize the rate-limiting enzyme in cholesterol biosynthesis.** Reduced cholesterol synthesis spurs a compensatory increase in hepatic uptake of plasma cholesterol mediated by an increase in the number of LDL receptors. The net effect of this is to lower the plasma levels of lipoproteins, especially LDL cholesterol. The effect on high-density lipoprotein (HDL) cholesterol is less pronounced. Although generally very well tolerated, **severe hepatotoxicity** has occurred, and monitoring of liver enzymes is mandatory while taking these medications. **Myalgia**① is a common side effect, but rarely severe, myositis and rhabdomyolysis have occurred. **Hepatotoxicity and myositis**② can occur while using an HMG-CoA reductase inhibitor alone, but they become more likely when combinations of medications are used.

Pharmacology of Lipid-Lowering Drugs

Objectives

1. Know the drugs used to treat hyperlipoproteinemias.
2. Know the adverse effects and toxicities of the drugs.
3. Know the therapeutic uses of each of the lipid-lowering agents.

Definitions

Hyperlipidemia③: An elevation in either plasma cholesterol or plasma triglycerides or both.

Myopathy[④]: General term for any disease of muscle.

Myositis: Muscle pain with increased creatinine kinase levels.

Rhabdomyolysis[⑤]: Muscle pain accompanied by a greater than 10-fold increase in creatinine kinase above upper limits of normal indicating serious muscle damage.

LDL cholesterol: Low-density lipoprotein. Atherogenic lipoprotein particle. Several subfractions have been identified, and the smallest are the most atherogenic. It contains apolipoproteins B_{100} (interacts with LDL receptor), apolipoprotein E (interacts with LDL receptor and Apo E receptor), and apolipoprotein C (activates lipoprotein lipase).

HDL cholesterol: High-density lipoprotein particle involved in transporting cholesterol from the periphery back to the liver. Has antiatherosclerotic activity. Contains apolipoproteins A, C, and D.

VLDL: Very-low-density lipoprotein, a triglyceride-rich lipoprotein particle synthesized in the liver.

Discussion of Class

Drugs that decrease plasma lipids are among the most commonly prescribed today. Some of these affect primarily cholesterol (e.g., the statins) and are useful in the treatment of hypercholesterolemia while other agents affect primarily triglycerides (e.g., gemfibrozil).

The National Cholesterol Education Program (NCEP) has classified levels of plasma cholesterol (Table 13-1). The LDL cholesterol treatment goal is determined by assessing the risk of cardiovascular disease of individual patients. The major risk factors that modify LDL goals are listed in Table 13-2.

Table 13-1

NATIONAL CHOLESTEROL EDUCATION PROGRAM (NCEP) LEVELS OF PLASMA CHOLESTEROL

LDL CHOLESTEROL (mg/dL)	CATEGORIZATION
<100	Optimal
100-129	Near/above optimal
130-139	Borderline high
160-189	High
>190	Very high
TOTAL CHOLESTEROL (mg/dL)	
<200	Desirable
200-239	Borderline high

续表

TOTAL CHOLESTEROL(mg/dL)	
>240	High
HDL CHOLESTEROL(mg/dL)	
<40	Low
>60	High

Table 13-2

RISK FACTORS FOR CARDIOVASCULAR DISEASE

Cigarette Smoking
Hypertension(BP >140/90 mmHg) or on an antihypertensive drug
Low HDL cholesterol(<40mg/dL)
Family history of premature coronary heart disease
Age(men >45years, women >55years)
Poor nutrition

Known CHD include patients who have had an infarction or angina or a surgical procedure for cardiovascular disease. In addition, patients with peripheral arterial disease, abdominal aortic aneurism, or symptomatic carotid artery disease or diabetes are considered to have known CHD or a high risk for CHD. The NCEP classification and the risk assessment are combined and used to modify the LDL cholesterol goals as illustrated in Table 13-3.

Table 13-3

CARDIOVASCULAR RISK AND LDL GOAL

RISK LEVEL	LDL GOAL(mg/dL)
Known CHD	<100
≥2 risk factors	<130
0-1 risk factors	<160

Agents Used for Hypercholesterolemia

Statins

Of the drugs that decrease plasma cholesterol, the statins have gained the widest use. The **statins**⑥ **are structural analogs of the substrate HMG-CoA that inhibit the activity of the enzyme HMG-CoA reductase** at nanomolar concentrations. 注This enzyme is required for the synthesis of isoprenoids and cholesterol. By inhibiting de novo biosynthesis of cholesterol, cellular uptake of cholesterol from plasma via the LDL receptor is increased, reducing plasma cholesterol levels. Because **statins have additional actions to inhibit the production of the triglyceride⑦-rich VLDL**, this makes them useful in the management of patients with hypertriglyceridemia; atorvastatin and rosuvastatin are particularly effective in this regard. There is evidence that statins also have antiinflammatory activity, and this may contribute to their reduction in cardiovascular events. **Statins may also reduce the rate of bone resorption and thereby lessen osteoporosis⑧**. This effect is thought to be caused by the inhibition of isoprenoid biosynthesis in osteoclast precursors, which inhibits their differentiation into mature osteoclasts. Six statins are approved in the United States: **lovastatin⑨, rosuvastatin⑩, fluvastatin⑪, atorvastatin⑫, pravastatin⑬, and simvastatin⑭**. They differ in efficacy: Rosuvastatin has been reported to reduce LDL cholesterol by more than 60 percent; atorvastatin, about 50 percent; and pravastatin and fluvastatin, about 35 percent. All of the statins are active orally.

Lovastatin and simvastatin are prodrugs that are converted to their active metabolite by the liver.

The two major adverse effects associated with statin use are hepatotoxicity and myopathy. Hepatotoxicity was initially thought to be as high as 1 percent with elevations in hepatic transaminases as high as three times the upper limits. Subsequent clinical trials indicate that the actual incidence of hepatotoxicity is much lower. Hepatic transaminase levels should be monitored on initiation of therapy and at least yearly thereafter. The myopathy associated with statin use occurs in less than 0.1 percent of patients. However, severe rhabdomyolysis has occurred rarely, and one statin, cerivastatin, was removed from the market after several rhabdomyolysis-associated deaths.

Bile-Acid-Binding Resins

The bile acid sequestrants are also useful in reducing plasma cholesterol. **Cholestyramine⑮**, colestipol, and colesevelam are ion-exchange resins that nonspecifically bind bile acids within the intestine and thereby reduce their enterohepatic circulation. This increases hepatic bile acid synthesis and the cholesterol for this synthesis comes, in part, from the plasma via the LDL receptor. **Bile acid sequestrants typically reduce plasma cholesterol by 15-20 percent with no effect on triglycerides**. Because they are not absorbed, the bile acid sequestrants are quite safe, and adverse effects are typically gastrointestinal and include bloating and constipation. In the intestine, these agents bind many molecules other than bile acids and they **impair the absorption of lipid soluble vitamins and many drugs including digoxin, furosemide, thiazides⑯, coumarin, and some statins**. Patient adherence with these drugs is poor.

Inhibitors of Cholesterol Absorption

Ezetimibe[17] is a **new class of cholesterol-lowering drug** that acts **within the intestine to reduce cholesterol absorption**. Cholesterol is absorbed from the small intestine by a process that includes specific transporters that have not been completely characterized. Ezetimibe **appears to block one or more of these cholesterol transporters, thereby reducing cholesterol absorption**. Ezetimibe used alone produces a reduction in plasma cholesterol of about 19 percent and about a 10 percent decline in triglyceride levels. When combined with a statin, reductions in plasma cholesterol as high as 72 percent have been reported in clinical trials. The complementary mechanisms—inhibition of cholesterol biosynthesis by statins and inhibition of cholesterol absorption by ezetimibe—may be useful in treating patients with refractory hypercholesterolemia. Few adverse effects have been reported with ezetimibe, but clinical experience is limited. The most frequently reported adverse effects are back and joint pain.

Nicotinic Acid

Niacin[18], at doses well beyond those used as a vitamin, has effects on all plasma lipids. It reduces LDL cholesterol by 20-30 percent and reduces **triglycerides** by 35-45 percent. It is the best agent available for **increasing** HDL. Niacin inhibits VLDL production in the liver by inhibiting both the synthesis and esterification of fatty acids. LDL levels are reduced as a consequence of the decline in VLDL synthesis. Niacin inhibits lipolysis in adipose tissue which reduces the supply of fatty acids to the liver, further decreasing VLDL synthesis. HDL levels are increased because niacin decreases the catabolism of apolipoprotein A1. Niacin is useful in treating hypertriglyceridemia as well as hypercholesterolemia especially in the presence of low HDL. The limiting adverse effect of niacin is **cutaneous flushing and itching**[19], **and dyspepsia** is common at the doses (1g/day) necessary to affect lipids. More medically serious adverse effects include hepatotoxicity and hyperglycemia. Niacin induces an **insulin-resistant state**[20] causing **hyperglycemia**[21]. For this reason niacin should not be used in diabetic patients.

Agents Used for Hypertriglyceridemia—Fibrates

The fibrates include clofibrate[22], **fenofibrate**[23], **ciprofibrate**[24], **bezafibrate**[25], **and gemfibrozil**[26]. These agents predominantly cause a decline plasma **triglycerides**[27] and a small decrease in LDL cholesterol[28]. HDL levels are increased. The fibrates[29] bind to a nuclear receptor peroxisomal proliferator-activator receptor γ (PPAR-γ) mostly in liver and skeletal muscle. Agonist-bound PPAR-γ induces lipoprotein lipase[30] (LPL), which increases the lipolysis of triglyceride-rich VLDL and chylomicrons. Fibrates reduce triglycerides by 35-50 percent and LDL cholesterol by 10-20 percent.

HDL levels are increased by 10-15 percent. All of the fibrates are orally active, but their absorption is decreased by food. The major adverse effect is gastrointestinal upset, cutaneous rash, and itching. Fibrates should not be used in patients with compromised renal function.

Comprehension Questions

[13.1] Lovastatin reduces plasma cholesterol by

A. Inhibiting $ApoB_{100}$ biosynthesis

B. Inhibiting cholesterol absorption

C. Inhibiting cholesterol biosynthesis

D. Interfering with bile acid reabsorption

[13.2] Which of the following is a usual effect of niacin?

A. Increases HDL
B. Increases LDL
C. Increases total cholesterol
D. Increases triglycerides

[13.3] A 33-year-old man has been prescribed medication for hyperlipidemia. He has been noted to have bleeding from his gums and easy bruisability. His prothrombin time is elevated. Which of the following agents is most likely to be involved?

A. Atorvastatin
B. Cholestyramine
D. Gemfibrozil
D. Niacin

Answers

[13.1] **C**. The statins are competitive inhibitors of HMG-CoA reductase and thereby inhibit de novo cholesterol biosynthesis.

[13.2] **A**. Niacin increases HDL, decreases total and LDL cholesterol, and decreases triglycerides.

[13.3] **B**. Cholestyramine interferes with the absorption of lipid soluble vitamins such as vitamin K, leading to decreased levels of vitamin K-dependent coagulation factors.

PHARMACOLOGY PEARLS

❖ The HMG-CoA reductase inhibitors, the statins, are the initial choice of drug for the treatment of hypercholesterolemia.

❖ The statins are structural analogs of the substrate HMG-CoA (3-hydroxy-3-methylglutaryl-coenzyme A) that inhibit the activity of the enzyme HMG-CoA reductase.

❖ The two major adverse effects associated with statin use are hepatotoxicity and myopathy.

❖ Bile acid sequestrants impair the absorption of lipid soluble vitamins and many drugs including digoxin, furosemide, thiazides, coumarin, and some statins.

❖ The fibrates including clofibrate, fenofibrate, ciprofibrate, bezafibrate, and gemfibrozil predominantly cause a decline in plasma triglycerides.

❖ **Niacin** has effects on all plasma lipids and has side effects of flushing and itching.

REFERENCES

National Cholesterol Education Program (NCEP) Expert Panel on Detection, Evaluation, and Treatment of High Blood Cholesterol in Adults (Adult Treatment Panel III). Third report of the national cholesterol education program (NCEP) expert panel on detection, evaluation, and treatment of high blood cholesterol in adults (adult treatment panel III) final report. Circulation 2002; 106 (25): 3143-421

Wierzbicki AS, Mikhailidis DP, Wray R. Drug treatment of combined hyperlipidemia. Am J Cardiovasc Drugs 2001; 1(5): 327-36.

词汇

1. Myalgia[肌痛]
2. hepatotoxicity and myositis[肝毒性及肌炎]
3. hyperlipidemia[高脂血症]
4. myopathy[肌病]
5. rhabdomyolysis[横纹肌溶解症]
6. statins[他汀类药物]
7. triglyceride[甘油三酯]
8. osteoporosis[骨质疏松症]
9. lovastatin[洛伐他汀]
10. rosuvastatin[罗苏伐他汀]
11. fluvastatin[氟伐他汀]
12. atorvastatin[阿托伐他汀]
13. pravastatin[普伐他汀]
14. simvastatin[辛伐他汀]
15. cholestyramine[消胆胺]
16. thiazides[噻嗪类利尿剂]
17. ezetimibe[依泽替米贝]
18. niacin[烟酸]
19. itching[瘙痒]
20. insulin-resistant state[胰岛素抵抗状态]

21. hyperglycemia[高血糖症]
22. clofibrate[氯贝特]
23. fenofibrate[非诺贝特]
24. ciprofibrate[环丙贝特]
25. bezafibrate[苯扎贝特]
26. gemfibrozil[吉非贝齐]
27. triglycerides[甘油三酯]
28. cholesterol[胆固醇]
29. fibrate[纤维化]
30. lipoprotein lipase[脂蛋白脂肪酶]

注

他汀类药物是降低总胆固醇和低密度脂蛋白胆固醇的一线药物，该药有一定程度的降低甘油三酯作用。即使对伴有甘油三酯轻中度升高(1.7～4.5mmol/L)的患者，他汀类药物仍可作为首选。他汀类药物一般在晚饭后或睡前服用效果较好，该类药物副作用较少，耐受性好，偶可出现肝酶升高和肌病，肝酶升高多为轻度升高，停药后可恢复正常，肌病表现为肌肉疼痛、乏力和肌酸激酶(CK)升高。为及时发现副作用，在使用8～12周左右，监测肝酶[谷丙转氨酶(ALT)和谷草转氨酶(AST)]，以后每年监测一次或多次，禁用于有活性和慢性肝病患者。病人在服药时如出现肌痛、肌无力(排除其他原因)及时报告医生，并查肌酸激酶。他汀类药物有多种，各种药物在体内的代谢过程不完全相同，调脂效果也有所差别，在使用时医生根据病人的血脂水平、合并的疾病和用药(其他药物)以及经济承受能力选择用药。

点评

目前，在临床上常用的降脂药物有许多，归纳起来大体上可分为五大类。(1)他汀类药物是目前治疗高胆固醇血症的主要药物。该类药物最常见的不良反应主要是轻度胃肠反应、头痛。与其他降脂药物合用时可能出现肌肉毒性。(2)贝特类药物的主要适应证为：高甘油三酯血症或以甘油三酯升高为主的混合型高脂血症。该药常见的不良反应为胃肠反应、恶心、腹泻，严重者可导致肝损害。(3)烟酸类药物属B族维生素，当用量超过其作为维生素作用的剂量时，可有明显的降脂作用。该类药物的适用范围较广，可用于除纯合子型家族性高胆固醇血症，及Ⅰ型高脂蛋白血症以外的任何类型高脂血症。但是，该药的速释制剂不良反应大，我们一般不单独应用。对于烟酸的降脂作用机制，目前医学界尚不十分明确。缓释制剂大大减少，主要为颜面潮红。(4)胆酸螯合剂，这类药物也称为胆酸隔置剂。有考来烯胺(Cholestyramine)，常用药物有降胆宁。该药常见的不良反应为胃肠反应、恶心、便秘或腹泻，肠梗阻或头痛等。(5)胆固醇吸收抑制剂，此类药物主要通过抑制肠道内饮食和胆汁中胆固醇的吸收，来达到降低血脂的目的。目前，该类药物上市很少。

李 清

❖ CASE 14

A 19-year-old man is brought to the office by his very concerned mother. He has been kicked out of the dormitory at college for his "bizarre[①]" behavior. He has accused several fellow students and professors of spying on him for the CIA[②]. He stopped attending his classes and spends all of his time watching TV because the announcers are sending him secret messages on how to save the world. He has stopped bathing and will only change his clothes once a week. In your office you find him to be disheveled[③], quiet, and unemotional. The only spontaneous statement he makes is when he asks why his mother brought him to the office of "another government spy." His physical examination and blood tests are normal. A drug screen is negative. You diagnose him with acute psychosis secondary to schizophrenia, admit him to the psychiatric unit of the hospital, and start him on haloperidol.

◆ **What is the mechanism of therapeutic action of haloperidol?**

◆ **What mediates the extrapyramidal side effects (EPSs) of the antipsychotic agents?**

◆ **Which autonomic nervous system receptors are antagonized by antipsychotic agents?**

ANSWERS TO CASE 14: Antipsychotic Drugs

Summary: A 19-year-old man with acute psychosis from schizophrenia is prescribed haloperidol.

- **Mechanism of therapeutic action of haloperidol**: Antagonist of postjunctional dopamine D_2-receptors in the mesolimbic and mesocortical areas of the brain. [注1]

- **Mechanism of Extrapyramidal[④] Side Effects (EPSs)**: Antagonist activity of dopamine receptors in the basal ganglia and other dopamine receptor sites in the central nervous system (CNS).

- **Autonomic nervous system receptors blocked by antipsychotics[⑤]**: α-adrenoceptors and muscarinic[⑥] cholinoreceptors[⑦].

CLINICAL CORRELATION

Schizophrenia is a chronic thought disorder that often presents in adolescence or early adulthood. [注2] It is characterized by the presence of "positive symptoms" which include delusions[⑧], hallucinations[⑨], and paranoia[⑩], and "negative symptoms," which include blunt affect, withdrawal, and apathy[⑪]. The therapeutic effects of the antipsychotic agents result from their antagonist actions on postjunctional dopamine D_2-receptors in the mesolimbic and mesocortical areas of the brain, although their benefits may also be related to antagonist activity at other dopamine receptor; additionally, atypical antipsychotic agents have efficacy at serotonin receptors. The dopamine receptor antagonist activity of antipsychotic agents at multiple sites in the CNS, and their antagonist activity at various other receptors in the CNS and throughout the body, contributes to presence of numerous adverse effects. Among these are the **extrapyramidal side effects, acute dystonia[⑫], akathisia[⑬], and Parkinson's syndrome**, as well as **tardive[⑭] dyskinesia[⑮]**, an often **irreversible facial movement disorder**, that are mediated by the antagonist activity of antipsychotic agents at dopamine D_2-receptors in the basal ganglia. **Autonomic system effects** include **orthostatic[⑯] hypotension, related to α-adrenoceptor blockade, and dry mouth, urinary retention and tachycardia[⑰], caused by muscarinic cholinoreceptor blockade**. The presence of so many, and frequently severe, side effects makes patient compliance with long-term antipsychotic therapy an important clinical issue. However, newer, "atypical" agents are now available with greater specificity for the receptors that mediate antipsychotic actions than for the receptors that mediate adverse effects.

Pharmacology of Antipsychotic Drugs

Objectives

1. List the classes and specific drugs that have antipsychotic activity.
2. Describe the mechanism of therapeutic action of antipsychotic agents.
3. Describe the common side effects of antipsychotic agents and indicate the receptors that mediate them.

Definitions

Acute dystonia: Sustained painful muscle spasms producing twisting abnormal posture usually shortly after taking a medication such as an anti-psychotic medication.

Akathisia: Characterized by feelings of intense muscle restlessness or strong desire to move about, related to exposure to antipsychotic medications, usually during the first 2 weeks of treatment.

Parkinson syndrome: Characterized by flat affect, shuffling gait, joint rigidity, and tremor that occurs weeks to months after treatment.

Neuroleptic malignant syndrome: Characterized by the acute onset of hyperthermia, muscle rigidity, tremor, tachycardia, mental status changes, diaphoresis, labile blood pressure, and exposure to a neuroleptic. This syndrome is associated with a significant mortality rate and usually occurs within the first few weeks of therapy.

Discussion of Class

Antipsychotic drugs can be classified according to chemical structure as **phenothiazines**, **thioxanthenes**, **butyrophenones**, and an important group with diverse **atypical structures**. The phenothiazines are further subdivided according to side-chain constituents: **aliphatic**, **piperidine**, **and piperazine** (Table 14-1).

Although very similar in their therapeutic efficacy, the "low-(oral-) potency" aliphatic and piperidine phenothiazines have a somewhat different adverse effect profile than the "high-potency" agents that include the piperazine phenothiazines, and also thiothixene, and haloperidol.

The newer, atypical agents have generally unique structures and have been documented to have greater therapeutic efficacy in some studies, particularly with regard to the negative symptoms of schizophrenia. They also have been documented to have superior adverse effect profiles. They are now considered the drugs of choice for initial management of the disease. Nevertheless, individual patient response to antipsychotic agents varies widely and often dictates drug selection.

Table 14-1
REPRESENTATIVE ANTIPSYCHOTIC DRUGS(SIDE CHAINS)

Phenothiazines	
	Chlorpromazine(aliphatic)
	Thioridazine, mesoridazine(piperidine)
	Fluphenazine, perphenazine, prochlorperazine, trifluoperazine(piperazine)
Thiozanthene	
	Thiothixine
Butyrophenone	
	Haloperidol
Atypical	
	Clozapine
	Risperidone
	Olanzapine
	Quetiapine

Administration of the low potency antipsychotic agents is more likely to result in **autonomic adverse effects** that include **orthostatic**⑯ **hypotension** caused by **α-adrenoceptor blockade, and dry mouth, urinary retention, and tachycardia**⑰ **resulting from blockade of muscarinic cholinoreceptors**. Their blockade of **histamine H_1-receptors in the CNS** results in **sedation**⑱. The still widely used high-potency agents, for example, **haloperidol**, are more likely to result in adverse neurological effects. Among these are the **EPSs, acute dystonia, akathisia, and Parkinson syndrome,** which occur relatively early in therapy and are thought to be primarily mediated by blockade of **dopamine D_2-receptors** in the nigrostriatal dopamine pathway of the basal ganglia. A **late-occurring tardive dyskinesia** that is often irreversible and that may be a result of the slow development of dopamine receptor supersensitivity also in the basal ganglia, is more or less likely to occur with all antipsychotic agents except clozapine. A **potentially fatal neuroleptic**⑲ **malignant syndrome is another serious adverse effect of antipsychotic agents in sensitive patients(1%)**. Also, **hyperprolactinemia**⑳ in women may occur as a result of enhanced prolactin release from the posterior pituitary㉑, because of antipsychotic drug blockade(except clozapine and possibly olanzapine) of dopamine D_2-receptors of the tuberoinfundibular dopaminergic pathway, which may lead to amenorrhea㉒, galactorrhea㉓, gynecomastia㉔, and decreased libido㉕. Weight gain is also a likely effect of many of these antipsychotic agents.

The **atypical agents** are **less likely** than the conventional agents to result in adverse **EPSs**. However, **weight gain** (clozapine, olanzapine), hypotension (risperidone), and **sedation**(clozapine, olanzapine) are not uncommon events. **Seizures**㉖ (2%-5%)

and **agranulocytosis**[27] (2% risk, 10% fatality) that must be monitored for with **weekly leukocyte counts** limit the use of **clozapine** to patients unresponsive to other agents.

Mechanism of Action

All clinically useful antipsychotic drugs **block postjunctional dopamine D_2-receptors**, although the degree of blockade among the drugs varies greatly in relation to their action on other neuroreceptors, particularly serotonin 5-hydroxytryptamine 2A (5-HT_{2A})-receptors and certain other dopamine receptor subtypes. Antipsychotic drugs appear to exert their therapeutic effect, at least in part, by **inhibition of dopamine's action in the mesocortical and mesolimbic dopaminergic pathways of the CNS**.

Administration

All antipsychotic agents can be administered by either the oral or parenteral route or both. Chlorpromazine and prochlorperazine can also be administered as an oral sustained-release or rectal preparation. Fluphenazine decanoate and haloperidol decanoate are available as parenteral depot preparations.

Pharmacokinetics

Most antipsychotic agents are readily but incompletely absorbed. They are highly lipid soluble and have longer clinical duration of action than would be expected from their plasma half-life, probably as a consequence of their deposition in fat tissue.

Thioridazine, which is metabolized to mesoridazine, is the exception to the rule that hepatic metabolism of the antipsychotic agents results in less active metabolites.

Concurrent use of certain antipsychotic agents with other drugs that also block cholinoreceptors may result in additive peripheral and CNS dysfunction.

Comprehension Questions

[14.1] Haloperidol-induced Parkinson's syndrome is a result of haloperidol's action in the

A. Mesocortical tract
B. Mesolimbic tract
C. Nigrostriatal tract
D. Tuberoinfundibular tract

[14.2] The therapeutic effect of haloperidol is mediated, at least in part, by its blockade of

A. α-adrenergic receptors
B. Dopamine D_2-receptors
C. Histamine H_1-receptors
D. Muscarinic receptors

[14.3] Compared to the low-potency phenothiazine antipsychotic agents, haloperidol is more like to causes which of the following adverse effects?

A. Akathisia B. Orthostatic hypotension
C. Sedation D. Urinary retention

Answers

[14.1] **C.** Haloperidol induced Parkinson's syndrome is a result of inhibition of dopamine D_2-receptors in the nigrostriatal tract of the CNS.

[14.2] **B.** Antipsychotic drugs like haloperidol exert their therapeutic effect, at least in part, by inhibition of dopamine's action at dopamine D_2-receptors in the mesocortical and mesolimbic dopaminergic pathways of the CNS. A number of adverse effects of these drugs are caused by inhibition of dopamine action in the nigrostriatal and tuberoinfundibular dopaminergic pathways of the CNS; blockade of histamine, muscarinic cholinergic, and α-adrenergic receptors in the CNS and the peripheral nervous system are also contributory.

[14.3] **A.** Haloperidol is most likely to cause dystonia, akathisia, and Parkinson syndrome, whereas the low-potency phenothiazines are more likely to cause autonomic adverse effects that include orthostatic hypotension, sedation, and urinary retention.

PHARMACOLOGY PEARLS

- The low-potency antipsychotic agents are more likely to result in autonomic adverse effects that include orthostatic hypotension as a consequence of α-adrenoceptor blockade, as well as dry mouth, urinary retention, and tachycardia resulting from blockade of muscarinic cholinoreceptors, and sedation (histamine H_1-receptor blockade).
- High-potency agents, for example, haloperidol, are more likely to result in EPSs, acute dystonia, akathisia, and Parkinson syndrome, mediated by blockade of dopamine D_2-receptors in the nigrostriatal dopamine pathway of the basal ganglia.
- A late-occurring tardive dyskinesia is often irreversible and is a serious effect of many antipsychotic agents.
- A potentially fatal neuroleptic malignant syndrome is another serious adverse effect of antipsychotic agents in sensitive patients (1%).
- Hyperprolactinemia in women may occur as a result of enhanced prolactin release from the posterior pituitary, as a result of antipsychotic drug blockade.
- Agranulocytosis may occur in patients treated with clozapine and warrants weekly leukocyte counts.

REFERENCES

Ananth J, Burgoyne KS, Gadasalli R, et al. How do atypical antipsychotics work? J Psychiatry Neurosci 2001; 26(5): 385-94.

Freedman R. Schizophrenia. N Engl J Med 2003; 349(13): 1738-49.

Thacker GK, Carpenter, WT. Advances in schizophrenia. Nature Med 2001; 7(6): 667-71.

词汇

1. bizarre[稀奇古怪的]
2. central intelligence agency(CIA)[(美)中央情报局]
3. disheveled[散乱的;蓬乱的]
4. extrapyramidal[锥体束外的]
5. antipsychotic[抗紧张剂,抗精神病药物]
6. muscarinic[毒蕈碱的]
7. cholinoreceptor[胆碱受体]
8. delusion[妄想,幻想]
9. hallucination[幻觉]
10. paranoia[偏执狂,妄想狂]
11. apathy[无情感,情感淡漠]
12. dystonia[张力障碍]
13. akathisia[静坐不能]
14. tardive[迟发性,延迟性]
15. dyskinesia[运动障碍]
16. orthostatic[体位性的]
17. tachycardia[心动过速,心搏过速]
18. sedation[镇静作用,镇静状态]
19. neuroleptic[抑制精神的,精神抑制药]
20. hyperprolactinemia[高催乳素血症]
21. pituitary[垂体后叶素]
22. amenorrhea[闭经]
23. galactorrhea[乳溢]
24. gynecomastia[男子乳腺发育]
25. libido[性欲]
26. seizure[癫痫发作]
27. agranulocytosis[粒细胞缺乏]

注 1

氟哌啶醇是第一个合成的丁酰苯类药物，是这类药物的典型代表。它能选择性阻断 D2 样受体，有很强的抗精神病作用。口服后 2 ~ 6h 血药浓度达高峰，作用可持续 3 天。可显著控制各种精神运动兴奋，对慢性症状也有较好疗效。但是，其锥体外系副作用发生率高、程度严重。

注 2

精神分裂症病因有许多假说，目前比较公认的，认为精神分裂症是由于脑内中脑-边缘通路和中脑-皮层通路中多巴胺(DA)系统功能亢进所致。典型抗精神病药物主要也是通过阻断上述两通路中的 D2 样受体而发挥疗效的。由于临床使用的大多数抗精神病药物是非选择性 D2 受体拮抗药，在发挥疗效时，同时阻断了黑质-纹状体通路的 D2 受体而不同程度引起了锥体外系的副作用。

点评

精神分裂症是以思维、情感、行为之间不协调，精神活动与现实脱离为主要特征的最常见的一类精神病。根据临床症状，将精神分裂症分为Ⅰ型和Ⅱ型，前者以阳性症状(幻觉和妄想)为主，后者则以阴性症状(情感淡漠、主动性缺乏等)为主。抗精神病药主要用于治疗精神分裂症，对Ⅰ型疗效较好。这类药物大多是强效多巴胺受体拮抗药，因此，在发挥治疗作用的同时，也引起精神运动迟缓和运动障碍等锥体外系不良反应。抗精神分裂症药分为四类：吩噻嗪类、硫杂蒽类、丁酰苯类和其他。

颜光美

❖ CASE 15

A 30-year-old woman presents to your office for the evaluation of fatigue[1]. For the past 2 months she has felt run down. She says that she doesn't feel like participating in activities that she previously enjoyed, such as her weekly softball games. She has not been sleeping well and has not had much of an appetite. On questioning, she admits to feeling "down in the dumps[2]" most of the time and has found herself crying frequently. She has never gone through anything like this before. She denies any thoughts of wanting to hurt herself or anyone else. Other than becoming tearful during her interview, her physical examination is normal. Her blood tests, including a complete blood count and thyroid function, are normal. A serum pregnancy test is negative. You diagnose her as having a major depression and, along with referring her for counseling, start her on fluoxetine[3].

◆ **What is the mechanism of action of fluoxetine**?

◆ **What are the common side effects of fluoxetine**?

ANSWERS TO CASE 15: Antidepressant Agents

Summary: A 30-year-old woman with major depression is prescribed fluoxetine.

- **Mechanism of action of fluoxetine**: Inhibition of the reuptake of serotonin (5-hydroxytryptamine, or 5-HT) at the prejunctional④ nerve terminal. 注1

- **Common side effects**: Headaches, nausea, agitation, insomnia, and sexual dysfunction (loss of libido and erectile dysfunction). 注2

CLINICAL CORRELATION

Selective serotonin⑤ reuptake inhibitors (SSRIs) are the most frequently prescribed antidepressant medications. **They act by inhibiting the reuptake of serotonin by the prejunctional nerve terminal, allowing more serotonin to interact with postjunctional neurons in the central nervous system (CNS).** This is thought to mediate their therapeutic effect. They have been highly effective in the treatment of major depressive disorders and have an excellent safety profile. Unlike tricyclic antidepressants⑥ (TCAs), which have multiple severe and potentially fatal effects in an overdose, SSRIs have relatively few severe toxicities and a very low potential for fatality in an overdose. SSRIs do have several side effects of clinical significance. They often cause headaches and gastrointestinal side effects such as nausea. In some cases, agitation, anxiety, and insomnia can be exacerbated. Many of these SSRI side effects tend to be temporary and can often be improved with dose reduction. Another common side effect of SSRIs is **sexual disturbance**. Decreased libido and erectile dysfunction occur frequently and do not generally spontaneously resolve while continuing SSRI therapy, often leading to reduced patient compliance.

Pharmacology of Antidepressant Drugs

Objectives

1. List the classes of antidepressant agents.
2. Contrast the mechanisms of action of the antidepressant agents.
3. Contrast the adverse effects and toxicities of the antidepressant agents.
4. Describe the indications and contraindications to antidepressant drug use.

Definitions

Major (endogenous) depression: Unexplained, long-term difficulty coping with life events characterized by an inability to experience pleasure, abnormal sleep, decreased libido and appetite, feelings of guilt, and suicidal ideation⑦.

Discussion of Class

Drugs used to treat depression are classified as **tricyclic antidepressants** (**TCAs**) , **heterocyclic**(**second-and third-generation**) **agents**, **selective serotonin reuptake inhibitors**(**SSRIs**), and **monoamine oxidase inhibitors** (**MAOIs**). Other conditions for which certain antidepressant agents are used include panic disorder, obsessive-compulsive disease(OCD)[⑧], chronic pain, and enuresis.

SSRIs are the most extensively prescribed antidepressant agents because, unlike tricyclic and heterocyclic agents, they produce **less sedation**, **have fewer antimuscarinic cholinoreceptor effects**, and are **safer** in overdose. Nevertheless, they **may cause sexual dysfunction**, **gastrointestinal dysfunction**, **insomnia**, **tremor**, **and anxiety**. TCAs may cause sedation, tremor, insomnia, blurred vision, constipation urinary hesitancy, weight gain, and sexual disturbances. The MAOI phenelzine may cause weight gain, sexual disturbances, and sleep disturbances. The adverse effects of heterocyclic agents vary depending on the agent. **Bupropion is contraindicated in patients with seizure disorders(Table 15-1)**.

Drug interactions include additive sedative effects of TCAs with other sedatives, particularly alcohol. **Phenelzine**, by increasing catecholamine[⑨] stores, sensitizes patients to indirectly acting sympathomimetic agents, including **tyramine** that is contained in many **fermented foodstuffs**(**red wine or aged cheese**), and which together can result in a severe and sometimes **fatal hypertensive episode**[⑩]. **MAOIs and SSRIs can interact to cause a potentially lethal "serotonin syndrome"**, similar to malignant hyperthermia, that includes **tremor**, **hyperthermia**, **muscle rigidity**, **and cardiovascular collapse**[⑪].

Structure

Tricyclic antidepressants(TCAs) have a three-ring nucleus similar to that of the antipsychotic phenothiazine agents. The monoamine oxidase inhibitors are subclassified as hydrazides(phenelzine) or nonhydrazides (tranylcypromine).

Mechanism of Action

All of the available therapeutic antidepressant agents work, at least in part, through actions on norepinephrine and serotonin.

The TCAs block, to one degree or another, the prejunctional neuronal reuptake pumps in the CNS, which terminate norepinephrine and serotonin neurotransmission thus allowing increased activity at their respective receptors.

Table 15-1

ANTIDEPRESSANT AGENTS

ANTIDEPRESSANT AGENTS	SELECTED ADVERSE EFFECTS
Tricyclic Agents Amitriptyline Desipramine Doxepin Imipramine Nortriptyline Protriptyline Trimipramine	Sedation, tremor, insomnia, blurred vision, constipation[12], urinary hesitancy[13], weight gain, and sexual disturbances
Heterocyclic Agents (second and third generation) Amoxapine Bupropion Maprotiline Mirtazapine Nefazodone Trazodone Venlafaxine	Amoxapine, maprotiline: Like TCAs. *Bupropion*: CNS stimulation, seizures at high doses (up to 0.4%) *Mirtazapine*: Sedation, weight gain *Nefazodone*: Mild sedation, drug-drug interactions *Trazodone*: Sedation, dizziness, orthostatic hypotension, priapism[14] *Venlafaxine*: Like SSRIs
Selective Serotonin Reuptake Inhibitors Citalopram Escitalopram Fluoxetine Fluvoxamine Paroxetine Sertraline	Sexual dysfunction, gastrointestinal dysfunction, insomnia, tremor, anxiety
Monoamine Oxidase Inhibitors Phenelzine Tranylcypromine	Weight gain, sexual disturbances, sleep disturbances

The heterocyclic agents have a variety of pharmacodynamic effects. Some act similarly to the TCAs and MAOIs, whereas others act as inhibitors at certain subtypes of the serotonin receptor (trazodone, mirtazapine, nefazodone). Mirtazapine also blocks the prejunctional α_2-adrenoceptor to enhance serotonin and norepinephrine neurotransmission.

As the name implies, SSRIs selectively block the prejunctional neuronal reuptake pumps in the CNS that terminate serotonin neurotransmission thus allowing increased activity at serotonin receptors.

The MAOI hydrazide, phenelzine, irreversibly binds to and inhibits the activity of monoamine oxidase (A and B forms). The nonhydrazide, tranylcypromine, also has a long duration of action even though it does not bind monoamine oxidase irreversibly. In either case, new enzyme must be synthesized to restore activity. As a result of their actions, both drugs prevent prejunctional metabolism of norepinephrine and serotonin, thus allowing more to accumulate and to be released on nerve stimulation.

The neurochemical and biochemical actions described for the antidepressant agents occur soon after their administration. However, the therapeutic effect of these drugs may not be apparent for up to several weeks with continued administration. Thus, considerable attention has been devoted to discovering the long-term neurochemical and biochemical actions of the antidepressant agents that may correlate better with their clinical effectiveness. Decreased numbers of β-adrenoceptors and decreased cyclic adenosine monophosphate (cAMP) concentrations are two such long-term effects of the antidepressant agents that initially increase norepinephrine levels. Enhanced serotonin transmission, either directly, perhaps through increased sensitivity of serotonin 5-HT_{1A} receptors, or indirectly, is also implicated in the therapeutic action of antidepressant agents with their chronic administration.

The antidepressant agents also produce a myriad of adverse effects that, depending on the agent, may be caused by blockade of histamine receptors, adrenoceptors, and cholinoreceptors in the peripheral and central nervous systems.

Administration

Dosing, which may be by the oral or parenteral[15] routes, is determined empirically in relation to the therapeutic response and the patient's tolerance of adverse effects.

Pharmacokinetics

Monodemethylation by the liver of the tertiary amines tricyclic antidepressants amitriptyline and imipramine results in, respectively, the active metabolites nortriptyline and desipramine. Venlafaxine has an active metabolite, *O*-desmethyl-venlafaxine.

Metabolism of the selective serotonin reuptake inhibitor fluoxetine results in an active metabolite, norfluoxetine, that has a long half-life. Fluoxetine inhibits a number of liver microsomal enzymes, particularly P450 2D6, which has resulted in clinically significant drug-drug interactions. Nefazodone inhibits cytochrome P450 3A4, which can result in increased levels of other drugs dependent on this metabolic pathway.

Comprehension Questions

[15. 1] Which of the following agents is contraindicated in a patient with epilepsy?

A. Bupropion B. Fluoxetine
C. Mirtazapine D. Venlafaxine

[15. 2] The antidepressant action of imipramine is thought to be caused by

A. Blockade of prejunctional α_2-adrenoceptors
B. Blockade of prejunctional neuronal norepinephrine and serotonin reuptake pumps in the CNS
C. Increased numbers of β-adrenoceptors
D. Inhibition of monoamine oxidase

[15. 3] Which of the following antidepressant agents inhibits hepatic microso-mal enzymes to cause clinically significant drug-drug interactions?

A. Fluoxetine B. Imipramine
C. Phenelzine D. Trazodone

Answers

[15. 1] **A.** Bupropion causes seizures in a small but significant number of patients. This number is reduced with use of the slow-release form.

[15. 2] **B.** Imipramine and other TCAs block prejunctional neuronal norepinephrine and or serotonin reuptake pumps in the CNS. Phenelzine and tranylcypromine inhibit monoamine oxidase. The heterocyclic agent mirtazapine blocks prejunctional α_2-adrenoceptors to enhance serotonin and norepinephrine neurotransmission.

[15. 3] **A.** The SSRI fluoxetine (and paroxetine, and to a lesser extent, sertraline, as well as the heterocyclic agent nefazodone) inhibits cytochrome P450 and therefore can significantly elevate the level of other drugs metabolized by these hepatic enzymes.

PHARMACOLOGY PEARLS

- SSRIs are the most commonly prescribed antidepressants because of their favorable side effect profile. Sexual dysfunction and gastrointestinal (GI) effects are common, however.
- Tricyclic antidepressants may lead to toxicity as a result of cardiac arrhythmias.
- The antidepressant agents are roughly equivalent in their therapeutic action. However, individual patients may respond better to one than another.
- Beginning with small doses of many antidepressant agents is usually preferred because tolerance may occur to some of their adverse effects.
- Bupropion is contraindicated in patients with seizure disorders.

REFERENCES

Ables AZ, Baughman OL. Antidepressants: Update on new agents and indications. Am Fam Physician 2003; 67(3): 547-54.

American Psychiatric Association. Practice guidelines for the treatment of patients with major depressive disorder(revision). Am J Psychiatry 2000; 157(suppl 4): 1-45.

Feighner JP. Mechanism of action of antidepressant medications. J Clin Psychiatr 1999; 60(5): 4-11.

词汇

1. fatigue[疲劳]
2. dumps[抑郁]
3. fluoxetine[氟西汀,百忧解]
4. prejunctional[接头前的]
5. serotonin[5-羟色胺,血清素]
6. tricyclic antidepressant[三环抗抑郁剂]
7. ideation[观念作用]
8. obsessive-compulsive disease(OCD)[强迫性神经失调]
9. catecholamine[儿茶酚胺,邻苯二酚胺]
10. hypertensive episode[高血压性发作]
11. cardiovascular collapse[心血管性虚脱]
12. constipation[便秘]
13. urinary hesitancy[排尿犹豫]
14. priapism[阴茎异常勃起]
15. parenteral[肠胃外]

注 1

氟西汀又名百忧解，是一种强效选择性 5-羟色胺(5-HT)摄取抑制剂，比抑制 NE 摄取作用强 200 倍，抑制这两种递质的重摄取增加突触间隙的浓度而发挥抗抑郁作用。

注 2

氟西汀的不良反应有厌食、恶心呕吐，头晕头痛、乏力失眠，体重下降，性欲减退，震颤、惊厥。“5-羟色胺综合征”发生在氟西汀与 MAO 抑制剂合用时，表现为不安、激越、恶心、呕吐或腹泻，随后高热、强直、肌阵挛或震颤、自主神经功能紊乱、心动过速、高血压、意识障碍、昏迷，严重者可致死。

点评

抑郁症是一种情感精神障碍性疾病，临床表现为情绪低落、抑郁消极。发病机制可能与脑内 5-羟色胺(5-HT)降低同时伴有去甲肾上腺素能神经功能(NE)降低。目前临床使用的抗抑郁药有：三环类抗抑郁症药、NE 再摄取抑制药、5-HT 再摄取抑制药以及其他抗抑郁症药。

颜光美

❖ CASE 16

A 29-year-old man is brought to the emergency center in a drunken stupor[①].. He is accompanied by his wife, who states that he hasn't been himself at all for the past few months. According to his wife, he was evaluated for depression by his personal physician about 3 months ago and started on a **selective serotonin reuptake inhibitor** (SSRI). He responded quite well to this therapy over the subsequent 2 months. He started feeling so good and so energetic that he stopped taking his medication. He found that he needed less and less sleep, to the point where he is now only sleeping 2-3 hours a day. He has been showering his wife with very expensive gifts and has hit the maximum limit on all of their credit cards. He has been extremely romantic and more interested in sexual relations than at any time before. He has also started drinking heavily and has passed out drunk more than once. His work has suffered, and his boss said that he is in danger of being fired if things don't straighten out. Other than being drunk, his physical examination and blood tests are normal. He is admitted to the psychiatric unit with a diagnosis of bipolar disorder and started on lithium[②].

◆ **What is the mechanism of action of lithium?**

◆ **What are the common side effects of lithium?**

◆ **What is the mechanism of action of lithium-induced polyuria[③]?**

ANSWERS TO CASE 16: Lithium

Summary: A 29-year-old man is diagnosed with bipolar disorder and is started on lithium.

- **Mechanism of action of lithium**: Not entirely known but may be related to inhibition of membrane phospholipid turnover with a reduction in key second messengers important in the overactivity of catecholamines[④] thought to be related to mood swings characteristic of bipolar disorder. [注1]
- **Common side effects of lithium**: Nausea, vomiting, diarrhea, tremor, edema, weight gain, polydipsia[⑤], and polyuria.
- **Mechanism of lithium induced polyuria**: Renal collecting tubule becomes resistant to antidiuretic[⑥] hormone.

CLINICAL CORRELATION

Lithium(Li^+) is an effective treatment for bipolar disorder. It is administered orally as lithium carbonate and eliminated almost entirely through the kidney. **Lithium has a narrow therapeutic window.** Frequent monitoring of blood levels is critical. There are potentially serious adverse effects at high levels. These include **confusion, dizziness, ataxia[⑦], and vomiting with mild elevations** and progress to **seizures, circulatory collapse[⑧], and coma with greater elevations.** [注2] The risks in an overdose are very high. Lithium also has significant drug interactions that may increase its blood levels. Increased sodium clearance or depletion, such as caused by thiazide diuretics, some nonsteroidal antiinflammatory drugs[⑨] (NSAIDs; but not aspirin or acetaminophen), or severe vomiting and diarrhea can lead to the increased renal reabsorption of lithium, thus causing toxicity. Even at therapeutic levels, there are frequent side effects. These include **gastrointestinal(GI) side effects, tremor, edema, polydipsia, and polyuria**, as well as diabetes insipidus[⑩] and weight gain. It can cause a **benign thyroid enlargement** and even overt **hypothyroidism**[⑪] (5%). It has been associated with congenital malformations when used during pregnancy.

Pharmacology of Lithium

Objectives

1. Describe the mechanism of action of lithium.
2. List other pharmacological agents used to treat bipolar disease.

Definitions

Bipolar affective (manic-depressive) disorder: Bipolar disorder is characterized by paranoid[12] thoughts, hyperactivity, and grandiosity[13], alternating in a cyclic fashion with symptoms of depression that often requires concomitant use of antidepressant agents.

Discussion of Class

In addition to Li^+, the antiepileptic[14] drugs valproic acid and carbamazepine are also first-line drugs that are effective for the treatment of the manic component of bipolar disease, often in patients unresponsive to lithium. These agents are referred to as mood stabilizers. Their adverse effect profiles when used to treat manic-depression[15] are generally milder than for lithium.

Structure

Lithium is a small, monovalent cation that is similar in its properties to sodium and that enters cell through Na^+ channels.

Mechanism of Action

Lithium has a number of actions that may have some relatifonship to its therapeutic activity, including its effects on the synthesis and release of the neurotransmitters norepinephrine, serotonin, and dopamine. It also **inhibits adenylyl cyclase activity**. Lithium's most common and best-studied effect is on the membrane recycling of phosphoinositides. It inhibits the key inositol[16] phosphatase enzymes with depletion of free inositol, which is necessary for the regeneration of phosphatidylinositol-4,5 bisphosphate(PIP_2), the precursor of the second messengers inositol trisphosphate(IP_3) and diacylglycerol (DAG)[17], which mediate the cellular actions(activation of adenylyl cyclase and protein kinase C) of G-protein-coupled muscarinic cholinoreceptors, α-adrenoceptors and serotonin 5-HT_2 receptors.

Administration

Lithium, as lithium carbonate, carbamazepine, and valproic acid are administered orally.

Pharmacokinetics

Lithium has a relatively slow onset of therapeutic action(valproic acid's effects can be achieved in a few days).

Lithium is associated with thyroid enlargement; hypothyroidism; diabetes insipidus; diarrhea, nausea, and vomiting; and weight gain. It has been associated with congenital malformations when used in pregnancy.

More than 90 percent of Li^+ is excreted into the urine, but only 20 percent is cleared. Lithium is actively reabsorbed in the proximal tubule in competition with and at the same sites as Na^+. Sodium depletion as a result of a low Na^+ diet, as well as diarrhea, concomitant use of diuretics, or even sweating, can lead to increased Li^+ retention and toxicity.

Because the renal clearance of lithium increases during pregnancy and then decreases following delivery, careful monitoring of lithium concentrations is necessary to avoid toxicity.

Comprehension Questions

[16.1] The therapeutic action of Li^+ is thought to be caused by direct inhibition of

A. Inositol phosphatase

B. Inositol triphosphate (IP_3)

C. Phosphatidylinositol-4,5 bisphosphate (PIP_2)

D. Phospholipase C

[16.2] The renal clearance of Li^+ may increase with

A. Diarrhea B. Diuretics

C. NSAIDs D. Pregnancy

[16.3] Which of the following is the most likely adverse effect of Li^+ at therapeutic doses?

A. Gastrointestinal dysfunction B. Hyperthyroidism

C. Oliguria D. Thrombocytopenia

Answers

[16.1] **A.** The therapeutic action of Li^+ is thought to be caused by direct inhibition of inositol phosphatases. Its effects on PIP_2, IP_3, and phospholipase C are an indirect consequence of this inhibition.

[16.2] **D.** The renal clearance of Li^+ may increase with pregnancy, which may lead to a reduction in its therapeutic effect. Diarrhea, certain NSAIDs, and diuretics that result in hyponatremia decrease the renal clearance of Li^+, which may result in more severe adverse effects.

[16.3] **A.** Gastrointestinal dysfunction, polydipsia (and polyuria), and hypothyroidism are adverse effects of Li^+ that may occur at therapeutic doses.

PHARMACOLOGY PEARLS

- Measurement of serum lithium concentrations are used routinely to carefully monitor treatment and to evaluate the likelihood of toxicity.
- Lithium is associated with thyroid enlargement; hypothyroidism; diabetes insipidus; diarrhea, nausea, and vomiting; and weight gain. It has been associated with congenital malformations when used in pregnancy.
- Lithium has a relatively slow onset of therapeutic action, and therefore antipsychotic drugs or benzodiazepines are used acutely to calm seriously ill patients.
- Tricyclic antidepressant agents may precipitate mania and induce more rapid cycling in some patients.

REFERENCES

Manji HK, Potter WZ, Lenox RH. Signal transduction pathways. Molecular targets for lithium's action. Arch Gen Psychiatry 1995; 52(7): 531-43.

Price LH, Heninger, GR. Lithium in the treatment of mood disorders. N Engl J Med 1994; 331 (9): 591-8.

词汇

1. stupor[木僵,昏呆]
2. lithium[锂]
3. polyuria[多尿症]
4. catecholamine[儿茶酚胺,邻苯二酚胺]
5. polydipsia[烦渴,多饮]
6. antidiuretic[抗利尿剂,抗利尿的]
7. ataxia[共济失调]
8. circulatory collapse[循环性虚脱,休克,循环衰竭]
9. non-steroidal antiinflammatory drugs[非甾体抗炎病]
10. insipidus[尿崩症]
11. hypothyroidism[甲状腺功能减退,甲状腺机能减退]
12. paranoid[妄想狂样的,偏执狂样的]
13. grandiosity[夸大]
14. antiepileptic[抗癫痫药,抗癫痫]
15. manic depression[躁狂忧郁]
16. inositol[肌醇]
17. diacylglycerol[二酰基甘油,甘油二酯,二酯酰甘油]

注 1

碳酸锂(lithium carbonate)临床用于治疗躁狂症。其中主要是锂离子发挥药理作用，其作用机制可能是抑制脑内去甲肾上腺素和多巴胺神经递质的释放，并促进其再摄取，使突触间隙中两种递质浓度下降所致。

注 2

碳酸锂的常见副作用：恶心、呕吐、腹泻，头晕、乏力、肢体震颤，口干、多尿，一般在用药初期出现，1～2 周减轻或消失。

点评

29 岁男性患者，3 个月前曾诊为抑郁症，并用选择性 5-羟色氨再摄取抑制剂（SSRI）治疗两月余，出现睡眠需要减少，一天只 2～3 小时。有挥霍，性欲亢进等躁狂症状及酒精滥用。考虑双相障碍可能性大。

锂盐为双相障碍的有效治疗手段。锂盐治疗起效较慢，有效剂量范围较窄，应监测血锂浓度。治疗浓度锂即可有胃肠道反应，可有肢体震颤，水肿，烦渴，多尿，尿崩症，体重增加等。高浓度锂可引起意识模糊，眩晕，共济失调，呕吐，兴奋甚至癫痫发作，休克与昏迷。锂盐有致畸作用。

锂盐治疗无效有可用丙戊酸和卡马西平。

颜光美

❖ CASE 17

A 66-year-old man comes in to your office for evaluation of a tremor[1]. He has noticed a progressively worsening tremor in his hands for the past 6 months. The tremor is worse when he is resting and improves some when he reaches for an object or is using his hands. He has also noticed that it is harder to "get started" when he stands up to walk. He takes several small, "shuffling[2]" steps before he can reach his full stride. He has no significant medical history and takes only an aspirin a day. On exam you note that his face is fairly expressionless, he has a pill-rolling[3] type tremor of his hands at rest and has cogwheel[4] rigidity of his arms. You diagnose him with Parkinson disease and prescribe a combination of levodopa[5] (L-dopa) and carbidopa.

◆ **What is the most common cause of the symptoms of idiopathic[6] Parkinson disease?**

◆ **What is the mechanism of action of L-dopa?**

◆ **Why is L-dopa usually given in combination with carbidopa?**

ANSWERS TO CASE 17: Drugs Used to Treat Parkinson Disease

Summary: A 66-year-old man is diagnosed with idiopathic Parkinson disease and started on L-dopa and carbidopa therapy.

- **Cause of symptoms of idiopathic Parkinson disease**: Degeneration of dopamine producing neurons in the substantia nigra[⑦].
- **Mechanism of action of L-dopa**: Decarboxylated in prejunctional neurons in the central nervous system (CNS) to restore dopamine (DA) activity in the corpus striatum. DA interacts with postjunctional dopamine D_2-receptors to activate inhibitory G-protein (Gi) and inhibit the activity of adenylyl cyclase.[注1]
- **Reason L-dopa is given with carbidopa**: Carbidopa inhibits peripheral but not central dopa-decarboxylase metabolism of L-dopa, thus allowing more of it to enter the CNS.[注2]

CLINICAL CORRELATION

Parkinson disease is a progressive, degenerative movement disorder. Symptoms of idiopathic Parkinson disease are caused by the degeneration of dopamineproducing neurons in the substantia nigra. This causes an imbalance in the actions of dopamine and acetylcholine[⑧], which, respectively, inhibit and excite the release of gamma (γ)-aminobutyric acid (GABA) from GABAergic neurons in the corpus striatum. These neurons affect motor activity via pathways leading to the thalamus[⑨] and cerebral cortex and regulate dopamine output by a feedback loop. The overall physiologic effect is to reduce excitation of the motor neurons of the spinal cord. The clinical effect is the classic parkinsonian movement disorder. These symptoms include a resting tremor, bradykinesia[⑩], masked facies, loss of postural reflexes[⑪], and rigidity[⑫]. Replacement of dopamine can help to restore the balance of activity of dopamine and acetylcholine. Dopamine, however, does not cross the blood-brain barrier into the CNS. Levodopa (L-dopa) can pass into the CNS where, as its immediate precursor, it is decarboxylated in the CNS to dopamine, which can then interact with postjunctional dopamine D_2-receptors to inhibit GABAergic neuron activity in the striatum[⑬]. L-dopa, however, is rapidly converted to dopamine in the periphery by the enzyme dopa-decarboxylase. If given by itself, high doses of L-dopa would be needed to provide a beneficial clinical effect in the CNS. **For that reason, L-dopa is usually given in combination with carbidopa**, which itself **does not cross the blood-brain barrier**, and which **inhibits peripheral, but not CNS, dopa-decarboxylase**. This allows therapeutic levels of L-dopa to enter the CNS at lower doses than would otherwise be necessary, and has the added benefit of reducing the incidence and severity of peripherally mediated adverse effects that would occur with L-dopa alone.

Nevertheless, the combination of L-dopa and carbidopa has many clinically important adverse effects. **Involuntary dyskinesias**[14], perhaps caused by developing dopamine receptor supersensitivity, are common (up to 90% of patients) and often limit the use of this therapy. The end of dose and on-off akinesias[15] may require more frequent dosage intervals or the use of sustained-release preparations. **Behavioral effects are also common, including depression, insomnia, nightmares, and changes in mood. Nausea, vomiting, anorexia**[16], and **orthostatic hypotension**[17] are not uncommon.

Pharmacology of Drugs Used to Treat Parkinson Disease

Objectives

1. List and explain the mechanisms of action, major adverse effects, and contraindications to the use of L-dopa and carbidopa combination (Sinemet) to treat Parkinson disease.
2. List other drugs or drug classes used to treat Parkinson disease, and describe their mechanism of action, benefits, and adverse effects.

Definitions

Tremor: Rhythmic oscillations of some body part, usually at a joint. In Parkinson disease tremor is present when there is minimal voluntary activity (tremor at rest).

Dyskinesia: Repetitive involuntary choreiform movements of the tongue, limbs, hands, and trunk.

Akinesia: Decreased voluntary movement.

On-off effect: Sudden onset of Parkinsonian symptoms with a usual therapeutic dose of L-dopa that may be the result of progression of the disease with loss of dopamine nerve terminals in the striatum.

Discussion of Class

In addition to L-dopa just described, there are several other drugs or drug classes used to treat Parkinson disease, including the **dopamine agonists, bromocriptine, pergolide, pramipexole, and ropinirole; the selective monoamine oxidase inhibitor, selegiline, the catechol-O-methyltransferase (COMT) inhibitors, entacapone and tolcapone; the antiviral drug, amantadine;** and several relatively selective centrally acting muscarinic cholinoreceptor blocking agents, such as benztropine, biperiden, orphenadrine, procyclidine, and trihexyphenidyl (Table 17-1).

Table 17-1

SELECTIVE LIST OF PARKINSON AGENTS

DRUGS FOR PARKINSON DISEASE	ADVERSE EFFECTS
L-dopa	Dyskinesias, depression, insomnia, nightmares, changes in mood, nausea, vomiting, anorexia, orthostatic hypotension
Dopamine Agonists Bromocriptine Pergolide Pramipexole Ropinirole	Like L-dopa
Selegiline	Serotonin syndrome, insomnia
COMT Inhibitors Entacapone Tolcapone	Gastrointestinal disturbances, dyskinesias, sleep disturbances, orange discoloration of the urine, hepatotoxicity(tolcapone)
Amantadine	Restlessness, insomnia, hallucinations, depression, livedo reticularis
Muscarinic cholinoreceptor blockers Benztropine Biperiden Orphenadrine Procyclidine Trihexyphenidyl	Dry mouth, blurred vision, mydriasis⑱, urinary retention, drowsiness, confusion, hallucinations

Dopamine agonists may be used alone or as an adjunct to L-dopa. Alone, there is a lower incidence of dyskinesia and response fluctuations. With L-dopa/carbidopa, dopamine agonists can be used to compensate for the diminishing effect of L-dopa that occurs after 3-5years, presumably because of progressive destruction of the substantia nigra and loss of dopaminergic neurons. Adverse effects, which are less severe with pramipexole and ropinirole, include gastrointestinal disturbances, postural hypotension, dyskinesias, and behavioral dysfunction. They are contraindicated in patients with psychosis⑲.

Selegiline, an **antiviral agent** which delays the metabolism of dopamine by monoamine oxidase B in the CNS, is used primarily as adjunctive therapy with L-dopa and carbidopa, generally in the later-stages of Parkinson disease. Its adverse effects are minimal, insomnia the most notable. It should not be taken with tricyclic antidepressants(TCAs), selective serotonin reuptake inhibitors(SSRIs), or the opioid meperidine because of potential development of a "serotonin syndrome[20]" with CNS stimulation, hyperpyrexia[21], and coma.

Entacapone, a COMT inhibitor, is used as an adjunct to L-dopa and carbidopa to **reduce response fluctuations**. It is preferred over tolcapone which is associated with hepatotoxicity. Other adverse effects of this class of drugs include GI disturbances, enhanced dyskinesias that may require a reduction in the dose of L-dopa, sleep disturbances, and an orange discoloration of the urine.

Amantadine, may be used early in the therapy of Parkinson disease to ameliorate its symptoms, possibly for only a few weeks before its effects wear off, or as an adjunct to L-dopa and carbidopa. **Adverse effects** include **restlessness**, **insomnia**, **hallucinations**[22], **depression** and, among many others, **livedo reticularis**[23] that results in **discoloration of the skin.**

Muscarinic cholinoreceptor blocking agents with some selectivity for CNS cholinoreceptors may be used alone to initially **diminish tremor and rigidity** (little effect on bradykinesia). Their adverse effects are those typically described for this class of agents and include dry mouth, blurring of vision, mydriasis, urinary retention, as well as certain behavioral effects including drowsiness, confusion, and hallucinations. **They are to be avoided in patients with angle-closure glaucoma**[24] **and prostatic hypertrophy**[25] and with other drugs that have muscarinic cholinoreceptor-blocking properties.

Structure

Bromocriptine and pergolide are ergot alkaloid[26] derivatives with activity at both dopamine D_1-and D_2-receptors. Pramipexole and ropinirole are nonergots with greater selectivity for dopamine D_2-receptors.

Mechanism of Action

L-dopa is decarboxylated in the striatum to dopamine which like the dopamine receptor agonists, interacts with postjunctional dopamine D_2-receptors to activate inhibitory G-proteins (Gi) and inhibit adenylyl cyclase activity in GABAergic neurons.

Selegiline is a selective monoamine oxidase inhibitor that delays the metabolism and prolongs the activity of the dopamine that is synthesized from L-dopa.

Entacapone inhibits the peripheral activity of the enzyme catechol-*O*-methyltransferase (COMT), which decreases the metabolism of L-dopa and thus increases its bioavailability and transport to the brain and prolongs its duration of action. Tolcapone also inhibits COMT in the CNS, which reduces the metabolism of dopamine and prolongs its duration of action. Amantadine's mechanism of action is unsure, but may be related to a change in the metabolism of dopamine that potentiates its action.

Muscarinic cholinoreceptor-blocking agents inhibit the activity of acetylcholine in the striatum thus restoring to some degree the balance of stimulatory activity with the already reduced inhibitory levels of dopamine in patients with Parkinson disease.

Administration

All antiparkinsonian drugs are administered by the oral route.

Pharmacokinetics

The absorption of L-dopa is rapid but is delayed by food and also by certain amino acids that compete for its transport in the gastrointestinal tract and transport from blood to the brain. The concomitant administration of carbidopa can decrease the peripheral metabolism of L-dopa by up to 75 percent.

Comprehension Questions

[17.1] Carbidopa reduces

A. Dopa-decarboxylase activity in the CNS

B. The L-dopa dose necessary to achieve a therapeutic effect

C. The severity of L-dopa associated dyskinesias

D. The time to onset of L-dopa's therapeutic effects

[17.2] Which of the following is the most common limiting adverse effect of L-dopa?

A. Depression

B. Dyskinesia

C. Nausea

D. Orthostatic hypotension

[17.3] Entacapone inhibits

A. Dopamine D_2-receptors

B. Catechol-*O*-methyltransferase

C. Monoamine oxidase B

D. Muscarinic cholinoreceptors

Answers

[17.1] **B.** Carbidopa, which does not penetrate the brain, reduces peripheral dopa decarboxylase activity and the metabolism of L-dopa. The therapeutic effect of L-dopa can be achieved at a lower dose than would be possible without carbidopa.

[17.2] **B.** The most common limiting adverse effect of L-dopa is dyskinesia that may occur in up to 90 percent of patients. Orthostatic hypotension, depression, and nausea are also adverse effects but can be more readily managed and tolerated by patients.

[17.3] **B.** Entacapone (and tolcapone) inhibits COMT. Selegiline inhibits monoamine oxidase B. Muscarinic cholinoreceptors are inhibited by biperidin and benztropine among others. Blockade of dopamine D_2-receptors would exacerbate the symptoms of Parkinson disease.

PHARMACOLOGY PEARLS

- ❖ Levodopa may exacerbate symptoms in psychotic patients.
- ❖ In the absence of carbidopa, pharmacological doses of pyridoxine (vitamin B_6) will increase the peripheral metabolism of L-dopa and thereby reduce its therapeutic effect.
- ❖ Signed patient consent is required for use of tolcapone, as is continuous evaluation of liver function.

REFERENCES

Koller WC, Tolosa E, eds. Current and emerging drug therapies in the management of Parkinson's disease. Neurology 1998; 50(6suppl 6): 51.

Frucht SJ. Parkinson disease: an update. Neurologist 2004; 10(4): 185-94.

词汇

1. tremor[震颤]
2. shuffling[慢慢移动]
3. pill-rolling[滚丸,搓丸,搓丸式]
4. cogwheel[钝齿轮,木齿铁轮]
5. levodopa[左旋多巴]
6. idiopathic[自发性的,原发性的,特发性的]
7. substantia nigra[(拉)黑质]
8. acetylcholine[乙酰胆碱]
9. thalamus [(复 thalami)丘脑]
10. bradykinesia[运动过慢,身心反应迟钝,运动徐缓]
11. postural reflex [姿势反射]
12. rigidity[僵硬]
13. striatum[纹状体]
14. dyskinesia[运动障碍]
15. akinesia[运动不能,暂时性肌麻痹]
16. anorexia[食欲缺乏,厌食症]
17. orthostatic hypotension[直立性低血压,起立性低血压]
18. mydriasis[瞳孔放大,瞳孔散大]
19. psychosis[精神病]
20. serotonin syndrome[血清素综合征]
21. hyperpyrexia[高热,温度过高]
22. hallucination[幻觉]
23. livedo reticularis[网状青斑,网状窒息]
24. angle-closure glaucoma[闭角型青光眼]
25. prostatic hypertrophy[前列腺肥大]
26. ergot alkaloid[麦角生物碱]

注 1

左旋多巴(L-dopa)是多巴胺的前体，通过血脑屏障后，被脑内多巴胺能神经元脱羧转变为多巴胺，补充纹状体中多巴胺的不足而发挥治疗帕金森病(PD)的作用。

注 2

临床上治疗 PD 时，通常是左旋多巴与卡比多巴联合应用。卡比多巴又称左旋多巴增效药，它是外周氨基酸脱羧酶抑制药，合用时能抑制左旋多巴在外周脱羧，从而进入中枢的左旋多巴增加，可减少左旋多巴用量，提高疗效，减轻不良反应。

点评

老年患者，有典型的静止性震颤表现，搓丸样震颤，静止时加重，随意运动时减轻；姿势步态异常，起步困难，下肢拖曳，小步态。检查手臂呈齿轮样强直，面无表情，典型帕金森病表现。帕金森病是由于中脑黑质多巴受能神经元变性，导致纹状体系统多巴胺含量降低，从而引起一系列症状和体征。表现为静止性震颤，运动迟，“面具脸”，姿势反射消失和肌强直。治疗帕金森病用左旋多巴和卡比多巴联合应用。左旋多巴通过血脑屏障后，被脑多巴胺能神经元脱羧变为多巴胺。为增强疗效，减少副作用，左旋多巴与外周多巴脱羧酶抑制剂卡比多巴合用。

颜光美

❖ CASE 18

An 18-year-old man is brought to the emergency department by paramedics[①] after a series of grand-mal[②] seizures. He required repeated doses of IV lorazepam to finally control the episode. A family member with him states that he has had epilepsy[③] since childhood. He is supposed to take phenytoin, but often forgets or refuses. His last seizure[④] was about 3 months ago. In the emergency room he is confused and combative but has an otherwise normal neurological examination. Blood tests show an undetectable phenytoin[注1] level. You give him an IV loading dose of fosphenytoin and restart him on his oral phenytoin.[注2]

◆ **What is the mechanism of action of phenytoin**?

◆ **How is phenytoin metabolized**?

ANSWERS TO CASE 18: Antiepileptic Drugs

Summary: An 18-year-old man presents with grand-mal seizures and is given phenytoin.

- **Mechanism of action of phenytoin**: Blocks sodium channels and inhibits the generation of action potentials.
- **Metabolism of phenytoin**: Parahydroxylation and glucuronide⑤ conjugation by hepatic microsomal enzymes.

CLINICAL CORRELATION

Phenytoin is one of the most widely used drugs for the treatment of tonicclonic (grand-mal) seizures⑥. It is also a major first-line drug used to treat partial seizures. It works by binding to and prolonging the inactive state of the Na^+ channel thus blocking use-dependent Na^+ conductance and the generation of action potentials. It can be given orally, and its long half-life allows for once-a-day dosing. Phenytoin is metabolized in the liver by microsomal enzymes through parahydroxylation and glucuronide conjugation. Rates of oral absorption and metabolism can vary significantly from one patient to the next. At very low doses elimination is first-order; however, even within the therapeutic range, the liver enzymes responsible for its metabolism near saturation, resulting in an increase in its half-life. Because of this inability to reach steady state and **phenytoin's low therapeutic index**, dosing of this drug must be individualized and plasma levels closely monitored. **Common side effects include nystagmus⑦, ataxia⑧, confusion⑨, hirsutism⑩, and gingival⑪ hyperplasia⑫** in children (up to 50%). **Idiosyncratic⑬ reactions include skin rashes**. Its use should be avoided, if possible, during **pregnancy because it is teratogenic⑭**. **Phenytoin induces hepatic metabolism by microsomal enzyme induction** and can lower plasma levels of other drugs. Phenytoin's level can be increased by drugs that inhibit its hepatic metabolism. Caution and close monitoring of blood levels of phenytoin must be undertaken when phenytoin is used in combination with other drugs.

Pharmacology of Antiepileptic⑮ Agents

Objectives

1. List the major antiepileptic agents.
2. Describe the mechanism of action of major antiepileptic agents.
3. List and discuss the common adverse effects and toxicities of major antiepileptic agents.
4. List the therapeutic uses of major antiepileptic agents.

Definitions

Seizure: A nonrecurrent abnormal discharge from the brain.

Epilepsy: A chronic dysfunction of recurrent seizures.

Therapeutic index: A measure of the relationship (ratio) between the dose necessary to produce a therapeutic effect, usually expressed as the median effective dose (ED_{50}), and the dose necessary to produce an undesired effect, usually expressed as the median toxic dose (TD_{50}).

First-pass effect: The extensive metabolism of many drugs administered orally that in some instances may limit bioavailability to such an extent that an effective therapeutic dose cannot be achieved.

Discussion of Class

There is some degree of drug specificity relative to seizure type (Table 18-1). In addition to phenytoin, **carbamazepine** is another major first-line antiepileptic drug used to treat both partial seizures and generalized tonic-clonic seizures. A number of other available drugs for treating partial and generalized tonicclonic seizures (e. g., gabapentin, lamotrigine, tiagabine, vigabatrin) are also used as second-line or add-on therapeutic agents. First-line drugs available to specifically treat **generalized absence seizures** include **ethosuximide and valproic acid**. These may also be used as second-line or add-on therapeutic agents to treat other seizure types. The **benzodiazepines, diazepam and lorazepam**, also have important first-line use, along with phenytoin or fosphenytoin, for treating generalized tonic-clonic status epilepticus.

Table 18-1

SELECTED ANTISEIZURE AGENTS

Generalized Tonic-Clonic Seizures
Phenytoin
Carbamazepine
Partial Seizures
Phenytoin
Carbamazepine
Absence Seizures
Ethosuximide
Valproic acid
Status Epilepticus
Diazepam
Lorazepam
Phenytoin/Fosphentoin

Carbamazepine, a first-line drug for treating partial seizures and generalized tonic-clonic seizures, is also used therapeutically to treat bipolar disorder and trigeminal neuralgia. **Drowsiness**[16], **diplopia**[17], **and ataxia are common side effects**. Gastrointestinal disturbances, headache, dizziness, and sedation are also not uncommon effects (Table 18-2). **Idiosyncratic reactions include skin rash** and rarely a **severe hypersensitivity or fatal aplastic anemia**[18]. Carbamazepine may exacerbate or precipitate absence seizures.

Table 18-2

SELECTED ANTISEIZURE AGENTS AND ADVERSE EFFECTS

AGENT	SELECTED ADVERSE EFFECTS
Phenytoin	Nystagmus, ataxia, confusion, hirsutism[19], gingival hyperplasia in children (up to 50%), idiosyncratic reactions (e.g., skin rashes), teratogenicity
Carbamazepine	Drowsiness, diplopia, ataxia, gastrointestinal disturbances, headache, dizziness, sedation, idiosyncratic reactions (skin rash, aplastic anemia)
Ethosuximide	Gastrointestinal disturbances
Valproic Acid	Idiosyncratic hepatoxicity

Ethosuximide, a first-line drug to treat generalized absence seizures, has generally mild adverse effects related primarily to gastrointestinal disturbances.

Valproic acid, like ethosuximide, is a first-line drug used to treat generalized **absence** seizures. However, because of the potential for an **idiosyncratic hepatotoxicity**, it is reserved for patients with concomitant generalized tonicclonic seizures. It is also used to control myoclonic seizures[20] and for the treatment of bipolar disorder and for prophylaxis[21] of migraine[22] headache.

As for **phenytoin**, the **therapeutic index for these drugs is low**. Thus, serum drug levels need to be carefully monitored.

Mechanism of Action

Carbamazepine acts like phenytoin.

Ethosuximide reduces low threshold T-Ca^{++} current in the thalamus that appears to provide pacemaker activity responsible for cortical generation of absence seizures.

Valproic acid may have more than one mechanism of action including an effect on Na^+ channels like phenytoin and carbamazepine, blockade of NMDA receptors, and increased activity of the neurotransmitter γ-aminobutyric acid (GABA)[23]. Its use in pregnancy is associated with an increased risk of **neural tube defects**[24].

The benzodiazepines, diazepam and lorazepam, potentiate GABA neurotransmission.

Administration

Phenytoin and valproic acid are available for both oral and parenteral (IV) administration[25].

Fosphenytoin is only available for parenteral administration, whereas carbamazepine and ethosuximide are only available for oral administration.

Phenytoin, because it may precipitate at its site of injection, has been replaced for intravenous injection by the more water-soluble fosphenytoin.

Both phenytoin and carbamazepine exist also in extended-release preparations.

Valproic acid is hydroscopic and therefore is available for oral administration as a capsule in corn oil or, for pediatric use, in syrup. It is also available as a more patient preferred enteric-coated tablet formulated as divalproex sodium, which is a 1∶1 compound of valproic acid and sodium valproic acid. It is also available for parenteral use.

Pharmacokinetics

Because phenytoin's liver metabolic enzymes become saturated at a low dose, relatively small changes in the dose can lead to very large changes in the plasma concentration and, with it, the development of toxicity.

With continuous administration, carbamazepine induces the synthesis of liver microsomal enzymes responsible for its own metabolism resulting in a substantially decreased half-life requiring significant dose adjustment. Through the same induction mechanism, carbamazepine can also alter the metabolism of a number of other drugs. Likewise, there are a number of drugs that can alter the metabolism of carbamazepine by induction of the appropriate microsomal enzymes. Oxcarbamazepine is a closely related anticonvulsant[26] that is less likely to induce microsomal enzyme[27] synthesis.

Valproic acid inhibits its own metabolism and the metabolism of other drugs, including phenytoin. It displaces phenytoin from its binding to plasma proteins.

Comprehension Questions

[18.1] Blockade of T-calcium currents is the major mechanism of action for which of the following drugs used to manage seizures?

A. Carbamazepine B. Diazepam
C. Ethosuximide D. Phenytoin

[18.2] Which of the following drugs used to manage seizures requires a significant dose adjustment with continuous administration?

A. Carbamazepine B. Diazepam
C. Ethosuximide D. Phenytoin

[18.3] For which of the following drugs used to manage epilepsy does a small change in its bioavailability result in a disproportionate increase in its blood levels?

A. Carbamazepine B. Diazepam

C. Ethosuximide D. Phenytoin

Answers

[18.1] **C.** The anticonvulsant activity of ethosuximide when used to treat absence seizures is is due to its blockade T-calcium currents in the thalamus. Carbamazepine and phenytoin, which are not used to treat absence seizures, block sodium channels. Diazepam, which is not a first-line drug for absence seizures, potentiates GABA neurotransmission.

[18.2] **A.** Carbamazepine induces the synthesis of liver microsomal enzymes responsible for its own metabolism, necessitating a significant dose adjustment with its continued administration.

[18.3] **D.** A small change in the bioavailability of phenytoin may result in a disproportionate increase in its blood level because its metabolic enzymes become saturated at therapeutic doses.

PHARMACOLOGY PEARLS

❖ Currently available antiepileptic drugs control seizures in about 80 percent of patients with epilepsy.

❖ Antiepileptic drugs increase the risk of congenital malformations, including the "fetal hydantoin syndrome" (phenytoin) and spina bifida (valproic acid).

❖ The main side effects of phenytoin are nystagmus, ataxia, confusion, hirsutism, and gingival hyperplasia.

❖ Phenytoin is metabolized by hepatic microsomal enzymes.

REFERENCES

Levy RH, et al. Antiepileptic drugs. Philadelphia: Lippincott Williams & Wilkins, 2002.

Lowenstein DH. Seizures and epilepsy. In: Harrison's principles of internal medicine, 15th ed. New York: McGraw Hill, 2000.

词汇

1. paramedic[随行医务人员,急救医士]
2. grand-mal[癫痫大发作]

3. epilepsy[癫痫,羊痫风]
4. seizure[发作,癫痫发作]
5. glucuronide[葡糖苷酸,葡萄糖醛酸苷,葡萄糖醛酸甙]
6. tonic clonic seizure[强直阵挛发作]
7. nystagmus[(希)眼球震颤,眼球震颤,眼震]
8. ataxia[共济失调]
9. confusion[散毛性,杂乱性]
10. hirsutism[多毛症]
11. gingival[牙龈的,龈(沟)液]
12. hyperplasia[超常增生]
13. idiosyncratic[特(异反)应性的,特异体质的]
14. teratogenic[畸形形成的]
15. antiepileptic[抗癫痫药,抗癫痫的]
16. drowsiness[困倦,昏昏欲睡]
17. diplopia[复视]
18. aplastic anemia[再生障碍性贫血]
19. hirsutism[多毛症]
20. myoclonic seizure[肌阵挛发作]
21. prophylaxis[预防]
22. migraine[偏头痛]
23. γ-aminobutyric acid(GABA)[γ-氨基丁酸]
24. neural-tube defect[神经管缺损]
25. parenteral administration[肠胃外投药,非经肠给药法]
26. anticonvulsant[抗惊厥剂,抗抽搐剂]
27. microsomal enzyme[微粒体酶]

注 1

苯妥英钠又称大仑丁，是常用的抗癫痫药。它具有膜稳定作用，可降低细胞膜对 Na^+ 和 Ca^{2+} 的通透性，抑制 Na^+ 和 Ca^{2+} 内流，导致动作电位不易产生，从而阻止癫痫病灶异常放电向周围正常组织扩散，来治疗癫痫。

注 2

苯妥英钠主要被肝药酶代谢为羟基苯基衍生物而失活，以原型由尿排出者不足 5%。静脉注射用于治疗癫痫持续状态，血药浓度低于 10μg/ml 时按一级动力学消除，t1/2 约 20h。高于此浓度时，则按零级动力学消除，血浆 t1/2 可延至 60h。药物羟化代谢能力受遗传基因影响，个体差异大，用药时注意剂量个体化。

点评

癫痫是大脑局部神经元异常高频放电并向周围正常组织扩散所引起的反复发作的慢性脑疾病，表现为突然发作，短暂的运动、感觉功能或精神异常。诊断主要依据病史，脑电图检查异常。全面性强直-阵挛发作(generalized tonic-clonic seizure)简称大发作(grand mall)是常见的发作类型。目前癫痫治疗仍以药物为主，用药的目的在于减少或阻止发作，不能有效的预防和治愈疾病。癫痫治疗往往是终身的。

颜光美

❖ CASE 19

An 18-year-old man is brought into the emergency department after being found on the street unresponsive.[注1] He is lethargic and does not answer questions. He has been given 1 ampule of Dextrose intravenously without result. On examination, his heart rate is 60 beats per minute, and respiratory rate is 8 per minute and shallow.[注2] His pupils are pinpoint and not reactive. There are multiple intravenous track marks on his arms bilaterally. The emergency physician concludes that the patient has had a drug overdose.

◆ **What is the most likely diagnosis?**

◆ **What is the most appropriate medication to be given?**

◆ **After he is given the medication to reverse the overdose, what symptoms may he have?**

ANSWERS TO CASE 19: Opioid Overdose

Summary: An 18-year-old unresponsive man presents with pinpoint pupils, shallow respirations, and multiple intravenous track marks on his arms bilaterally.

- **Most likely diagnosis**: Opioid overdose, likely heroin.
- **Most appropriate medication to be given**: Naloxone.
- **After reversal of the overdose, what symptoms may he have**?

  Withdrawal symptoms may include lacrimation, rhinorrhea, sweating, dilated pupils, diarrhea, abdominal cramping, and tremor.

CLINICAL CORRELATION

Opioids are drugs with morphine-like activity that reduce pain and induce **tolerance** and **physical dependence**. Individuals seek the euphoria obtained from the intravenous injection of opioids such as heroin. There are three different cell **receptors** specific for opioids: **mu, kappa, and delta**(μ, κ δ), all of which exist as multiple subtypes. This patient has the classic signs of **opioid overdose: somnolence**①, **respiratory depression**②, **and miosis**③. Stimulation of the mu receptor results in analgesia (supraspinal and spinal), respiratory depression, euphoria, and physical dependence. Stimulation of the kappa receptor result in analgesia, as well as miosis and sedation. Continuous, heavy use of opioids can result in tolerance where more drug is required to obtain the same euphoric "high" and also to physical dependence. Naloxone, a competitive antagonist of opioids, is used to treat opioid overdose. Its intravenous administration leads to an almost immediate reversal of all effects of the opioids.

In patients, or other individuals who are physically dependent ("addicts"), administration of naloxone will immediately precipitate **opioid withdrawal**, which consists of a constellation of signs and symptoms that include nausea and vomiting, muscle aches, lacrimation or rhinorrhea, diarrhea, fever, and dilated pupils. Likewise, when someone physically dependent on opioids ceases its administration there is a more slowly developing (hours or days) constellation of symptoms of opioid withdrawal that includes **sensitivity to touch and light**, **goose flesh**④, **autonomic hyperactivity**, **gastrointestinal distress**, **joint and muscle aches**, **yawning**⑤, **salivation**, **lacrimation**, **urination**, **defecation**, **and a depressed or anxious mood.** In general, physical dependence induced by opioids with a short half-life tend to result in a rapid severe withdrawal, while physical dependence induced by opioids with a long half-life tends to be associated with a less severe and more gradual course of withdrawal. Although very uncomfortable, opioid withdrawal is **generally not life-threatening**.

Clonidine, a nonopioid, has been used to **decrease the autonomic symptoms of opioid withdrawal, such as the hypertension, tachycardia, sweating, lacrimation, and rhinorrhea** (it may also reduce the subjective sensations or cravings for opioids that may exist). Blood pressure must be monitored carefully if this drug is to be used since an α-adrenoceptor agonist is thought to act on noradrenergic neurons of the locus ceruleus to reduce central sympathetic outflow.

The opioid methadone may be administered in a daily dose to individuals physically dependent on opioids, most notably heroin, as a "maintenance therapy" or to ameliorate the symptoms of opioid withdrawal.

Pharmacology of the Opioids

Objectives

1. Describe the mechanism of action of opioids as analgesics.
2. Explain how opioids reduce pain.
3. List the major opioid agonists and antagonists, their therapeutic uses, and their important pharmacokinetic properties.
4. Describe the adverse effects of opioids.

Definitions

Opioids[6]: Drugs with morphine-like activity, including the naturally occurring compounds derived from opium referred to collectively as opiates (e. g., morphine and heroin), as well as other semisynthetic and synthetic man-made drugs.

Endogenous Opioid Peptides[7]: Class of natural endogenous peptides that bind to human mu, delta, and kappa opioid receptors. Four classes of such peptides have been described: 1) the pentapeptide enkephalins (met and leu), 2) β-endorphin, 3) the dynorphins, all of which are proteolytically released from larger precursor molecules, and 4) the endomorphins. Together, they appear to modulate a number of important functions of the body (e. g., analgesia, reactions to stress and to anxiety).

Autonomic hyperactivity[8]: Symptoms of autonomic hyperactivity include tachypnea, hyperreflexia, tachycardia, hypertension, sweating, and hyperthermia.

Fasciculation[9]: Muscular twitching of contiguous groups of muscle fibers.

Lacrimation[10]: Secretion of tears from the eyes.

Rhinorrhea[11]: Mucous-like material that comes out of the nose.

Salivation[12]: Saliva flowing outside the mouth.

Discussion of Class

Morphine, the prototype opioid, is derived from opium, a crude material obtained from the seed pod of the opium poppy plant. The chemical structure of morphine is shown in Fig. 19-1. Many other derivatives of the opium plant (opiates) and other drugs with similar effects (opioids) have been discovered or synthesized. Chemical modifications of the morphine structure results in significant alterations in potency and in the ratio of agonist to antagonist effects (Table 19-1). However, no major improvement in the analgesic effect of this class of opioids has been achieved; morphine is still one of the most widely used opioids. The opioids are classified in several ways: (1) **strength of analgesic** effect (strong and weak agents); (2) ratio of **agonist to antagonist effects** (pure agonists, mixed agonist-antagonists, and partial agonists that act both as an opioid agonist and antagonist, and antagonists), and (3) **spectrum of action** (analgesics, antitussive, and antidiarrheal drugs).

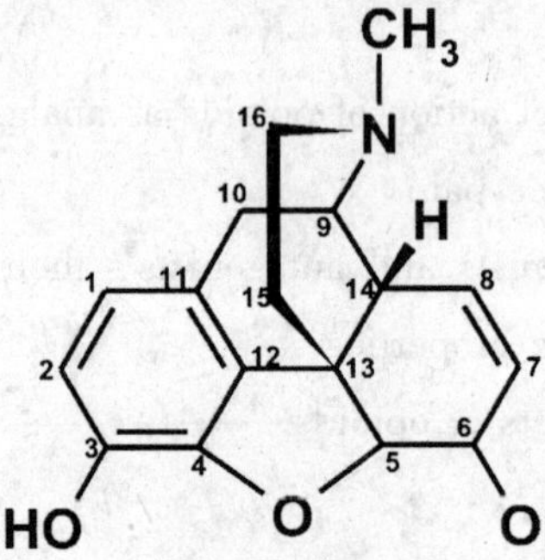

Ring Position

	3[1]	6[1]	17[2]	Substitution
Morphine	$-OH$	$-OH$	$-CH_3$	prototype
Codeine[3]	$-OCH_3$	$-OH$	$-CH_3$	methylmorphine
Heroin[4]	$-OCOCH_3$	$-OCOCH_3$	$-CH_3$	diacetyl morphine
Naloxone[5]	$-OH$	$=O$	$-CH_2CH=CH_2$	allyl
Thebaine[6]	$-OCH_3$	$-OCH_3$	$-CH_3$	dimethyl morphine

[1] Substitutions at the C-3 phenolic position and the C-6 hydroxyl position of morphine

[2] Modification of the methyl group on the nitrogen in the piperidine ring (N-17)

[3] Methyl substitution: decreased first pass effect, increased oral absorption in the brain to morphine

[5] Allyl substitution: antagonist

[6] Dimethyl substitution: convulsant

Figure 19-1. Structure-activity relationships of opioids.

The major therapeutic application for morphine and other **strong opioids** (e. g. , **meperidine, fentanyl, hydromorphone**) is the management of moderate to severe pain (e. g. , pain associated with trauma, burns, cancer, acute myocardial infarction, and renal or biliary colic). **Weaker opioids** such as **codeine** and **pentazocine** are used to

Table 19-1

SELECTED OPIOIDS

STRONG OPIOID AGONISTS	NOTES
Morphine (also hydromorphone, oxymorphone, heroin)	See above
Meperidine	Indications are similar to morphine. Used as an obstetrical anesthetic premedication. Overdose may cause CNS excitation (tremors, delirium, and hyperreflexia) and seizures as a result of formation of an N-demethylated metabolite, normeperidine. With MAO inhibitors may cause severe restlessness, excitement, fever, and seizures (serotonin syndrome). It has weak anticholinergic activity that may result in mydriasis (not miosis) and tachycardia. Meperidine has weak or no effect on the cough reflex.
Fentanyl (also alfentanil, sufentanil, remifentanil)	Has a shorter duration of action than morphine. Available for parenteral use only. Used as a preanesthetic medication and for pre- and postoperative pain. Fentanyl (or morphine) is used to supplement the analgesia and sedative-hypnotic effects of nitrous oxide and halothane equals "balanced anesthesia". Rapid IV administration of high doses may cause severe truncal muscle rigidity that can be reversed by naloxone.
Methadone	Used as an oral opioid substitute to treat opioid dependence. Its long duration of action and slow metabolism result in less severe withdrawal than with other shorter-acting opioids.
Codeine (also oxycodone, hydrocodone, dihydrocodeine)	Used for moderate pain. Has good bioavailability by the oral route (compared to morphine); 10% converted to morphine. Causes little respiratory depression and less dependence liability than morphine. An overdose may cause seizures. Codeine and other weak opioid agonists are often used in combination with other analgesics such as aspirin (Percodan) or acetaminophen (Percocet).

续表

WEAK OPIOID AGONISTS	NOTES
Diphenoxylate, Loperamide	Used for the symptomatic treatment of diarrhea. Insolubility of diphenoxylate limits its absoption across the GI tract. Loperamide does not cross the blood-brain barrier. Minimal dependence liability or other centrally mediated opioid effects. To limit its parenteral use, diphenoxylate is only available combined with atropine.
MIXED OPIOID AGONIST-ANTAGONISTS/ PARTIAL AGONISTS	
Pentazocine, Buprenorphine (also nalbuphine, butorphanol, dezocine, tramadol)	Pentazocine has agonist activity at the kappa receptor and agonist activity at the mu receptor. Buprenorphine is a partial agonist at the μ-receptor. They are used for moderate pain. Buprenorphine is used for heroin detoxification. They have less dependence liability than morphine, although they can precipitate withdrawal in an opioid-dependent person. High doses may cause sweating, dizziness, and nausea, and, occasionally, dysphoria, hallucinations, and depersonalization.
OPIOID ANTAGONISTS	
Naloxone and Naltrexone (also nalmefene)	Competitive antagonists at opioid receptors which can precipitate opioid withdrawal. Naloxone is administered IV because of poor oral absorption. It is used to treat acute opioid overdose. Because of its short duration of action, multiple dosing may be necessary. Naltrexone is FDA approved for use in chronic alcoholics to reduce craving for alcohol.
ANTITUSSIVE AGENTS	NOTES
Dextromethorphan	Dextromethorphan, a nonopioid drug, is nearly as effective as codeine as an antitussive agent but with less constipating effect. It has no or limited analgesic activity or dependence liability. It may cause some dizziness, nausea, or drowsiness. Opioids other than codeine are not commonly used because of their dependence liability.

manage mild to moderate pain. Other important therapeutic uses include the management of **diarrhea** (e. g. , **codeine**, **diphenoxylate**, **loperamide**), dyspnea associated with pulmonary edema secondary to acute left ventricular failure, suppression of the cough reflex (codeine, **dextromethorphan**), and maintenance and withdrawal therapy for opioid dependence (**methadone**, **buprenorphine**). The antitussive (cough suppressant) action and antidiarrheal action of the opioids are at least partially separable from their analgesic action. Separate drugs have been developed to exploit these effects.

The sites of opioid action include areas in the central nervous system (CNS) where they **raise the threshold to pain** (i. e. , decrease the sensation of pain) including 1) the ***spinal cord***, where opioids act directly on **receptors** on the **terminals of primary afferent sensory neurons** in the **dorsal horn of the spinal cord** to inhibit release of excitatory transmitters like **substance P**, 2) the ***thalamus***, where opioids act on **ascending pathways** to **directly inhibit pain transmission from the spinal cord to higher centers of the brain** (via the spinothalamic tract and spinoreticular tract), and 3) the ***midbrain*** periaqueductal gray area and rostral ventral medulla (nucleus raphe magnus) where opioids **activate descending *inhibitory* neurons to the spinal cord**, thus preventing pain transmission. Opioids also act on the cerebral cortex, amygdala, and hippocampus to decrease the emotional reactivity to pain (i. e. , decrease the perception of pain). There is also a direct inhibitory effect of opioids on sensory nerve endings. In addition to the CNS, opioids also act on other organs including, notably, the GI tract and kidney.

The most commonly observed effects when the opioids are used for the relief of pain are **sedation**, **nausea and vomiting**, **and constipation**⑬. Large doses regularly induce **respiratory depression and euphoria**⑭ or mental clouding. The major adverse effects of selected opioids are presented in Table 19-2.

Tolerance⑮ to some effects of the opioids (Table 19-3) occurs gradually (days) with repeated administration such that a larger dose is necessary to produce the same initial effect. The tolerance is because of a direct action of opioids on neurons (i. e. , cellular tolerance) rather than to an increase in their metabolism (metabolic tolerance). Tolerance does not occur to all the effects of the opioid agonists or to the action of antagonists (see Table 19-3). Tolerance to one opioid agonist can confer tolerance to other opioid agonists, that is, cross-tolerance. However, there is no cross-tolerance between opioid agonists and other nonopioid drugs that act on the CNS such as the benzodiazepines, barbiturates, ethanol, stimulants, etc.

Opioid-induced **respiratory depression** may be potentiated in the presence of sedative-hypnotics agents, antipsychotic agents, or antidepressant agents. Opioids, particularly **meperidine**, may interact with **monoamine oxidase inhibitors** (MAOIs; tranylcypromine, phenelzine) to cause a "**serotonin syndrome**⑯".

Table 19-2

ADVERSE EFFECTS OF OPIOIDS

(Generally Extensions of Pharmacological Activity)

ADVERSE EFFECT: CAUSE	NOTES
Respiratory depression (major limiting effect) caused by direct inhibition of respiratory center in the brain stem that results in decreased sensitivity to hypoxic drive by carbon dioxide.	Occurs at therapeutic doses of morphine. Tolerance develops that parallels tolerance to analgesia. Respiratory depression is generally not a serious clinical problem except in several special circumstances where opioids may be contraindicated: 1. decreased respiratory reserve (e. g., emphysema, obstructive lung disease); 2. head injury or CNS tumors; and 3. pregnancy (to avoid fetal respiratory depression). Respiratory depresson is a serious and potentially fatal consequence of opioid overdose.
Sedation/drowsiness	A decreased ability to concentrate. Ambulatory patients and elderly are at risk for accidents. A paradoxical dysphoria and increased anxiety may occur in children and women.
Nausea (30%), vomiting (10%): Caused by direct stimulation of the CTZ in the area postrema of the medulla which activates the vomiting center.	More likely to occur in ambulatory patients. Self-limiting with continued administration because of subsequent direct inhibition by morphine of the vomiting center.
Dependence	See clinical correlation.
Pneumonia: May result from inhibition of cough reflex.	Increased likelihood in patients whose respiration is already seriously compromised.
Miosis: Stimulation of the Edinger-Westphal nucleus of the oculomotor nerve (III) results in contraction of the pupillary sphincter with constriction with of the pupils ("pin-point" pupils).	Occurs at therapeutic doses. Pupils do not dilate, even in the dark. Parasympathetic pathways involves release of ACh in the ciliary ganglion; miosis can be blocked by atropine. Sign of opioid (e. g., heroin) overdose.
Hypotension: Opioids inhibits the (tonically active) vasomotor center in the brain stem to cause some peripheral arterial and venous vasodilation.	Usually not a clinical problem but is a relative contraindication for patients in shock or who have low blood pressure or who are hypovolemic (reduced blood volume). The elderly are particularly susceptible.

续表

ADVERSE EFFECT: CAUSE	NOTES
Constipation (delayed fecal movement/increased absorption of water): Mechanism is uncertain, but probably due to peripheral action on the enteric nervous system to inhibit acetylcholine release. Effect is to increase GI tone with a concomitant decrease in coordinated propulsive activity and motility. Opioids also increase anal sphincter tone and decrease attention to the defecation reflex.	A major complaint of patients receiving opioids for analgesia. There is no clinically significant tolerance in humans. Stool softeners are used to treat (mineral oil/glycerin suppositories).
Urine retention: Opioids decrease urinary output due to decreased renal plasma flow, possible increased release of ADH from pituitary, decreased coordinated contractility of the ureters and bladder, increased urethral spincter tone, and inattention to the urinary reflex.	Usually not a clinical problem except in patients with enlargement of the prostate. Catheterization may be necessary. More common in elderly. Increased tone of the ureters may result in a paradoxical increase in pain. A similar effect may occur when opioids are used to treat the pain of biliary colic.

Table 19-3

RELATIVE DEVELOPMENT OF TOLERANCE TO OPIOIDS

SUBSTANTIAL	MINIMAL
Analgesia	Constipation
Respiratory depression	Seizures (meperidine, codeine)
Euphoria	Antagonist activity (naloxone, naltrexone)
Sedation	Miosis
Nausea and vomiting	

Structure

Opioids may be full agonists (e. g. , morphine, heroin) or partial agonists (e. g. , buprenorphine, pentazocine). Morphine is a phenanthrene alkaloid with a phenylmethyl-piperidine ring structure. Simple chemical substitutions can markedly alter its pharmacological properties (see Fig. 19-1).

Mechanism of Action

Opioid agonists bind to G-protein-coupled neural receptors (**mu**, **delta**, **kappa**) to **reduce adenylyl cyclase activity**, to reduce prejunctional calcium conductance, which causes a decrease in neurotransmitter release, and to enhance postjunctional potassium conductance, which causes a decreased cell responsiveness to excitatory neurotransmitters. Together, these actions are thought to result in analgesia.

Administration

Opioids are usually administered orally, but some like morphine can also be administered rectally or parenterally.

Specialized administration

Patient controlled analgesia (PCA): By infusion (morphine/meperidine/hydromorphone).

Regional analgesia: Epidural route is favored because it produces fewer adverse effects. May also be administered into subarachnoid or intrathecal spaces. There may be delayed respiratory depression, nausea, and vomiting that can be reversed with naloxone.

Transdermal fentanyl patch: Used for chronic pain.

Buccal fentanyl lozenge/lollipop

Butorphanol nasal spray

Pharmacokinetics

Most opioids are absorbed well. Morphine, given orally, shows variable but significant first-pass metabolism (glucuronide conjugation) with a low oral to parenteral potency ratios (25%). It is usually given parenterally. Codeine and methadone are well absorbed after oral administration (approximately 60%) because of limited first pass metabolism.

All opioids are metabolized by the liver. Metabolism usually results in more polar metabolites and frequently involves conjugation of the phenolic hydroxyl with glucuronic acid. Excretion is primarily by way of the kidneys. In addition to inactive metabolites, morphine is conjugated in the liver to morphine-3-glucuronide, which has neuroexcitatory properties. Morphine is also metabolized (10%) to morphine-6-glucuronide which has analgesic potency greater than morphine itself. Codeine is metabolized, in part, to morphine. Heroin is also metabolized to morphine. Meperidine is metabolized to normeperidine that may be responsible for seizures in patients where it accumulates.

The fetal blood-brain barrier is readily crossed by the opioids, and infants born to mothers given (or self-administering) large doses of opioids may have severe respiratory depression.

Comprehension Questions

[19.1] Morphine produces analgesia through which of the following actions?

A. Activation of neuronal adenylyl cyclase

B. Increased prejunctional neurotransmitter release

C. Reduction of postjunctional neuronal potassium conductance

D. Reduction of prejunctional neuronal calcium conductance

[19.2] Which of the following opioid agonists is metabolized to an active agent with analgesic activity?

A. Clonidine

B. Codeine

C. Meperidine

D. Naloxone

[19.3] The antitussive agent dextromethorphan

A. Activates mu, delta, and kappa receptors

B. Has analgesic activity in addition to its antitussive activity

C. Has no dependence liability

D. Is more constipating than codeine

Answers

[19.1] **D**. Opioid agonists bind to G-protein-coupled receptors to reduce adenylyl cyclase activity, to reduce prejunctional calcium conductance, which results in a decrease in neurotransmitter release, and to enhance postjunctional potassium conductance, which results in decreased responsiveness to excitatory neurotransmitters.

[19.2] **B**. Codeine is metabolized, in part, to morphine. Naloxone is an opioid antagonist. Clonidine is not an opioid. Meperidine is metabolized to normeperidine that may result in seizures.

[19.3] **C**. Dextromethorphan is a nonopioid drug that is nearly as effective as codeine as an antitussive agent but with less constipating effect. It has no analgesic activity or dependence liability.

PHARMACOLOGY PEARLS

- Seeking the relief of pain is one of the most common reasons for patient visit.
- Up to 75 percent of hospitalized patients who receive opioids for their pain still report severe or moderate distress as result of under-dosing, often because clinicians are afraid of causing physical dependence or addiction.
- A patient, particularly a terminally ill patient, should never agonize or wish for death because of a physician's reluctance to use adequate doses of opioids!
- Seizures may occur in patients with renal failure because of the action of the morphine metabolite morphine-3-glucuronide.
- An accentuated action of morphine may occur in patients with renal failure as a consequence of the action of the active morphine metabolite morphine-6-glucuronide.

REFERENCES

Ferrante FM. Principles of opioid pharmacotherapy: practical implications of basic mechanisms. J Pain Symptom Manage 1996; 11(5): 265-73.

Julius D, Basbaum AI. Molecular mechanisms of nociception. Nature 2001; 413(6852): 203-10.

Loeser JD, ed. Bonica's management of pain. Philadelphia: Lippincott Williams Wilkins, 2001.

词汇

1. somnolence[嗜睡]
2. respiratory depression[呼吸抑制]
3. miosis[瞳孔缩小]
4. goose flesh[鸡皮疙瘩]
5. yawning[呵欠]
6. opioid[阿片类药物]
7. endogenous opioid peptide[内源性阿片肽]
8. autonomic hyperactivity[自主性活动亢进]
9. fasciculation[肌束震颤]
10. lacrimation[流泪]
11. rhinorrhea[鼻漏]
12. salivation[流涎]
13. constipation[便秘]
14. euphoria[欣快]
15. tolerance[耐受性]
16. serotonin syndrom[5-HT 综合征]

注 1

病史中未提及患者是否有饮酒，应用吗啡的患者如同时饮用含酒精的饮料，有发生吗啡过量的危险。因此如服用吗啡类镇痛药应避免饮酒。

注 2

遇到有吸毒史的昏迷患者，如呼吸浅促则应高度怀疑重度海洛因戒断综合征，可静脉推注吗啡 5～10mg，病情常迅速缓解；若用纳洛酮静注，常可致病情加重。

点评

本病例患者发病前具有明确的吸毒史，并具有昏迷、呼吸抑制与瞳孔缩小等典型急性重度海洛因中毒表现，因此考虑阿片类药物（可能是海洛因）中毒的可能性大。急性海洛因中毒是严重危及生命的急症，及时、适量静注纳洛酮及有效人工呼吸，综合救治，积极改善呼吸，纠正低氧血症，大多数中毒者预后良好。

陈建国

❖ CASE 20

A 22-year-old woman is brought in the emergency department via ambulance because of a suicide attempt. Soon after a "night on the town," she called her boyfriend saying that she took a handful of sleeping tablets[注1]. On examination, she appears lethargic, but groans and moves all her extremities to painful stimuli. Her blood pressure is 110/70 mmHg, heart rate is 80 bpm, and oxygen saturation is 99 percent. Her pupils are of normal size and reactive to light. Her deep tendon reflexes[①] are normal bilaterally. In the field, she was given an intravenous bolus of dextrose and an ampule of naloxone[注2] without response. Her boyfriend, with whom she had an argument, brings in the bottle of sleeping medication which reads "lorazepam".

- **What is the danger of an overdose with this class of medication?**

- **What is the cellular mechanism of action of this class of medication?**

- **What pharmacological agent can be used to treat this patient, and what is its mechanism of action?**

ANSWERS TO CASE 20: Benzodiazepines

Summary: A 22-year-old woman is brought to the emergency department because of an suicide attempt overdose with lorazepam. She is hemodynamically stable, has no focal neurological deficits, but is lethargic. Intravenous dextrose and naloxone have been given without response.

- **Danger of an overdose with this class of medication**: Lorazepam is a benzodiazepine that belongs to a class of agents known as sedativehypnotics that can depress the activity of the central nervous system (CNS). An overdose of a benzodiazepine, particularly in the presence of another CNS depressant like alcohol, can lead to sedation, hypotension, respiratory depression, coma, and death.
- **Cellular mechanism of action of lorazepam**: Binds to a distinct benzodiazepine receptor site on the γ-aminobutyric acid (GABA) receptor-chloride channel complex to allosterically increase the affinity and frequency of GABA interactions with neuronal GABA-A receptors.
- **Pharmacological agent used to treat benzodiazepine overdose and its mechanism of action**: Flumazenil is a competitive antagonist at benzodiazepine receptors. It is used clinically to reverse the symptoms of benzodiazepine overdose.

CLINICAL CORRELATION

This 22-year-old woman ingested numerous tablets of lorazepam, a benzodiazepine, and exhibits the **classic signs of overdose: drowsiness**[2], **confusion**[3], **and amnesia**[4]. In general, an overdose of benzodiazepines is not fatal, which is a major advantage over previous classes of drugs used for their sedative-hypnotic[5] properties, such as the barbiturates. Symptoms of benzodiazepine overdose may include **drowsiness**, **confusion**, **amnesia**, **hypotension**, and, in the absence of compromised pulmonary function, **mild respiratory depression**. However, in the presence of other sedative-hypnotic agents like ethanol, which is suspected in this case, there may be **enhanced sedation** and respiratory depression that can result in **coma and even death**.

Benzodiazepines are drugs used to treat a variety of disorders including, most notably, anxiety (their sedative action) and insomnia (their hypnotic action), as well as status epilepticus and drug or toxin-induced seizures. They are also used clinically as muscle relaxants, as preanesthetic medications, and as amnestic agents for short medical and surgical procedures (Table 20-1).

Chronic use (weeks) of the benzodiazepines (BZ) can result in **tolerance**[6] (a decreased response with continued drug administration) and **physical dependence**[7] with an

Table 20-1
CLINICAL USES OF BENZODIAZEPINES

Anxiety disorders
Insomnia
Convulsive disorders
Acute status epilepticus
Amnestic (before surgery)
Spastic disorder or muscle spasm
Involuntary movement disorder (such as restless leg syndrome)
Detoxification from alcohol
Other psychiatric conditions (e.g., acute mania, impulse control disorders)
Other uses (e.g., surgery, imaging studies, endoscopy, chemotherapy)

identifiable **withdrawal syndrome**⑧ that includes **severe anxiety and insomnia** and less frequently, as seen with alcohol **withdrawal**, **tremulousness**, **tachycardia**, **hypertension**, **hallucinations**, **and seizures** that **can be life-threatening.** Withdrawal from shorter-acting and intermediate-acting BZ occurs more quickly and is more severe than from longer-acting drugs, and is usually managed with tapered dose reduction⑨ of the drug. Alternatively, because of the phenomenon of cross-tolerance⑩, benzodiazepines with longer half-lives (e.g., diazepam) can be substituted for shorter-acting benzodi-azepines or other sedative-hypnotic drugs, like ethanol and the barbiturates, to stabilize the patient and to reduce the severity of the withdrawal syndrome.

Flumazenil, **a competitive inhibitor at benzodiazepine receptors**, will quickly reverse the effects of the benzodiazepines. In dependent individuals it can induce symptoms of withdrawal. It is used to treat significant CNS depression because of benzodiazepine overdose such as in this clinical case.

Mechanism of Action

Like the barbiturates (another class of sedative-hypnotic agents), the benzodiazepines bind to the **GABA-A receptor-chloride channel complex** (Fig. 20-1). However, unlike the barbiturates, which increase the *duration* of GABA-mediated chloride channel opening, the benzodiazepines, which bind to a different site, increase the affinity of the complex for GABA and the *frequency* of GABA-stimulated chloride channel opening. This results in **increased chloride conductance with cell hyperpolarization**. Because GABA is the principal inhibitory neurotransmitters of the brain, its increased action, facilitated by a benzodiazepine, will lead to a reduced neuronal stimulation by excitatory neu-rotransmitters. The outcome, among others, is sedation and hypnosis.

Flumazenil competitively inhibits the action of benzodiazepines at their receptors on the GABA receptor-chloride channel complex.

Pharmacokinetics

Benzodiazepines are well absorbed from the gastrointestinal tract, although clorazepate, a prodrug⑪, is first decarboxylated in gastric juice to the long-acting(>50 hr) **active metabolite**⑫ **N-desmethyldiazepam**. Because the lipid solubility⑬ of the benzodiazepines varies more than 50-fold, there is considerable variation in their onset of action(diazepam and triazolam > chlordiazepoxide and lorazepam). The **most highly lipid soluble benzodiazepines have a short duration of action** after a low *single dose* because of their rapid redistribution from brain to peripheral tissues(e. g. , flurazepam, diazepam, triazolam). However, under most circumstances, the duration of action of the benzodiazepines(Table 20-2) is related to their biotransformation by:

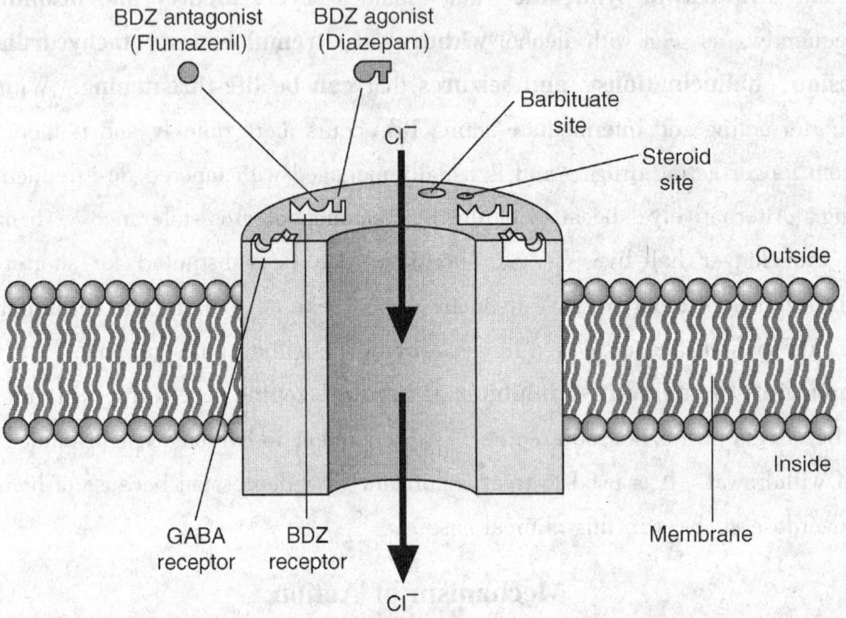

Figure 20-1. Chloride channel showing benzodiazepine receptor on cell membrane. From Case Files: Psychiatry, with permission.

Dealkylation to the long acting(>50 hr) active metabolites desmethyldiazepam(e. g. , diazepam, chlordiazepoxide) or desalkylflurazepam(flurazepam).

Oxidation to short-intermediate acting metabolites(alprazolam, triazolam).

Rapid conjugation to metabolites with no intrinsic activity (e. g. , oxazepam, lorazepam).

Clearance of the benzodiazepines is **decreased significantly in the elderly**, or in patients with **liver disease**. Thus these populations should, in general, be administered reduced dosages. **Elderly patients** may also be susceptible to **paradoxical agita-**

tion[14] and insomnia[15]. The benzodiazepines should be **avoided in pregnancy**, because **neonates may develop withdrawal symptoms.**

Table 20-2

SELECTIVE BENZODIAZEPINES

BENZODIAZEPINE	ONSET OF ACTION	HALF-LIFE OF PARENT (hours)	HALF-LIFE OF METABOLITE (hours)	COMPARATIVE ORAL DOSE
Short Acting				
Midazolam (Versed)	Rapid IV	0. 5-1	Inactive	None
Trazolam (Halcion)	Intermediate	1-4	Inactive	0. 5 mg
Intermediate Acting				
Alprazolam (Xanax)	Intermediate	6-20	Inactive	0. 5 mg
Clonazepam (Klonopin)	Intermediate	20-40	Inactive	0. 25 mg
Lorazepam	Intermediate (po) Rapid (IV)	10-20	Inactive	1 mg
Oxazepam (Serax)	Slow	10-20	Inactive	15 mg
Temazepam (Restoril)	Slow	10-20	Inactive	30 mg
Long Acting				
Chlordiazepoxide (Librium)	Intermediate(po)	5-30	3-100	10 mg
Diazepam (Valium)	Rapid (po,IV)	20-50	3-100	5 mg
Flurazepam (Dalmane)	Rapid	Inactive	50-100	30 mg

Source: Bosse GM. Benzodiazepines. In: Tintinalli JE, Kelen GD, Stapczynski JS, eds. Emergency Medicine. New York: McGraw-Hill; 2004: 1005-1057.

Comprehension Questions

[20. 1] An 18-year-old male is having difficulty sleeping because of the death of his grandfather. He is given a benzodiazepine that

A. Binds to serotonin 5-HT_1 receptors

B. Binds to GABA-A receptors

C. Is an antagonist at α-adrenoceptors

D. Is an antagonist at dopamine D_2-receptors

[20. 2] A 22-year-old woman is diagnosed with a generalized anxiety disorder. Which of the following is a contraindication for the use of a benzodiazepine to treat this patient?

A. Cigarette smoking

B. Seizure disorder

C. Diabetes mellitus

D. Sleep apnea

[20. 3] A 35-year-old man complains of seeing giant spiders in the hospital room. He is tremulous and agitated, hypertensive, and admits to heavy alcohol use at home. Which of the following actions of the benzodiazepines is the main rationale for their use to manage this patient?

A. Vasodilation

B. Hypnosis

C. Cross-tolerance with alcohol

D. Elevation of mood

[20. 4] An 18-year-old man is brought into the emergency department with a seizure that has lasted 15 minutes without resolution. After administering oxygen, which pharmacologic agent is most appropriate to arrest the seizure?

A. Lidocaine

B. Lorazepam

C. Chlordiazepoxide

D. Triazolam

Answers

[20. 1] **B**. Benzodiazepines bind to GABA-A receptors to increase chloride influx and to decrease stimulation of neurons by excitatory neurotransmitters.

[20. 2] **D**. Sleep apnea is a condition of relaxed soft tissue of the posterior pharynx, which occludes the airway during sleep. Family members usually note loud snoring and episodes of apnea of affected individuals. Sedatives, alcohol, and muscle relaxants are contraindicated in these patients, because severe apnea and death may ensue.

[20. 3] **C**. Because there is cross-tolerance between them (they both interact with the GABA-A receptor), a long-acting benzodiazepine can be used to ameliorate the symptoms associated with alcohol withdrawal.

[20. 4] **B**. A short-acting benzodiazepine such as lorazepam is usually the best choice in the acute setting to arrest status epilepticus. Triazolam is used as a hypnotic agent.

PHARMACOLOGY PEARLS

- ❖ Benzodiazepines bind to the GABA-A receptor, increasing chloride influx, rendering the cell less excitable. Because alcohol and barbiturates also bind to the GABA-A receptor complex, there is cross-tolerance among these agents.
- ❖ Benzodiazepine overdose causes sedation, hypotension, and respiratory depression. Alcohol and barbiturates can potentiate these effects and also lead to coma and death.
- ❖ Acute benzodiazepine withdrawal can cause tremor, anxiety, tachycardia, hallucinations, and life-threatening seizures.
- ❖ Flumazenil is a competitive inhibitor of benzodiazepines and will quickly reverse its effects, sometimes inducing withdrawal symptoms.

REFERENCES

Longo LP, Johnson B. Addiction: Part I. Benzodiazepines-side effects, abuse risk and alternatives. Am Fam Physician 2000; 61(8): 2121-8.

Maczaj M. Pharmacological treatment of insomnia. Drugs 1993; 45(1): 44-55.

Ninan PT. New insights into the diagnosis and pharmacological management of generalized anxiety disorder. Psychopharmacol Bull, 2002; 36(2): 105-22.

词汇

1. deep tendon reflexes[深部腱反射]
2. drowsiness[困倦]
3. confusion[意识错乱]
4. amnesia[健忘]
5. sedative-hypnotic[镇静催眠药]
6. tolerance[耐受性]
7. physical dependence[生理依赖性]
8. withdrawal syndrome[戒断综合征]
9. tapered dose reduction[药量递减]
10. cross-tolerance[交叉耐受性]
11. prodrug[前体药物]
12. active metabolite[活性代谢物]
13. lipid solubility[脂溶性]
14. paradoxical agitation[反常的情绪激动]
15. insomnia[失眠]

注 1

镇静催眠药应用首先，应详细询问失眠原因，根据不同症状对症治疗，切忌盲目使用镇静催眠药物。躯体疾病影响睡眠者应首先治疗原发病；有精神因素者以心理治疗为主，并合理应用抗焦虑的苯二氮䓬类药物。如拟使用，应以短程为宜，待失眠原因解除后尽快停药。一般以单一用药治疗为主，应试用 2～3 天，无效后再考虑加量或换药。剂量和用法应以临床需要为准，最理想的是入睡时间缩短、睡眠较深、晨醒后药物作用消失。但催眠药过量可引起全身麻醉，更大剂量可引起呼吸和心血管运动中枢抑制进而导致昏迷，甚至死亡。

注 2

纳洛酮为阿片受体拮抗剂，对四种阿片受体亚型（μ-受体、δ-受体、κ-受体、б-受体）均有拮抗作用。对吗啡中毒者，小剂量(0.4～0.8mg)肌内或静脉注射，可迅速翻转吗啡的作用，1～3 分钟就可消除吗啡中毒引起的呼吸抑制、镇静、瞳孔缩小以及严重中毒引起的血压降低、昏迷等作用。对吗啡成瘾者可迅速诱发戒断综合征。纳洛酮还有抗休克作用，对抗休克时内啡肽的作用。对动物酒精中毒有促醒作用。

点评

本病例患者有自杀倾向，并服用大量催眠药，体检发现患者嗜睡，但对外界刺激有反应，血压、心率和氧饱和度正常，瞳孔大小和对光反射正常，深部腱反射对称，因此考虑该患者无明显器质性病变，催眠药过量的可能性较大。给予纳洛酮无效，因此考虑患者未服用吗啡类药物。后其男友证明该患者服用苯二氮䓬类药物劳拉西泮，因此除对症治疗外，可采用苯二氮䓬类受体拮抗药氟马西尼解救。

陈建国

❖ CASE 21

A 30-year-old woman presents to the office for treatment of an ingrown toenail①. For the past 3 weeks she has had progressively worsening redness, swelling, and pain from the area around the right great toenail. On examination you find that the distal, medial corner of the right great toenail is ingrown. The skin on the medial border or the nail is red and tender. There is a visible purulent drainage as well. You place her on a 1-week course of oral cephalexin[注1] and have her return to the office. On follow-up, the redness is markedly improved, and there is no further drainage. You surgically correct the ingrown toenail after achieving local anesthesia② with 2 percent lidocaine[注2] injected to infiltrate the digital nerves.

◆ **What is the mechanism of action of lidocaine as an anesthetic agent?**

◆ **Why does the treatment of infection increase the effectiveness of the local anesthetic?**

ANSWERS TO CASE 21: Local Anesthetics

Summary: A 30-year-old woman with an infected, ingrown toenail receives lidocaine as a local anesthetic.

- **Mechanism of action of lidocaine**: Time- and voltage-dependent blockade of the inactivated state of sodium channels on the inner axon membrane, which results in an increased refractory period and threshold for sensory nerve excitation.

- **Reason for treating infection prior to use of local anesthetic**: Infection and inflammation lower tissue pH, reducing the diffusion of the agent into the nerve, thus reducing its effectiveness.

CLINICAL CORRELATION

Local anesthetics produce a transient loss of sensation in a defined region of the body without producing a loss of consciousness. They may be used topically, for infiltration, for field block, for intravenous regional block, for nerve block, and for spinal and epidural anesthesia. Lidocaine and related local anesthetics work by inactivating Na^+ channels on axonal membranes, raising the threshold for axonal excitation. Nerves that carry pain and temperature signals are blocked before nerves that perform proprioception or motor functions. Some local anesthetics are effective topically, but most require injection into tissue, around nerves or into the subarachnoid or epidural space to be effective. Most local anesthetics are weak bases, and at physiologic pH, therefore, a greater proportion will be in their cationic charged form, which is thought to be the active form at their site of action. However, it is the uncharged form that is important for penetration of local anesthetics into biological membranes. When tissue pH is lowered by infection or inflammation, more of the anesthetic is in the cationic form. This reduces its diffusion into the nerve and can reduce its anesthetic effect. Lidocaine and related anesthetics are vasodilators[③]. Local anesthetics are frequently coadministered with dilute solutions of epinephrine, which produces vasoconstriction. This slows the absorption of the anesthetic, which prolongs its effect and lowers the risk of systemic toxicity. Epinephrine administration is contraindicated in areas supplied by end arteries, such as the digits, the tip of the nose, and the penis, as vasoconstriction of end arteries may result in tissue ischemia and necrosis.

Pharmacology of Local Anesthetics

Objectives

1. List the drugs used for local anesthesia.

2. Describe the metabolism, adverse effects, and toxicities of local anesthetics.

Discussion of Class

Depending on their structure, local anesthetics are classified as either **esters or amides** (Table 21-1). The choice of local anesthetic depends on the specific procedure and is usually based on the **desired duration of action** which may be **short** (procaine and chloroprocaine), **intermediate** (mepivacaine, lidocaine, prilocaine), or **long** (bupivacaine, etidocaine, ropivacaine, tetracaine). **Cocaine**, which has its own inherent vasoconstrictor④ properties, is used primarily for topical local anesthesia of the nose and throat.

Application of **very high levels of local anesthetics**, particularly lidocaine, may result in a **neurotoxicity**⑤ referred to as transient radicular irrigation. High systemic local anesthetic levels, usually from **accidental intravascular injection, may result in central nervous system (CNS) effects** that may include symptoms ranging from lightheadedness⑥ and visual disturbances⑦ to **nystagmus**⑧ and **muscle twitching**⑨ to tonic-clonic **seizures**⑩, **respiratory depression**, **and death.** Unlike other local anesthetics that may produce hypotension and decreased cardiac conduction, and in rare instances cardiovascular collapse, cocaine overdose produces vasoconstriction and hypertension and may result in cardiac arrhythmias. Bupivacaine, like cocaine, is also notable for being more cardiotoxic than other local anesthetics. **Ester-type local anesthetics** are metabolized to para-aminobenzoic acid derivatives and may result **in allergic reactions**⑪ in some patients.

Structure

Local anesthetics generally consist of some ionizable group connected through either an ester or an amide to a lipophilic group.

Table 21-1

LOCAL ANESTETHICS (route)

ESTERS	AMIDES
Cocaine[t]	Bupivacaine[p]
Benzocaine[t]	Lidocaine[p]
Procaine[p]	Mepivacaine[p]
Tetracaine[p,t]	Prilocaine[p]
	Ropivacaine[p]

p = parenteral, t = topical

Administration

Depending on the drug, local anesthetics may be administered by the parenteral route and topically.

The extent of systemic absorption of injected local anesthetics from the site of administration, and therefore the duration of their action, is modified by a number of factors. Vasoconstrictor agents like epinephrine are used to decrease local blood flow and thus extend the duration of anesthetic action, and reduce the toxicity, of such local anesthetics as lidocaine, procaine, and mepivacaine. In spinal analgesia, clonidine can also be used concomitantly with local anesthetics to enhance the activation by epinephrine of α_2-adrenoceptors, which reduces sensory nerve firing by inhibition of the release of substance P.

Pharmacokinetics

Ester-type local anesthetics[12] **are metabolized rapidly** by **nonspecific plasma cholinesterases**[13] and, generally, have **shorter half-lives** than amide-type local anesthetics.

Amide-type local anesthetics[14] are metabolized at various rates by **hepatic microsomal enzymes**[15]. In severe liver disease, toxicity is more likely. Likewise, metabolism may be slowed when amide-type local anesthetics are used with other drugs metabolized by the same enzymes.

Comprehension Questions

[21.1] Local anesthetic action is a result of blockade of the movement of which of the following ion channels?

A. Calcium
B. Chloride
C. Potassium
D. Sodium

[21.2] An allergic reaction is most likely to occur with which of the following local anesthetics?

A. Bupivacaine
B. Lidocaine
C. Mepivacaine
D. Procaine

[21.3] Which of the following agents is often combined with local anesthetics to prevent its systemic distribution from the site of injection?

A. Acetylcholine
B. Dopamine
C. Epinephrine
D. γ-aminobutyric acid (GABA)

Answers

[21.1] **D.** Local anesthetic action is a result of prevention of sodium movement caused by blockade of the inactivated state of neuronal sodium channels.

[21.2] **D**. An allergic reaction is most likely to occur with ester-type local anesthetics like procaine because of the metabolic formation of the allergen, para-aminobenzoic acid.

[21.3] **C**. Local anesthetics are often combined with the vasoconstrictor epinephrine to prevent their distribution from the site of injection and thus extend their duration of action and reduce their systemic toxicity.

PHARMACOLOGY PEARLS

- Use of a carbon dioxide saturated local anesthetic solution ("carbonation") to increase acidity can accelerate onset of anesthetic action.
- Ester-type local anesthetics are metabolized rapidly by nonspecific plasma cholinesterases and generally have shorter half-lives than amide-type local anesthetics.
- High systemic local anesthetic levels, usually from accidental intravascular injection, may result in CNS effects, tonic-clonic seizures, respiratory depression, and death.

REFERENCES

Butterworth JF, Strichartz GR. Molecular mechanisms of local anesthesia: a review. Anesthesiology 1990; 72(4): 711-34.

Smith C. Pharmacology of local anesthetic agents. Br J Hosp Med 1994; 52(9): 455-60.

Stoelting RK. Local anesthetics. In: Pharmacology and physiology in anesthetic practice, 3rd ed. New York: Lippincott-Raven, 1999.

词汇

1. ingrown toenail[嵌甲]
2. local anesthesia[局部麻醉]
3. vasodilator[血管扩张药]
4. vasoconstrictor[血管收缩药]
5. neurotoxicity[神经毒性]
6. light-headedness[头晕目眩]
7. visual disturbances[视觉障碍]
8. nystagmus[眼球震颤]
9. muscle twitching[肌肉颤搐]
10. tonic-clonic seizures[强直阵挛发作]
11. allergic reactions[过敏反应]
12. ester-type local anesthetics[酯类局部麻醉药]
13. cholinesterase[胆碱酯酶]
14. amide-type local anesthetics[酰胺类局部麻醉药]
15. hepatic microsomal enzymes[肝微粒体酶]

注 1

头孢氨苄属第一代头孢菌素，除肠球菌属、甲氧西林耐药葡萄球菌外，肺炎链球菌、溶血性链球菌、产或不产青霉素酶葡萄球菌的大部分菌株对本品敏感。本品对奈瑟菌属有较好抗菌作用，但流感嗜血杆菌对本品的敏感性较差；本品对部分大肠埃希菌、奇异变形杆菌、沙门菌和志贺菌有一定抗菌作用。其余肠杆菌科细菌、不动杆菌、铜绿假单胞菌、脆弱拟杆菌均对本品呈现耐药。适用于敏感菌所致的急性扁桃体炎、咽峡炎、中耳炎、鼻窦炎、支气管炎、肺炎等呼吸道感染、尿路感染及皮肤软组织感染等。本品为口服制剂，不宜用于重症感染。

注 2

利多卡因主要用于口咽和气管内表面麻醉；硬膜外阻滞或臂丛、颈丛神经阻滞和抗室性心律失常。口咽和气管内表面麻醉用 2%～4% 溶液。硬膜外阻滞或臂丛神经阻滞用 1%～2% 溶液，成人一次最大用量 400 mg。本品吸收快，易发生毒性反应，故应用中勿误入血管。加入 1/20 万肾上腺素作神经阻滞可减少毒性作用发生率，延长作用时效。

点评

本病例患者具有典型的嵌甲病史，右脚趾周围出现严重的红、肿、热、痛，并出现甲下脓肿，因此考虑嵌甲合并感染。一旦发生嵌甲感染，轻者局部涂抹碘酒或新洁尔灭湿敷浸泡，并应用抗生素控制感染，重者红肿疼痛剧烈伴化脓，除加强抗感染外，必要时作局部切开引流，以减压缓解疼痛，引流通畅使炎症消退。待感染控制后采用 2% 利多卡因自拇指根部行神经阻滞麻醉后，施行嵌甲矫形术，从根本上解决甲片卷曲生长的问题。

陈建国

❖ CASE 22

A 35-year-old man is in the surgical holding area being evaluated prior to a scheduled hernia① repair. He asks the anesthesiologist about the type of "anesthetic gas"[注1] to be used, because he recalls that his mother developed severe liver problems from general anesthesia for a hysterectomy② performed 2 years previously. The patient asks whether nitrous oxide③[注2] might be used, because he has heard that it was a safe agent. To allay the patient's anxiety, the anesthesiologist proposes spinal anesthetic for the surgery.

◆ **What is the probable general anesthetic agent used for the patient's mother?**

◆ **What is the disadvantage of nitrous oxide as an inhalation anesthetic agent?**

ANSWERS TO CASE 22: Inhalation Anesthetic Agents

Summary: A 35-year-old man is in the surgical holding area being evaluated prior to a scheduled hernia repair. The patients' mother developed severe liver problems from general anesthesia. The patient asks whether nitrous oxide might be used.

- **Probable inhalation anesthetic agent[4] used for the patient's mother**: A halogenated agent, such as halothane.
- **Disadvantage of nitrous oxide as an inhalation anesthetic agent**: Lack of anesthetic potency requires large amounts to be used as a single agent, associated with postoperative nausea and vomiting.

CLINICAL CORRELATION

Patients such as the one described in the case are often nervous about "being put to sleep" because of fear about not having sufficient anesthesia and feeling pain, or about "never waking up". However, this is highly unlikely because the expertise in the field of anesthesia and the knowledge of the anesthetic agents is better today than ever before. This patient relates a story of how his mother developed severe liver problems as a result of a general anesthetic agent[5]. Halothane-related mild type I hepatotoxicity is benign, self-limiting, and relatively common, affecting up to 25 percent of individuals, and is characterized by mild, transient increases in serum transaminase and by altered postoperative drug metabolism. However, halothane-related type II hepatotoxicity is associated with massive centrilobular liver cell necrosis often leading to fulminant liver failure. The patient clinically has fever, jaundice, and a grossly elevated serum transaminase level that is probably immune mediated. Approximately 20 percent of halothane is oxidatively metabolized compared to only 2 percent of enflurane and 0.2 percent of isoflurane. Halothane-induced hepatotoxicity may result from the anaerobic formation of reductive reactive intermediates during halothane metabolism, including trifluoroacetic acid(TFA), that cause direct liver damage or initiate an immune response in genetically predisposed individuals. The occurrence of type II hepatotoxicity after enflurane or isoflurane administration is extremely rare, approximately 1 in 35,000 individuals.

Pharmacology of Inhalation Anesthetic Agents

Objectives

1. List the characteristics of the ideal general anesthetic agent.
2. Describe the pharmacokinetic parameters of inhalation anesthetics that influence the onset of and recovery from anesthesia.

3. List the advantages and disadvantages of the commonly used inhalation anesthetic agents.
4. List the commonly used intravenously administered anesthetic agents and adjunct agents used in a "balanced anesthesia".

Definitions

Minimum alveolar concentration (MAC)[⑥]: Anesthetic dose of an inhalation anesthetic agent at 1 atmosphere, expressed in terms of alveolar tension (mmHg), which produces immobility in 50 percent of individuals exposed to a noxious stimulus, such as a standardized skin incision.

Blood-gas partition coefficient[⑦]: The solubility of an inhalation anesthetics in blood relative to air at 37℃ (98.6℉).

Second gas effect[⑧]: The rate of rise of alveolar tension and inflow of an inhalation anesthetic gas can be increased in the presence of high concentrations another anesthetic gas, usually nitrous oxide.

Discussion of Class

Inhalation anesthetics, as the name implies, are administered via the pulmonary route, often by assisted ventilation. The **ideal anesthetic agent** should be able to induce **unconsciousness**, **analgesia**[⑨], **amnesia**[⑩], **skeletal muscle relaxation**, and **inhibition of autonomic and sensory reflexes**. However, in practice, a combination of drugs ("balanced anesthesia"), including anesthetic agents that are administered intravenously, is used to provide a more satisfactory anesthesia than is possible with any one anesthetic agent alone, and to minimize their individual adverse effects (Table 22-1).

The **minimum alveolar concentration, or MAC**, of an inhalation anesthetic that is necessary to achieve effective anesthetic concentrations is usually expressed as the mole fraction of the gas.

Mole fraction equals partial pressure of anesthetic agent as percentage of total gas pressure (760 mmHg). For example,

$$\text{Halothane's MAC} = 5.7\ \text{mmHg}/760\ \text{mmHg} \times 100 = 0.75\%$$

MAC is an indicator of anesthetic potency, the **lower the MAC** the **more potent** is the agent (Table 22-2). It is used only as a guide. For example, the anesthesiologist might use either multiples of an inhalation anesthetic agent's MAC or a fraction of an inhalation anesthetic agent's MAC to achieve clinical anesthesia depending on whether or not the agent is used alone (rare for volatile anesthetics), in combination, and with other intravenously administered anesthetic agents or preanesthetic agents (Table 22-3).

Most halogenated inhaled anesthetic agents reduce peripheral vascular resistance

with the possibility of reflex tachycardia. Halothane is a notable exception in that it has both vascular constrictor and relaxation activity and blocks reflex sympathetic stimulation of the heart. However, it does sensitize the heart to catecholamine-induced arrhythmias⑪.

Table 22-1

ADVANTAGES AND ADVERSE EFFECTS OF INHALATION ANESTHETIC AGENTS

ANESTHETIC AGENTS[1]	ADVANTAGES	ADVERSE EFFECTS
Nitrous Oxide (N_2O; for minor surgery, used with volatile or intravenous anethetics)	Odorless Rapid induction Minimal cardiovascular effects	Postoperative nausea and vomiting Synergistic respiratory depression with other drugs (opioids, benzodiazepines)
Desflurane (used to maintain anesthesia after induction with another agent)	Very rapid recovery Cardiac output maintained Heart is not sensitized to catecholamines Minimal metabolism to toxic products	Objectionable odor Irritates respiratory tract Decreases blood pressure Tachycardia
Sevoflurane	Pleasant odor Very rapid induction and recovery	Decreases cardiac output Decreases blood pressure Reflex tachycardia
Enflurane	Pleasant odor	Decreases cardiac output Marked decrease in blood pressure Tachycardia Sensitized heart to catecholamine-induced arrhythmias Depresses neuromuscular transmission Can induce seizures
Isoflurane	Rapid induction and recovery Cardiac output maintained Heart is not sensitized to catecholamines Preserves tissue perfusion Very little metabolism to toxic products	Objectional odor Decreases blood pressure Transient tachycardia Depresses neuromuscular transmission

续表

ANESTHETIC AGENTS[1]	ADVANTAGES	ADVERSE EFFECTS
Halothane[2] (used primarily in pediatrics	Pleasant odor Rapid induction and recovery	Depresses respiratory function Decreases cardiac output and arteria Decreases blood pressure Sensitizes heart to catecholamine-induced arrhythmias Increases cerebral blood flow with increased intracranial pressure Toxic metabolites that may cause hepatotoxicity

[1] Although available for use, the inhalation anesthetic methoxyflurane is considered obsolete because of potential renal and nephrotoxicity.

[2] Use is declining.

Table 22-2

MAC VALUES(%)[1] AND BLOOD: GAS PARTITION COEFFICIENTS OF SELECTED INHALATION ANESTHETIC AGENTS

ANESTHETIC AGENT	MAC	PARTITION COEFFICIENT
Nitrous Oxide	>100.00[2]	0.47
Desflurane	6.00	0.42
Sevoflurane	2.00	0.69
Enflurane	1.70	1.80
Isoflurane	1.40	1.40
Halothane	0.75	2.30

[1] Expressed as a percentage of lung gases at 1 atmosphere.

[2] MAC values greater than 100 indicate that hyperbaric conditions are necessary to produce anesthesia. MAC = minimum alveolar concentration.

Table 22-3

SELECTED INTRAVENOUS ANESTHETIC AGENTS AND PRE-ANESTHETIC AGENTS

ANESTHETIC AGENTS	PREANESTHETIC AGENTS
Barbiturates (e. g., thiopental)	Sedative-hypnotics
Benzodiazepines (e. g., diazepam midazolam, lorazepam)	Opioids
	Muscle relaxants
Opioids (e. g., fentanyl, sulfentanil, alfentanyl, remisentanil)	Anticholinergic agens
	Local anesthetics
Ketamine	
Propofol	
Etomidate	

Malignant hyperthermia[12] is a **life-threatening, autosomal-dominant disorder** that develops during or after general anesthesia with volatile anesthetics and muscle relaxants(e. g. ,succinylcholine). It's incidence is 1:10,000. Symptoms include a rapidly occurring hypermetabolic state of **tachycardia**, **hypertension**, **severe muscle rigidity**, **hyperthermia**, **acidosis**, **and hyperkalemia.** The biochemical basis of malignant hyperthermia is compromised regulation of calcium flux with increased intracellular concentrations of calcium in skeletal muscle. Treatment includes dantrolene, which prevents release of calcium from the sarcoplasmic reticulum, and supportive measures such as procedures to reduce body temperature and restore electrolyte balance.

Structure

With the exception of nitrous oxide, the major inhalation anesthetic agents in current use today are **halogenated hydrocarbons**[13]. They are either gaseous(nitric oxide) with boiling points below room temperature, or volatile liquids that at room temperature vaporize to the extent necessary to achieve anesthetic concentrations.

Mechanism of Action

The mechanism of action of inhalation anesthetics is not well understood. Current theories suggest that anesthetics directly interact with proteins at hydrophobic sites on ligand-gated ion channels at neural synapses to inhibit the activity of excitatory receptors(e. g. , *N*-methyl D-aspartic acid[NMDA], nicotinic, serotonin 5-HT_3) or potentiate the activity of inhibitory receptors(e. g. ,GABA-A, glycine).

Pharmacokinetics

The concentration of an inhaled gas in the brain sufficient to achieve anesthesia depends on a number of factors, including the anesthetic agent's concentration in the inspired air, its **solubility** in blood relative to air, the **arteriovenous concentration gradient**, as well as **pulmonary blood flow and pulmonary ventilation rate**[14].

The concentration(as a percentage) of an inhaled anesthetic in the inspired air directly affects the rate of induction of anesthesia by influencing the rate of transfer of the agent into blood. In clinical practice, an inhaled anesthetic may be administered initially at a relatively high concentration to speed the rate of induction, following which the concentration in the inspired air would be reduced to a level that maintains the anesthetic state.

The solubility of an inhalation anesthetics in blood relative to air at 37℃(98.6°F), is described by their **blood: gas partition coefficients**[15] (see Table 22-2), is an important factor in determining the rate of rise of their arterial tension in the arterial blood, which influences directly their rate of equilibration with the brain and rate of onset of action. For anesthetic agents with low blood solubility the partial pressure, and therefore the arterial tension, rises relatively quickly. The partial pressure and arterial tension rise more slowly with anesthetic agents of moderate to high solubility.

The greater the difference in the arterial and venous anesthetic concentrations, which is a reflection of the uptake of an anesthetic agent by the tissues, particularly muscle, kidney, liver, and splanchnic bed (which in turn is a reflection of, among other factors, blood flow, and tissue solubility relative to blood), the more time it will take for an inhaled anesthetic agent to equilibrate with brain tissue and to induce surgical anesthesia.

Pulmonary blood flow also affects the rate of induction of anesthesia. Although counterintuitive, the higher the blood flow (and the higher the cardiac output), the slower the rate of rise of arterial tension, an effect that is most notable for inhaled anesthetics of moderate to high blood solubility. The opposite occurs with a decrease in blood flow, as might occur during shock.

An increase in **pulmonary ventilation rate** (i. e., minute ventilation), for example, by mechanical hyperventilation, increases anesthetic gas tension and the speed of induction, most notably for inhalation anesthetic agents with moderate to high blood solubility. Depression of unassisted respiration will have the opposite effect.

The **second gas effect** can also be taken advantage of to increase the rate of rise of alveolar tension of an inhalation anesthetic gas.

Following termination of its administration, recovery from anesthesia depends on the rate of elimination of an anesthetic agent from the brain, which can be influenced by pulmonary blood flow and pulmonary ventilation, and by the tissue solubility and the blood solubility of the anesthetic agent. Clearance by the lungs is the major route of elimination of inhalation anesthetic agents, with perhaps metabolism playing a contributing role for halothane.

Comprehension Questions

[22. 1] Which of the following is most important to quickly achieves a partial pressure of an inhalation anesthetic that is sufficient to induce anesthesia?

A. A decrease in pulmonary ventilation rate of an inhalation anesthetic agents of high blood solubility

B. Coadministration of dantrolene

C. Low blood and tissue solubility

D. Low MAC

[22. 2] An anesthesiologist administers an inhalation agent with a low MAC (minimum alveolar concentration). Which of the following is most likely to be correct regarding this agent?

A. It is likely to require high partial pressures to have an effect.

B. It is likely to lower oil-gas partition coefficient.

C. It is likely to be hydrophilic.

D. It is likely to have high potency.

[22.3] A 34-year-old woman is undergoing general anesthesia for a cholecystectomy. After the completion of the case, the anesthesiologist turns off the gas, and notes that the patient is recovering from the anesthetic agent very quickly. What are likely properties of this inhalation anesthetic?

A. Associated with decreased pulmonary circulation

B. Associated with an unpleasant odor

C. High MAC

D. High solubility

Answers

[22.1] **C.** The alveolar partial pressure of an inhalation anesthetic with low blood and tissue solubility will rise quickly. Under these conditions, blood and brain will equilibrate, and anesthesia will be induced, rather quickly. An inhalation anesthetic with a low MAC will equilibrate with brain tissue rather slowly. An increase, not decrease, in pulmonary ventilation rate will increases anesthetic gas tension and the speed of induction, particularly for inhalation anesthetic agents with moderate to high blood solubility. Dantrolene is not an anesthetic agent. It is used to counter the effects of malignant hyperthermia.

[22.2] **A.** An agent with a low MAC is highly potent, usually has a low oilgas partition coefficient, and high lipid solubility.

[22.3] **B.** Agents that have a rapid onset of action and rapid recovery have a low solubility. One such agent is desflurane, which has an unpleasant odor.

PHARMACOLOGY PEARLS

❖ Modern day inhalation anesthetic agents cause a rapid progression through the classical Guedel stages of anesthesia (analgesia, loss of consciousness, surgical anesthesia, and respiratory and cardiovascular depression).

❖ Although independent of gender and weight, MAC may be decreased (increased potency) with age, pregnancy hypothermia, and hypotension.

❖ MAC may increase (decreased potency) with central nervous system (CNS) stimulants.

REFERENCES

Campagna JA, Miller KW, Forman SA. Mechanisms of action of inhaled anesthetics. N Engl J Med 2003; 348(21): 2110-24.

Wiklund RA, Rosenbaum SH. Anesthesiology. N Engl J Med 1997; 337(16): 1132-41; 1215-9.

词汇

1. hernia[疝气]
2. hysterectomy[子宫切除术]
3. nitrous oxide[氧化亚氮]
4. inhalation anesthetic agent[吸入性麻醉药]
5. general anesthetic agent[全身麻醉药]
6. minimum alveolar concentration(MAC)[最低肺泡浓度]
7. blood-gas partition coefficient [血气分配系数]
8. second gas effect[第二气体效应]
9. analgesia[镇痛]
10. amnesia[记忆缺失]
11. catecholamine-induced arrhythmias[儿茶酚胺所致心律失常]
12. malignant hyperthermia[恶性高热]
13. halogenated hydrocarbons[卤代烃]
14. pulmonary ventilation rate[肺换气率]
15. blood: gas partition coefficient[血:气分配系数]

注 1

与静脉麻醉药相比，使用吸入麻醉药有两个优点：(1)能通过呼吸有效地调节血中麻醉药浓度(或分压)，特别是能迅速将吸入麻醉药从身体“洗出”；(2)通过测定呼气末浓度可估计吸入麻醉药在其作用部位(中枢神经系统)的浓度(分压)。

注 2

氧化亚氮(笑气)是一种毒性小的吸入性镇痛或麻醉气体，为无色、略带甜味的惰性无机气体，理化性质稳定，对呼吸道无刺激，在体内不经任何生物转化或降解，绝大部分仍以原药随呼气排出体外，仅小量由皮肤蒸发，无蓄积作用。通过抑制中枢神经系统兴奋性神经递质的释放和神经冲动的传导及改变离子通道的通透性而产生药理作用，其显著特点是镇痛作用强而麻醉作用弱。

点评

本病例患者母亲全麻行子宫切除术后，出现严重的肝损伤，考虑为吸入性麻醉药氟烷所致的肝损伤。氟烷引起肝损害的机制可能与中间代谢产物的毒性作用，细胞缺氧、脂质过氧化及免疫功能紊乱有关。氟烷麻醉术后不明原因的发热是一个警告信号，尤应注意。与氟烷同类的麻醉剂甲氧氟烷和氟甲氧氟烷也可引起这种肝损伤。氧化亚氮虽然不良反应少，但麻醉效能较低，主要用于诱导麻醉或与其他全身麻醉药配伍使用。为了减轻患者对全身麻醉的焦虑心理，因此将麻醉方法改为区域阻滞麻醉。

陈建国

❖ CASE 23

A 50-year-old salesman was admitted to the hospital with acute appendicitis[①]. He has no significant medical history, takes no medications, does not smoke cigarettes, and has an alcoholic beverage "once in a while with the boys". He underwent an uncomplicated appendectomy. On the second hospital day you find him to be quite agitated[②] and sweaty. His temperature, heart rate, and blood pressure are elevated. A short time later he has a grand-mal seizure[③]. You suspect that he is having withdrawal symptoms[注1] from chronic alcohol abuse[④] and give IV lorazepam[注2] for immediate control of the seizures and plan to start him on oral chlordiazepoxide when he is more stable.

◆ **What are the acute pharmacologic effects of ethanol?**

◆ **What are the chronic pharmacologic effects of ethanol?**

◆ **How is alcohol metabolized?**

◆ **What is the pharmacological basis of benzodiazepines lorazepam and chlordiazepoxide for the treatment of alcohol withdrawal?**

ANSWERS TO CASE 23: Drugs of Abuse

Summary: A 50-year-old man is displaying symptoms and signs of acute alcohol withdrawal.

- **Symptoms of acute ethanol toxicity**: Disinhibited behavior and judgment, slurred speech, impaired motor function, depressed and impaired mental function, respiratory depression, cutaneous vasodilation⑤, diuresis⑥, gastrointestinal side effects, and impaired myocardial contractility.
- **Symptoms of chronic ethanol toxicity**: Alcoholic fatty liver, alcoholic hepatitis, cirrhosis, liver failure, peripheral neuropathy, alcohol amnesic syndrome, pancreatitis, gastritis, fetal alcohol syndrome, nutritional deficiencies, cardiomyopathy, cerebellar degeneration.
- **Metabolism of alcohol**: Oxidized in the liver, stomach, and other organs to acetaldehyde by the cytosolic enzyme alcohol dehydrogenase⑦ (ADH) and by hepatic microsomal enzymes⑧; acetaldehyde is oxidized to acetate by hepatic mitochondrial aldehyde dehydrogenase.
- **Benzodiazepines in alcohol withdrawal⑨**: Both alcohol and benzodiazepines enhance the effect of γ-aminobutyric acid (GABA) on GABA-A neuroreceptors, resulting in decreased overall brain excitability. The cross-reactivity of benzodiazepines alleviates the alcohol withdrawal symptoms.

CLINICAL CORRELATION

Ethanol is the most widely used central nervous system (CNS) depressant. It is rapidly absorbed from the stomach and small intestine and distributed in total body water. Its exact mechanism of action is not known, but may be caused by its generally disruptive effects on cell membrane protein functions throughout the body, including effects on signaling pathways in the CNS. At low doses it is oxidized by cytoplasmic ADH. At higher doses it is also oxidized by liver microsomal enzymes, which may be induced by chronic use. These enzymes are rapidly saturated by the concentrations of alcohol achieved by even one or two alcoholic drinks, so its rate of metabolism is independent of plasma concentration. Tolerance to the intoxicating effects of alcohol can develop with chronic use. Cross-tolerance with barbiturates and benzodiazepines may also develop. Because of this cross-tolerance effect, benzodiazepines are the most commonly used agents for the treatment of alcohol withdrawal, a potentially life-threatening syndrome commonly seen 2-3 days after the abrupt cessation of alcohol use by a chronic abuser. A long-acting benzodiazepine can be taken, and gradually tapered, to mitigate this effect. Disulfiram is also used on occasion to manage alcoholism. It is a drug that inhibits aldehyde dehydrogenase that in the presence of alcohol causes an accumulation of acetaldehyde, which results in a highly aversive reaction⑩ consisting of flushing, severe headache, nausea and vomiting, and confusion. Naltrexone, an opioid antagonist, is yet another drug used to manage alcoholism.

Pharmacology of Ethanol

Objectives

1. Define drug abuse, drug tolerance, drug dependence, and drug addiction.
2. List the common drugs of abuse and their properties.
3. List the adverse effects of the common drugs of abuse.

Definitions

Drug abuse⑪: Nonmedical use of a drug taken to alter consciousness or to change body image that is often regarded as unacceptable by society. Not to be confused with drug misuse.

Drug tolerance⑫: Decreased response to a drug with its continued administration that can be overcome by increasing the dose. A cellular tolerance develops to certain drugs of abuse that act on the CNS because of a poorly understood biochemical or homeostatic adaptation of neurons to the continued presence of the drug. Also, in addition to a cellular tolerance, a metabolic tolerance can develop to the effects of some drugs because they increase the synthesis of enzymes responsible for their own metabolism (alcohol, barbiturates).

Drug dependence⑬: Continued need of the user to take a drug. Psychological dependence⑭ is the compulsive behavior of a user to continue to use a drug no matter the personal or medical consequences. Inability to obtain the drug activates a "craving" that is very discomforting. Physical or physiological dependence⑮ is a consequence of continued drug use and following drug abstinence results in a constellation of signs and symptoms that are often opposite to the initial effects of the drug and to those sought by the user. Psychological dependence generally precedes physical dependence but, depending on the drug, does not necessarily lead to it. The development of physical dependence, the degree of which varies considerably for different drugs of abuse, is always associated with the development of tolerance, although the exact relationship is unclear.

Drug addiction⑯: A poorly defined, imprecise term with little clinical significance that indicates the presence of psychological and physical dependence.

Discussion of Class

In addition to alcohol, the major drugs of abuse are nicotine, marijuana(Δ9-tetrahydrocannabinol), heroin, and the CNS stimulants, notably cocaine and amphetamine and its derivatives(Table 23-1).

Table 23-1

DRUGS OF ABUSE

	NICOTINE	MARIJUANA	COCAINE/ AMPHETAMINE
Route of administration	Smoking.	Smoking.	Smoking, oral IV.
Mechanism of action	Mimics action of acetylcholine.	Interacts with G-protein coupled cannabinoid receptors among other actions.	Cocaine binds the dopamine reuptake transporter. Amphetamine increases release of neuronal catecholamines, including dopamine.
Pharmacological effects	Stimulant and depressant actions on the CNS and cardiovascular system.	Euphoria uncontrollable laughter, introspection, loss of sense of time sleepiness, loss of concentration.	Euphoria, excitation, increased alterness an orgasmic-like "rush".
Tolerance and dependence	Tolerance develops rapidly. Strong psychological dependence. Withdrawal syndrome indicative of physical dependence.	Arguably, some tolerance and very mild physical dependence.	Rapid development of tolerance. Withdrawal syndrome characterized by increased appetite, depression, and exhaustion.
Therapeutic uses	None.	Nausea and vomiting of cancer. Appetite stimulation in AIDS (dronabinol).	Local anesthesia (cocaine). ADHD (methylphenidate). Narcolepsy (modafinil).

续表

	NICOTINE	MARIJUANA	COCAINE/ AMPHETAMINE
Adverse effects	Cancer, obstructive lung disease, cardiovascular disease.	Bronchitis, increased pulse rate, reddening of conjunctiva.	Paranoid schizophrenia. Amphetamine-specific necrotizing arteritis. Cocaine-related arrhythmias, seizures, respiratory depression, hypertension, stroke, increased fetal mortality, and abnormalities.
Treatment of abuse	Nicotine gum and transdermal patch.	Behavioral modification.	Antipsychotic agents. Antidepressant agents.

Comprehension Questions

[23.1] Alcohol is oxidized by

A. Acetate oxidase
B. Alcohol dehydrogenase
C. Aldehyde dehydrogenase
D. Monoamine oxidase

[23.2] Which of the following is most commonly found in an individual with chronic ethanol toxicity?

A. Cirrhosis
B. Cutaneous vasodilation
C. Disinhibited judgment
D. Respiratory depression

[23.3] A drug of abuse that binds the dopamine reuptake transporter is

A. Alcohol
B. Cocaine
C. Marijuana
D. Nicotine

Answers

[23.1] **B**. Alcohol is oxidized in the liver, stomach and other organs to acetaldehyde by the cytosolic enzyme alcohol dehydrogenase (ADH) and the hepatic microsomal enzymes. Acetaldehyde is oxidized to acetate by mitochondrial hepatic aldehyde dehydrogenase.

[23.2] **A.** Liver cirrhosis is an effect of chronic alcohol use. Disinhibited judgment, respiratory depression and cutaneous vasodilation are acute effects of alcohol.

[23.3] **B.** Cocaine is a drug of abuse that binds the dopamine reuptake transporter.

Ethanol may nonspecifically disrupt cell membrane protein functions. Marijuana interacts with G-protein coupled cannabinoid receptors. Nicotine mimics the action of acetylcholine.

REFERENCES

Cami J, Farre M. Mechanisms of disease: Drug addiction. N Engl J Med 2003; 349(10): 975-86.

Lieber CS. Medical disorders of alcoholism. N Engl J Med 1995; 333(16): 1058-65.

Swift RM. Drug therapy for alcohol dependence. N Engl J Med 1999; 340(19): 1482-90.

词汇

1. acute appendicitis[急性阑尾炎]
2. agitated[激动的]
3. grand-mal seizure[癫痫大发作]
4. alcohol abuse[酒精滥用]
5. cutaneous vasodilation[皮肤血管扩张]
6. diuresis[利尿]
7. alcohol dehydrogenase[乙醇脱氢酶]
8. hepatic microsomal enzymes[肝微粒体酶]
9. alcohol withdrawal[戒酒]
10. aversive reaction[厌恶反应]
11. drug abuse[药物滥用]
12. drug tolerance[药物耐受性]
13. drug dependence[药物依赖性]
14. psychological dependence[精神依赖性]
15. physiological dependence[生理依赖性]
16. drug addiction[药物成瘾性]

注 1

酒精戒断症状是指一周以上连续多量饮酒之后，急剧地减少或中断 5 ~ 10 小时以上而出现一系列的临床综合征。包括自律神经系统的亢进(出汗、脉速、发热)、手指颤抖、睡眠障碍、恶心呕吐、一过性幻视、幻听、运动亢进、精神不安、癫痫大发作等。戒断症状的出现是因为具有神经系统抑制作用的酒精减少(或缺乏)而诱发，在治疗时选择在药理学上与酒精具有交叉耐药性，而且半衰期比酒精长的药物来缓和其缺乏而发生的一系列病理生理学反应。从这个目的出发可选择的镇静药有很多种，但在安全性方面考虑苯环类药物比较好，如苯二氮䓬类。该药在开始使用即可明显地抑制戒断期的癫痫发作及震颤谵妄等作用。

注 2

劳拉西泮作用与地西泮相似，但抗焦虑作用较地西泮强，诱导入睡作用明显。口服用于治疗焦虑症和失眠，治疗癫痫持续状态必须采取肌内或静脉注射。

点评

本病例为一中年患者，有饮酒史，无吸烟史，无脑炎及脑外伤等病史，无神经局灶病变体征，而术后第二天表现出癫痫大发作，因此考虑患者在对酒精高度耐受的基础上，突然戒酒所引起的精神症状，主要表现为癫痫发作，治疗首选苯二氮䓬类药物来控制症状，对于酒精中毒所致的精神障碍，给予中、小剂量的抗精神病药物治疗，同时给予配合躯体支持治疗以及心理治疗。

陈建国

❖ CASE 24

An 8-year-old girl is brought in by her mother for evaluation[①] of allergies[②]. Each year in the spring the child develops a runny[③] nose; itchy[④], watery[⑤] eyes; and sneezing[⑥]. She has been treated in the past with diphenhydramine,[注1] but the child's teacher says that she is very drowsy during school. She has no other medical problems and is on no chronic medications. Her examination is unremarkable today. You diagnose her with seasonal allergic rhinitis[注2] and prescribe fexofenadine.[注3]

◆ **What is the mechanism of action of antihistamine medications?**

◆ **What are the common side effects of antihistamine medications?**

◆ **What is the pharmacological basis of switching to fexofenadine?**

ANSWERS TO CASE 24: Antihistamines⑦

Summary: An 8-year-old girl with seasonal allergic rhinitis is switched to fexofenadine because of the sedation caused by diphenhydramine.

- **Mechanism of action of antihistamines**: Competitive antagonist of histamine receptors.
- **Common side effects**: Sedation, dizziness, nausea, constipation⑧, diarrhea, loss of appetite, anticholinergic effects—dry mouth, dry eyes, blurred vision, urinary retention.
- **Rationale for switching to fexofenadine⑨**: Less central nervous system (CNS) penetration and less sedating than earlier antihistamines.

CLINICAL CORRELATION

Histamine is found in many tissues throughout the body. Most histamine is stored in mast cells and basophils. Histamine is primarily released from mast cells via the process of degranulation. Degranulation occurs when immunoglobulin E (IgE) fixates to mast cells, and there is a subsequent exposure to a specific antigen. Complement activation may also induce degranulation. When released, histamine becomes bound to specific membrane-bound histamine receptors. The therapeutic uses of antihistamine medications primarily involve the H_1 and H_2 receptor subtypes. **H_1 receptors are located in the brain, heart, bronchi, gastrointestinal (GI) tract and vascular smooth muscle.** Their activation increases phospholipase C activity, causing increases in diacylglycerol and intracellular calcium. Activation of H_1 receptors in the brain increases wakefulness. In blood vessels, activation causes vasodilation and increased permeability. H_1 receptor antagonists are competitive inhibitors at this receptor site. H_1 receptor antagonists are frequently used for the treatment of allergic rhinitis, urticaria, and hives. Some are used as prophylaxis for motion sickness and as sleep aids. Older, first-generation, antihistamines cross the blood-brain barrier, contributing to their potentially use-limiting side effect of sedation and can also have significant anticholinergic effects (dry mouth, dry eyes, blurred vision, urinary retention). They must be used with caution in the elderly and in combination with other sedating medications, because the effects can be additive. **Newer, second-generation antihistamines have significantly less penetration into the CNS and reduced anticholinergic activity.** This results in a lower incidence of sedation and fewer anticholinergic side effects. H_2 receptor activity is coupled to cyclic adenosine monophosphate (cAMP). **Activation of H_2 receptors in gastric parietal cells causes an increase**

in gastric acid production. Medications that are competitive antagonists of H_2 receptors are used to reduce gastric acid secretion. These are used clinically in the management of peptic ulcer disease, gastroesophageal reflux disease, heartburn, and acid hypersecretory syndromes.

Pharmacology of Histamine and Antihistamines

Objectives

1. Know the synthesis and mechanism of action of histamine.
2. Know the mechanism of action, uses, and adverse effects of antihistamine medications.

Definitions

Allergic rhinitis[10]: An antigen-mediated allergic reaction that causes nasal congestion, sneezing, itchy eyes, and bronchoconstriction; also called hay fever.

Discussion of Class

Histamine, β-aminoethylimidazole, is formed in many tissues by decarboxylation of the amino acid L-histidine by the enzyme histidine decarboxylase. Mast cells and basophils are the principal histamine-containing cells in most tissues. **Histamine is stored in vesicles in a complex with heparin** and **released by either an immunologic trigger** or following a **mechanical or chemical stimulus.** Once released, **histamine produces a number of responses including local vasodilation, transudation of fluid through endothelial cells, and stimulation of nerve ending, producing pain and itching.** In the lung, histamine is a **bronchoconstrictor**, and this action is magnified in patients with asthma. Histamine has actions in the GI tract and causes **contraction of smooth muscle**; it is also a potent secretagogue for gastric acid secretion, pepsin, and intrinsic factor. In the brain, histamine acts as a **neurotransmitter**[11].

The actions of histamine are mediated by four distinct membrane receptors that are **coupled to G-proteins**. The H_1 receptor, located in smooth muscle cells, endothelium, and brain, is coupled to increased diacylglycerol[12] and Ca^{2+} release. The H_2 receptor is located in gastric mucosa mast cells, immune cells, and brain, and is coupled to increased cAMP. There is no clinical pharmacology yet for H_3 (located in the brain and peripheral neurons) or H_4 (found on eosinophiles[13] and neutrophiles[14]) receptors.

Histamine itself has a variety of untoward effects and is useful only diagnostically to assess bronchial hyperreactivity.

Antihistamines

Compounds that block histamine H_1 receptors have been used for years and are widely marketed both as prescription and over-the-counter medications. The current group of available drugs can be divided into **first-generation and second-generation agents.** In general, **first-generation agents can cross the blood-brain barrier**, and they have a number of effects in the brain including sedation and reduction in nausea. Table 24-1 lists some currently used H_1 antagonists.

Table 24-1

CURRENTLY AVAILABLE ANTIHISTAMINES

CHEMICAL CLASS	DRUG	ANTI-CHOL ACTIVITY	COMMENT
First-Generation Antihistamines			
Ethanolamines	Diphenhydramine	+++	I
	Doxylamine		
	Carbinoxamine	+++	
Ethylamine diamines	Pyrilamine	+	
	Tripelennamine	+	
Piperazines	Cyclizine	nil	I
	Meclizine	nil	
	Hydroxyzine		
Alkalamines	Chlorpheniramine	+	I
	Brompheniramine	+	
Phenothiazines	Promethazine	+++	I
	Cyproheptadine	+	
Second-generation Antihistamines			
Piperidines	Fexofenadine	nil	
	Loratadine	nil	
Piperazines	Cetirizine	nil	
	Levocetirizine	nil	
Alkylamines	Acrivastine	nil	
Phthalazinones	Azelastine	nil	

I = available in an injection preparation; ANTI-CHOL = Anti-Cholinergic

All of these drugs are competitive antagonists of H_1 receptors, and they do not possess significant affinity for the H_2 receptor. However, many of the **first-generation agents** have **significant anticholinergic activity**, and this is responsible for a significant degree of their central effects. Second-generation agents are less lipid soluble and do not penetrate the blood-brain barrier and hence have much fewer central adverse effects.

The major use of antihistamines is in the treatment of allergic reactions. Histamine is released by IgE sensitized cells, especially mast cells and antihistamines can reduce the rhinitis, conjunctivitis, sneezing, and urticaria associated with this reaction. They are most effective in acute allergic reactions with a relatively low antigen burden, and effectiveness diminishes in chronic disorders. Antihistamines are not effective as monotherapy for bronchial asthma. Antihistamines are marketed for treatment of the common cold, but they have very limited effectiveness in this application and their adverse effects (e. g. , sedation) outweighs their benefit. Some of the first-generation agents, especially dimenhydrinate, meclizine, cyclizine, and promethazine, are useful for the prophylaxis of motion sickness and vertigo. **Promethazine** is the most potent in this regard but has pronounced sedative activity that limits its usefulness. The sedating action of some antihistamines has been exploited in their use as sleeping aids.

Diphenhydramine is the most commonly used antihistamine in sleeping preparations.

The **major adverse effect of the first-generation agents is sedation.** The **anticholinergic activity** produces atropine-like effects including dry mouth, urinary retention, and cough. Second-generation agents avoid these effects but do have adverse effects such as headache, back pain, and in the GI tract cause nausea, loss of appetite, and constipation or diarrhea. **Cetirizine** causes the highest incidence of fatigue and somnolence (approximately 10%); of the presently available second-generation antihistamines; loratadine appears to have the lowest incidence of this effect (approximately 1%-2%). These agents may produced cardiovascular adverse effects such as hypotension, brady- or tachycardia, and electrocardiograph (ECG) changes.

Administration

All of the agents listed in Table 24-1 are available for oral use, and some of the first-generation agents are available for parenteral use. Topical application of diphenhydramine is useful in the treatment of minor allergic dermatological reactions.

Pharmacokinetics

Following oral administration, the H_1 antagonists reach peak levels in about 2-3 hours and last 6-24 hours depending on the agent. Azelastine is administered by nasal spray.

H_2 Receptor Antagonists

Histamine is a potent gastric acid secretagogue and this action is mediated by histamine H_2 receptors. Cimetidine, ranitidine, nizatidine, and famotidine are H_2-specific antagonists and are used to treat gastroesophageal reflux disease and peptic ulcers.

Comprehension Questions

[24. 1] The major use of second-generation histamine H_1 receptor blockers is the treatment of

A. Cough associated with influenza
B. Hay fever
C. Motion sickness
D. Sleeplessness

[24. 2] You see a long-distance truck driver in the clinic who complains of serious allergic rhinitis. Which of the following would be the best antihistamine to prescribe?

A. Diphenhydramine
B. Fexophenadine
C. Meclizine
D. Promethazine

[24. 3] Which of the following statements is correct?

A. Antihistamine agents used for allergic rhinitis have antagonistic activity against both H_1 and H_2 receptors.
B. Antihistamine agents are generally useful in the treatment of asthma.
C. Antihistamines are the preferred agent in the treatment of acute anaphylaxis.
D. Second-generation antihistamines have fewer anticholinergic effects than first-generation antihistamines.

Answers

[24. 1] **B.** First-generation agents that cause sedation have been used as sleeping aids, and some have antiemetic effects.

[24. 2] **B.** The other agents are sedating.

[24. 3] **D.** Second-generation antihistamines have less sedating and anticholinergic side effects than first-generation agents.

PHARMACOLOGY PEARLS

❖ Second-generation antihistamines do not penetrate the blood-brain barrier and have little sedative effect.

❖ Antihistamines are of little or no benefit in treating the common cold.

REFERENCES

Borish L. Allergic rhinitis: systemic inflammation and implications for management. J Allergy Clin Immunol 2003 Dec; 112(6): 1021-31.

Quraishi SA, Davies MJ, Craig TJ. Inflammatory responses in allergic rhinitis: traditional approaches and novel treatment strategies. J Am Osteopath Assoc 2004; 104(5 suppl 5): S7-15.

词汇

1. evaluation[估计,评价]
2. allergies[变态反应]
3. runny[流鼻涕的]
4. itchy[痒的]
5. watery[潮湿的]
6. sneeze[喷嚏]
7. Antihistamine[抗组胺剂]
8. constipation[便秘]
9. fexofenadine[非索非那定,抗组胺药]
10. rhinitis[鼻炎]
11. neurotransmitter[神经递质]
12. diacylglycerol[二酰甘油]
13. eosinophiles[嗜红细胞]
14. neutrophiles[中性白细胞]

注 1

苯海拉明为第一代抗组胺药的代表药，该药能够通过血脑屏障而产生镇静，眩晕等副作用，还具有明显的抗胆碱能作用(口干,眼干,视力模糊,尿潴留)。

注 2

季节性变应性鼻炎(SAR)又称花粉症，是由变应原(花粉)激发的，由 IgE 介导的 I 型变态反应性疾病。抗组胺药对此类疾病疗效较好，可作为首选药物，现多用第二代抗组胺药。二代抗组胺药具有①大多长效；②无嗜睡作用；③对喷嚏、清涕和鼻痒效果好，而对鼻塞效果较差的特点。

注 3

非索非那定为第二代抗组胺药的代表药，与一代相比，该药的血脑屏障通透性及抗胆碱能作用明显减弱，副作用小。

点评

本病例中，患者有随季节变化规律性发作的流涕、流泪、鼻痒、打喷嚏等症状，因此考虑季节性变应性鼻炎的可能性大。患者曾服用苯海拉明治疗，服药期间有明显的思睡，困倦等症状，提示药物副作用明显，因此可采用二代抗组胺药非索非那定进行治疗，降低药物副作用，以达到良好的疗效。患者本人应远离花粉播散区，避免接触致敏变应原。

魏敏杰

❖ CASE 25

A 40-year-old woman presents for evaluation of her chronic① migraine② headaches③. She reports that approximately once a month she has a severe④, unilateral⑤ headache associated with nausea⑥ and extreme photophobia⑦. The headache will last for a full day if not treated. She has had success in reducing the severity of the headaches with opioid⑧ pain medications⑨, but usually she is too nauseous to take them. When she is able to tolerate⑩ them,[注1] she will have to sleep for several hours afterwards.[注2] She is missing about a day of work a month because of the headaches. She has no other significant medical history and takes no medications on a regular basis. Her examination today is normal. You decide to prescribe⑪ sumatriptan[注3] for her to try with her next migraine headache.

◆ **Which receptor is the site of action of sumatriptan?**

◆ **What is the mechanism of action of sumatriptan?**

ANSWERS TO CASE 25: Serotonin Receptor Agonists and Antagonists

Summary: A 40-year-old woman with migraine headaches is treated with sumatriptan.

- **Receptor site of action of sumatriptan**[12]: Serotonin 5-HT_{1D} and 5-HT_{1B} receptors
- **Mechanism of action of sumatriptan**: Receptor activation inhibits the activity of adenyl cyclase and decreases cyclic adenosine monophosphate (cAMP) accumulation that results in contraction of arterial smooth muscle, especially in carotid and cranial circulation.

CLINICAL CORRELATION

Migraine headaches are common causes of severe symptoms among patients and a leading cause of absenteeism from work and school. Sumatriptan was the first of a class of serotonin (5-HT) agonist medications for the treatment of migraines. Multiple subtypes of 5-HT receptors have been identified. Sumatriptan specifically acts at the 5-HT_{1D} and 5-HT_{1B} receptor subtypes that are coupled to an inhibition of cAMP. Stimulation of these receptors results in vasoconstriction in the carotid circulation that may directly oppose the vasodilation thought to be involved in migraine. At prejunctional sites, activation of these receptors results in decreased transmission of nociceptive signals in the trigeminal nerve. While being fairly specific for the carotid circulation, there can be activity at other vascular sites. Cerebrovascular[13], peripheral vascular, mesenteric arterial or coronary artery diseases are all contraindications to its use. Vasospastic coronary[14] disease is a contraindication as well.

Pharmacology of Serotonin Receptor Agonists and Antagonists

Objectives

1. Describe the activity of the different classes of serotonin receptors.
2. List the agents which act as serotonin agonists and describe their mechanisms of action and uses.
3. List the agents which act as serotonin antagonists and describe their mechanisms of action and therapeutic uses.

Definitions

Partial agonist: A drug that at full receptor occupancy produces less of a response than a full agonist. Partial agonists can competitively inhibit the response to a full agonist, including the physiological response to endogenously released hormones and neurotransmitters.

Discussion of Class

Other than the **triptans** (almotriptan, eletriptan, naratriptan, rizatriptan, sumatriptan, and zolmitriptan), which are the drugs of choice to treat acute, severe migraine headache, there are few clinically important agents that are directacting serotonin-receptor agonists. The **ergot**⑮ **alkyloids**(ergotamine[the prototype], dihydroergotamine, ergonovine, methylergonovine) act through the same mechanisms as the triptans are used **effectively clinically during the prodrome of a migraine attack**. **Diarrhea, nausea and vomiting and drowsiness** are their most common adverse effects. **Prolonged vasospasm** resulting from smooth muscle stimulation is a serious consequence of **overdose** that may result in **gangrene**⑯ **and amputation of arms, legs, or digits**. **Bowel infarction** has also been reported. They are **contraindicated** for patients with **obstructive vascular disease**.

Because of potential serious **cardiac arrhythmias**, **cisapride**, a 5-HT_4 receptor agonist that promotes release of acetylcholine from the myenteric plexus, is used only compassionately to treat gastroesophageal reflux and motility disease. It also causes gastrointestinal discomfort and diarrhea in a significant number of patients(about 15%).

Tegaserod, a partial agonist at 5-HT_4 receptors, is used to treat irritable bowel syndrome(IBS). Diarrhea is its major adverse effect.

The major clinical use of **selective serotonin**⑰ **receptor antagonists** is as first-line drugs for **treatment of nausea and vomiting** resulting from **vagal stimulation that is associated with surgery and cancer chemotherapy**. These agents, the prototype being **odansetron**(also granisetron, serotonin, dolasetron), act on 5-HT_3 receptors. Their most common adverse effects are **headache and constipation**. Dolasetron prolongs the QT interval and, therefore, should not be administered to patients with this condition or with other similarly acting drugs.

Alosetron⑱ is a 5-HT_3 receptor antagonist that is used to treat **IBS with diarrhea**. It is only approved for treatment of women because efficacy has not been documented for men. Its major adverse effects are constipation that may be severe and require discontinuation of therapy. **Ischemic colitis** (incidence about 0.3%), may be **fatal**⑲ and therefore precludes it's the use of alosetron except for patients who have not responded to other therapies.

Mechanism of Action

The **ergot alkaloids**(dihydroergotamine, ergonovine, ergotamine the prototype, methylergonovine) have **agonist and partial agonist activity at serotonin** ($5\text{-}HT_{1D}$ receptors and $5\text{-}HT_{1A}$ receptors) that, like the triptans (see above), are responsible for their therapeutic action. Their antagonist and agonist and partial agonist activity at α-adrenergic receptors and dopamine receptors are responsible for some adverse actions. Cisapride activation of $5\text{-}HT_4$ receptors on enteric neurons promotes release of acetylcholine that results in increased lower esophageal sphincter pressure. Tegaserod activation of $5\text{-}HT_4$ receptors results in release of neurotransmitters in the submucosal and myenteric plexuses in the gastrointestinal tract that promote peristalsis.

Odansetron and other selective serotonin antagonists act to inhibit nausea and vomiting through peripheral blockade of serotonin $5\text{-}HT_3$ receptors on intestinal vagal afferent nerves, and through central blockade of serotonin $5\text{-}HT_3$ receptors in the vomiting center and chemoreceptor trigger zone.

Alosetron is a selective serotonin receptor $5\text{-}HT_3$ antagonist that acts peripherally on enteric afferent and cholinergic neurons to reduce intestinal activity and visceral afferent pain. It also acts centrally on the same receptors to inhibit afferent nerve activation of the central nervous system (CNS).

Administration

Sumatriptan may be administered orally, as a subcutaneous injection, or as a nasal spray, making it particularly valuable for migraine patients with nausea and vomiting as symptoms. Ergotamines are available for oral, sublingual rectal, parenteral, and inhaler administration.

Selective serotonin receptor antagonists can be administered orally or IV. They are most effective against nausea and vomiting when administered IV prior to the administration of chemotherapeutic agents.

Pharmacokinetics

Cisapride is metabolized by microsomal enzymes that are inhibited by a wide variety of agents and can lead to large increases in cisapride serum levels and toxicity. Tegaserod is poorly absorbed and should be taken before meals. Severe hepatic or renal disease may significantly reduce its clearance.

Ergotamine tartrate may be administered combined with caffeine which facilitates its absorption.

Comprehension Questions

[25. 1] Sumatriptan

A. Causes vasoconstriction in the carotid and cranial circulation

B. Increases transmission of nociceptive signals in the trigeminal nerve

C. Increases adenylyl cyclase activity

D. Is an antagonist at the 5-HT_{1D} receptor subtype

[25.2] The major clinical use of odansetron is

A. Compassionate treatment of gastroesophageal reflux and motility disease

B. Major depression

C. Migraine headache

D. Nausea and vomiting that is associated with surgery and cancer chemotherapy

[25.3] Prolonged vasospasm is a serious consequence of

A. Alosetron B. Cisapride C. Ergotamine D. Odansetron

Answers

[25.1] **A.** Sumatriptan, a 5-HT_{1D} receptor agonist, inhibits the activity of adenylyl cyclase and decreases cAMP accumulation that results in contraction of arterial smooth muscle, especially in carotid and cranial circulation.

[25.2] **D.** The major clinical use of odansetron, a 5-HT_3 receptor antagonist, is for treatment of nausea and vomiting that is associated with surgery and cancer chemotherapy. Migraine is treated with triptans and ergot alkaloids. Cisapride, a 5-HT_4 receptor agonist, is used only compassionately to treat gastroesophageal reflux and motility disease. Selective serotonin reuptake inhibitors (SSRIs) act to block serotonin transporters and are used to treat major depression.

[25.3] **C.** Prolonged vasospasm caused by smooth muscle stimulation is a serious consequence of overdose with ergotamine. The most common adverse effects of odansetron are headache and constipation. Serious cardiac arrhythmia is a serious adverse effect of cisapride. The major adverse effect of alosetron, a 5-HT_3 receptor antagonist, is constipation.

PHARMACOLOGY PEARLS

❖ Because the vasoconstrictor activity of ergotamine is long-lasting, its dose and frequency of administration must be limited.

❖ Ergot alkyloid agents can cause vasoconstriction and should not be used in patients with occlusive vascular disease.

❖ The effects of selective serotonin receptor antagonists like odansetron seem to be enhanced with concomitant administration of dexamethasone.

REFERENCES

Lake AE，Saper JR. Chronic headache. New advances in treatment strategies. Neurology 2002；59：S8.

Peroutka SJ. Serotonin receptor subtypes. Their evolution and clinical relevance. CNS Drugs 1995；4：19.

Young WB，Silberstein SD，Dayno JM. Migraine treatment. Semin Neurol 1997；17：325.

词汇

1. chronic[慢性的,长期的]
2. migraine[偏头痛]
3. headache[头痛]
4. severe[严重的]
5. unilateral[单侧的]
6. nausea[恶心]
7. photophobia[畏光]
8. opioid[阿片样物质,类吗啡物质]
9. medication[药物治疗]
10. tolerate[忍受]
11. prescribe[开药方,开处方]
12. sumatriptan[舒马普坦(5-HT_1 受体激动药)]
13. cerebrovascular[脑血管的]
14. coronary[冠状的]
15. ergot[麦角]
16. gargrene[坏疽]
17. serotonin[血清素]
18. alosetron[阿洛司琼,5-HT 受体阻滞剂]
19. fatal[致命的,致死的]

注 1

阿片类药物可用于治疗严重头痛，能有效的缓解疼痛症状；而对于中-重度头痛，宜首选麦角衍生物类或曲普坦类。麦角胺能收缩血管，减少脑动脉搏动幅度，用于偏头痛的诊断和治疗；曲普坦类药物能收缩血管，降低血管调节系统神经元兴奋性，减少炎症性和血管扩张性神经肽的释放，是近年来研究最多的治疗偏头痛的药物。

注 2

患者头痛发作时，因严重恶心，呕吐而无法正常服药，在服用其他药物无效的情况下，可给予小剂量氯丙嗪，氯丙嗪是吩噻嗪类药物的典型代表，有较强的镇吐作用，小剂量时即可对抗多巴胺(DA)受体激动药引起的呕吐反应，大剂量的氯丙嗪可直接抑制呕吐中枢。

注 3

舒马普坦为5-HT_1 受体激动药，选择性激动 5-HT_{1D}和 5-HT_{1B}受体。导致颈动脉和颅内血管收缩，并减慢三叉神经疼痛信号的传导，从而起到减轻偏头痛症状的作用。但应注意该药还可以收缩其他部位的血管，脑血管、外周血管、肠系膜动脉及冠状动脉疾病均为使用该药的禁忌证。

点评

本病例具有典型的偏头痛病史，单侧头痛，伴有恶心，畏光等症状，大约每月发作一次，患者在服用阿片类药物后，头痛症状得到缓解，因此可以诊断为偏头痛。治疗采用舒马普坦，用于缓解头痛症状，此外，若患者头痛发作时，伴有严重恶心，呕吐，可给予小剂量氯丙嗪。

魏敏杰

CASE 26

You are called to see a 24-year-old G_3P_3 woman who approximately 1 hour ago underwent a vaginal delivery[①] of an 8 lb infant. The nurse is concerned that the patient is continuing to bleed more than would be expected, and that her uterine fundus[②] does not feel firm. A brief history from the nurse reveals that the patient required IV oxytocin[③] augmentation of her labor, but otherwise had an uncomplicated labor and delivery. Her placenta[④] delivered spontaneously and intact. She has no significant medical history. Examination of the patient reveals her to be comfortable and cooperative but she is mildly tachycardic[⑤]. Her uterine fundus is boggy[⑥] and nontender on palpation[⑦].[注1] Vaginal examination[⑧] shows no cervical[⑨] or vaginal lacerations[⑩], but there is a steady flow of blood from the still-dilated cervix[⑪].[注2] You diagnose the patient as having a postpartum hemorrhage[⑫] secondary to uterine atony[⑬] and order an immediate IM injection of methylergonovine[⑭].[注3]

◆ **What is the mechanism of action of methylergonovine?**

◆ **What are the common adverse effects of methylergonovine?**

ANSWERS TO CASE 26: Ergot Alkyloids

Summary: A 24-year-old woman has a postpartum hemorrhage secondary to uterine atony. She is given an IM injection of methylergonovine.

- **Mechanism of action of methylergonovine**: α-adrenoceptor agonist with activity on uterine smooth muscle, causing forceful and prolonged uterine contraction.
- **Side effects of methylergonovine**: Hypertension, headaches, nausea, vomiting.

CLINICAL CORRELATION

Methylergonovine is an amine ergot alkaloid with relatively selective activity at uterine smooth muscle. Ergot alkaloids[15] are structurally similar to norepinephrine, dopamine, and serotonin. They can have agonist or antagonist effects on α-adrenoceptors, dopamine receptors, and serotonin receptors. Methylergonovine acts primarily via α-adrenoceptors and 5-HT_2 receptors to cause tetanic uterine contraction. This provides its therapeutic benefit in the treatment of postpartum hemorrhage because of uterine atony. This drug can have other effects mediated by α-adrenoceptors, including acute hypertensive reactions and vasospasm. It is contraindicated in patients with uncontrolled hypertension. Other common side effects include headaches, nausea, and vomiting.

Pharmacology of the Ergot Alkaloids

Objectives

1. Know the mechanism of action of the ergot alkaloids.
2. Know the therapeutic uses and side effects of ergot alkaloids.

Definitions

Postpartum hemorrhage: Vaginal bleeding exceeding 500 mL after a vaginal delivery or 1000 mL after a cesarean[16] delivery. The most common etiology[17] is uterine atony.

Migraine: A familial disorder marked by periodic, usually unilateral, pulsatile headaches that begin in childhood or early adult life and tend to recur with diminishing frequency in later life. There are two closely related syndromes[18] comprising what is known as migraine. They are classic migraine (migraine with aura[19]) and common migraine (migraine without aura).

Discussion of Class

The ergot alkaloids are produced by the fungi[20] *Claviceps purpurea*, There are two major families of ergots: the peptide ergots and the amine ergots, all contain the tetracyclic ergoline nucleus. The peptide ergots include ergotamine, α-ergocryptine and bromocriptine; the amine ergot ergots include lysergic acid, lysergic acid diethylamide, ergonovine, and methysergide. The ergots have agonist, partial agonist, and antagonist actions at α-adrenergic receptors and serotonin receptors, and agonist or partial agonist actions at central dopamine receptors.

Postpartum Hemorrhage

Ergonovine and its semisynthetic derivative, methylergonovine, cause **powerful contractions of smooth muscle**; the gravid uterus is especially sensitive to this drug. Postpartum hemorrhage is most often treated with oxytocin. In circumstances where oxytocin is not effective, methylergonovine causes forceful contractions of uterine smooth muscle that effectively stops the bleeding. This action appears to be mediated by agonist activity at α_1-adrenergic receptors and agonist action at 5-HT_2 receptors. Methylergonovine can be administered orally or IM; effects are seen in 3-5 minutes following IM administration. Acute administration of methylergonovine has few side effects.

Migraine Headache

Dihydroergotamine is useful in the management of migraines. It binds with high affinity to 5-$HT_{1D\alpha}$ and 5-$HT_{1D\beta}$ receptors. It also binds with high affinity to serotonin 5-HT_{1A}, 5-HT_{2A}, and 5-HT_{2C} receptors, noradrenaline α_{2A}, α_{2B}, and α receptors, and dopamine D_{2L} and D_3 receptors. The therapeutic activity of dihydroergotamine in migraine is generally attributed to the agonist effect at 5-HT_{1D} receptors. Two current theories have been proposed to explain the efficacy of 5-HT_{1D} receptor agonists in migraine. One theory suggests that activation of 5-HT_{1D} receptors located on carotid and intracranial blood vessels, including those on arteriovenous anastomoses, leads to vasoconstriction, which correlates with the relief of migraine headache. The alternative hypothesis suggests that activation of 5-HT_{1D} receptors on sensory nerve endings of the trigeminal system results in the inhibition of proinflammatory neuropeptide release. Adverse effects include gastrointestinal disturbances including diarrhea, vomiting, and vasospasm.

The triptans—sumatriptan, rizatriptan, almotriptan, and others—are selective 5-HT_{1D} and 5-HT_{1B} receptor agonists that are also useful for treating an acute migraine headache.

Methysergide is used for **prophylaxis** of migraine. It acts as a 5-$HT_{2A,C}$ antagonist to block in vascular smooth muscle. It is effective in preventing or reducing the frequency of migraines in about 60 percent of patients. Chronic use of methysergide is associated with **retroperitoneal fibroplasia and subendocardial fibrosis**. For this reason drug-free periods are recommended if it is used for chronically.

Endocrine Abnormalities

Bromocriptine is very effective in reducing the high levels of prolactin production that occur with certain pituitary tumors. It has also been used to suppress lactation. Bromocriptine is a potent dopamine receptor agonist, and its prolactin-suppressive action are mediated via interaction with this receptor. Side effects are dose related and range from nausea to Parkinson syndrome. Bromocriptine has been associated with postpartum cardiovascular toxicity.

Comprehension Questions

[26.1] Methylergonovine is useful in treating postpartum hemorrhage because it

A. Causes forceful contractions of the myometrium

B. Causes rapid production of thrombin

C. Is a potent vasoconstrictor

D. Stimulates the activity of antithrombin III

[26.2] Which of the following would be the best drug to reduce prolactin levels in a patient with a pituitary tumor?

A. Bromocriptine B. Ergonovine C. Ergotamine D. Methysergide

[26.3] A 35-year-old woman is noted to have dyspnea with exertion. Echocardiography identifies a restrictive cardiomyopathy with decreased flexibility of the heart. The cardiologist notes that one of his medications may be responsible. Which of the following agents is most likely the etiology?

A. Bromocriptine B. Ergonovine C. Ergotamine D. Methysergide

Answers

[26.1] **A.** Although methylergonovine does cause vasoconstriction, its action in postpartum hemorrhage is mediated by forceful clamping of the myometrium, which restricts blood flow.

[26.2] **A.** Bromocriptine is a dopamine receptor agonist that is used to treat prolactin secreting pituitary adenomas.

[26.3] **D.** Methysergide can induce a fibroelastosis of the heart, which leads to a restrictive cardiomyopathy.

PHARMACOLOGY PEARLS

❖ Methysergide is useful for prophylaxis of migraine headaches but has no effect on an acute episode.

❖ Bromocriptine is a dopamine receptor agonist and is used to treat prolactin secreting pituitary adenomas.

❖ Methylergonovine is used to treat postpartum hemorrhage caused by uterine atony and causes contraction of the uterine smooth muscle.

REFERENCES

de Groot AN, van Dongen PW, Vree TB, et al. Ergot alkaloids. Current status and review of clinical pharmacology and therapeutic use compared with other oxytocics in obstetrics and gynaecology. Drugs 1998 Oct; 56(4): 523-35.

Silberstein SD. Migraine. Lancet 2004; 363: 381-91.

词汇

1. vaginal delivery[阴道分娩]
2. uterine fundus[子宫底]
3. oxytocin[缩宫素]
4. placenta[胎盘瘤]
5. tachycardic[心搏过速的]
6. boggy[潮湿的]
7. palpation[触诊]
8. vaginal examination[阴道检查]
9. cervical[子宫颈的]
10. laceration[撕裂,裂伤]
11. cervix[子宫颈]
12. postpartum hemorrhage[产后出血]
13. uterine atony[子宫张力缺乏,子宫无力]
14. methylergonovine[甲基麦角新碱,甲麦角新碱,美占飞]
15. alkaloids[生物碱,植物碱]
16. cesarean[剖腹产术]
17. etiology[病因学,病原学]
18. syndrome[综合征,症候群]
19. aura[气味,香味]
20. fungi[菌类]

注 1

对病人检查发现，病人比较舒适并且查体合作，但是有些轻微的心动过速。触诊发现，病人子宫底潮湿并且缺乏张力。以上体格检查结果都表明，病人仍然有活动性出血，引起反射性心动过速。这种情况下，病人应该应用对子宫平滑肌产生收缩的药物，使血管收缩，抑制活动性出血，目前临床常用甲基麦角新碱 0.2mg 肌注。胎盘娩出以后要触诊子宫以判断是否存在子宫弛缓。如果存在子宫弛缓，应施行有力的子宫按摩术，如果按摩时仍有持续出血，进行双手子宫压迫常可控制出血。

注 2

行阴道检查没有发现子宫颈或阴道撕裂，但是仍然有稳定量的血流从仍处于扩张状态的子宫颈流出，说明出血不是由于产道裂伤造成，而是来自子宫颈。由此可见，对该病人行阴道检查尤为重要，通过体格检查有助于正确判断出血部位。临床上对于无子宫弛缓而持续出血的病人应怀疑是否有产道裂伤，应该做宫颈和阴道检查以排除产道裂伤。如果没有发现裂伤而仍然出血，应该进行用手检查以排除子宫破裂。

注 3

经诊断，病人为继发子宫张力缺乏性产后出血，应该立即肌肉注射甲基麦角新碱。该疾病为妇产科急症，在临床应采取有效措施，尽早确定出血部位，并密切观察病人呼吸、血压等临床表现，及早注射甲基麦角新碱。

点评

本病例为典型的经阴道分娩产妇，由于产后子宫张力缺乏造成的产后出血。经阴道分娩一小时后，子宫底不固定，触诊发现子宫底潮湿，子宫颈仍然扩张，说明仍然有活动性出血，在排除子宫及阴道撕裂的情况下，可以初步诊断为子宫张力缺乏，产后出血。治疗上应采用立即肌肉注射甲基麦角新碱。甲基麦角新碱为α-肾上腺素受体激动剂，属麦角生物碱类，能够对子宫平滑肌产生强力而持久的收缩作用。但是，甲基麦角新碱应用时可产生高血压、头痛、恶心、呕吐等副反应。故临床应用时应加以注意。

魏敏杰

❖ CASE 27

A 24-year-old G_3P_3 woman, now 90 minutes after vaginal delivery① and having received an injection② of methylergonovine③, continues to have postpartum bleeding④. Her uterus⑤ is firmer⑥ but still somewhat boggy⑦. Her heart rate⑧ remains mildly tachycardic⑨, but her blood pressure⑩ has gone up in response to the methylergonovine. [注1] Her examination is otherwise unchanged. You now order an IM injection⑪ of carboprost tromethamine⑫ (prostaglandin⑬ $F_{2\alpha}$, or $PGF_{2\alpha}$). [注2]

◆ **What is the therapeutic action of $PGF_{2\alpha}$ in postpartum hemorrhage?**

◆ **What is the effect of PGFs on vascular smooth muscle?**

◆ **What is the effect of PGFs on bronchial smooth muscle?**

ANSWERS TO CASE 27: Eicosanoids

Summary: A 24-year-old woman has continued postpartum hemorrhage despite ergot alkyloids.

- **Therapeutic action of $PGF_{2\alpha}$:** Causes contraction of uterine smooth muscle.
- **Effect on vascular smooth muscle:** Arteriolar[14] vasodilation and constriction of superficial veins.
- **Effect on bronchial smooth muscle:** Smooth muscle contraction.

CLINICAL CORRELATION

Eicosanoids are a large and varied group of autocoids with effects on most tissues in the body. They are derivatives of eicosanoic[15] acids and are synthesized throughout the body. They typically have short plasma half-lives and are catabolized in the lung. There is no common mechanism of eicosanoid action. Specific cell surface receptors mediate activities of each class of eicosanoid and many different second messenger pathways are involved. Prostaglandin $F_{2\alpha}$ ($PGF_{2\alpha}$) is produced via the prostaglandin H synthase (cyclooxygenase) pathway. It causes arteriolar vasodilation, superficial vein[16] constriction, and bronchial smooth muscle contraction and increases the rate of longitudinal muscle contraction in the gastrointestinal (GI) tract. It causes contraction of uterine smooth muscle in the pregnant uterus. This effect mediates its primary therapeutic use, the treatment of postpartum hemorrhage. Because of the risk of bronchospasm, its use is contraindicated in asthmatics. It can cause nausea, vomiting, diarrhea, and cramps as a result of its effect on the GI tract.

Pharmacology of the Eicosanoids

Objectives

1. Know the pathways of eicosanoid synthesis.
2. Know the actions of eicosanoids on tissues throughout the body.
3. Know the therapeutic uses, adverse effects, and contraindications to the use of eicosanoids.

Definitions

Eicosanoids: Metabolites of 20-carbon fatty acids.

Prostanoids[17]**:** Prostaglandins and thromboxanes[18].

COX: Cyclooxygenase, rate limiting enzymes (COX-1 and COX-2) in prostaglandin biosynthesis.

HETE: Hydroxyeicosatetraenoic acid.

EET: Epoxyeicosatrienoic acids.

Discussion of Class

The **eicosanoids** are **fatty acid metabolites** that include the **prostaglandins**, the **thromboxanes**, and the **HETEs** and the **EETs**. These small molecules affect nearly every physiologic system, including blood flow, especially in the kidney, airway diameter, inflammation, ovulation, and uterine smooth muscle tone. The eicosanoids are metabolites of the **20-carbon fatty acid arachidonic acid**. A substrate pool of arachidonic acid is stored as part of the lipids in the plasma membrane. Figure 27-1 outlines the two major biosynthetic routes of eicosanoic metabolites. Most of the free arachidonic acid in cells is liberated from the plasma membrane phospholipid by phospholipase A_2.

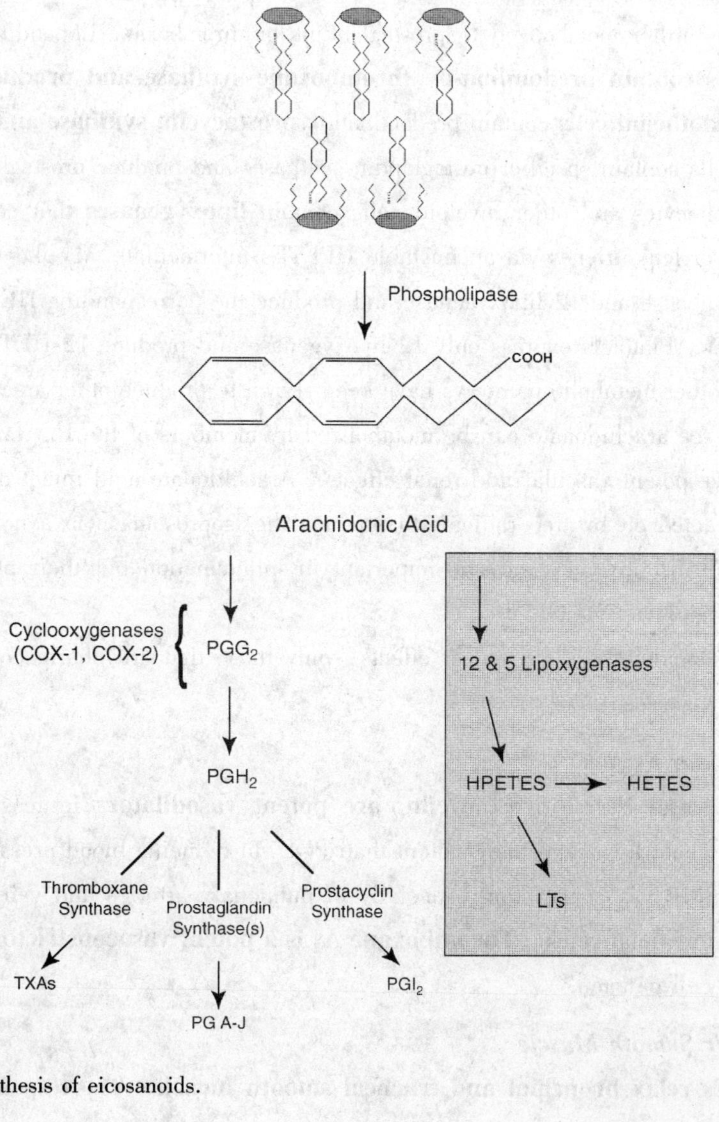

Figure 27-1. Synthesis of eicosanoids.

A minor amount can be liberated from phosphatidylinositides by the action of phospholipase C and diglyceride lipase. The free arachidonic acid is metabolized by either cyclooxygenase to form prostaglandins and thromboxane, or by **lipoxygenases** to form the **HETEs** and **leukotrienes**. There are two isoforms of cyclooxygenases that catalyze the same reaction.

Cyclooxygenase type 1 (COX-1) is fairly widely distributed in the **stomach, kidneys, and connective tissues**. COX-1 is expressed in a constitutive manner. **COX-2** is also expressed in numerous tissues including the **GI tract, kidneys, ovaries** and **connective tissues**. Basal COX-2 expression is very low, but it is highly induced by cytokines, growth factors, and serum factors. The cyclooxygenases perform two catalytic steps: a **cyclooxygenase reaction that introduces oxygen and a peroxidase**[19] reaction that yields **PGH_2**, the **immediate precursor to all prostaglandins and thromboxane**. PGH_2 is further metabolized to prostaglandins or thromboxane depending on the tissue. **Platelets contain predominantly thromboxane synthase and produce thromboxane A_2**; **endothelial cells** contain predominantly **prostacyclin synthase and produce PGI_2**; other cells contain specific prostaglandin synthases and produce prostaglandins A-J.

Lymphocytes and other myeloid cells contain **lipoxygenases** that convert PGH_2 into HETEs or leukotrienes via an unstable HPETEs intermediate. Leukocytes express both 5-lipoxygenase and 12-lipoxygenase and produce the corresponding HETEs and the leukotrienes. Platelets express only 12-lipoxygenase and produce 12-HETE.

Two other metabolic pathways have been shown to produce other arachidonate metabolites. Free arachidonate can be metabolized by members of the P_{450} family to the EETs that have potent vascular and renal effects. Arachidonate acid intact on a phospholipid can be acted on by free radicals to produce the isoprostanes via a nonenzymatic pathway. The isoprostanes may be important in inflammation but their physiologic role is still under investigation.

Eicosanoids have a myriad of effects; only those that are pharmacologically relevant will be discussed here.

Vascular System

PGE_2 and PGI_2 (prostacyclin) are potent vasodilators in most vascular beds. PGI_2 is about five times more potent than PGE_2 in reducing blood pressure. $PGF_{2\alpha}$ typically causes vasoconstriction especially in pulmonary arteries and veins, and vasoconstricts superficial veins. **Thromboxane A_2 is a potent vasoconstrictor** and is a smooth muscle cell mitogen.

Other Smooth Muscle

PGEs relax bronchial and tracheal smooth muscle. The response of the uterine myometrium is complex with low doses of PGE_2 causing contraction and high doses causing relaxation. In the GI tract, PGEs relax circular smooth muscle but the longitudinal muscle is contracted. $PGF_{2\alpha}$, PGD, and TXA_2 cause bronchoconstriction in the airways and contraction of gastrointestinal smooth muscle.

Gastrointestinal Secretion

PGEs and PGI_2 inhibit gastric acid and pepsin production and increase mucus production; these actions are cytoprotective in the upper GI tract.

Kidney

Prostaglandins are important local regulators of renal blood flow. PGEs and PGI_2 increase renal blood flow and diuresis without changing the glomerular filtration rate. TXA_2 decreases renal blood flow and glomerular filtration rate.

Pharmacologic Uses of Eicosanoids

PGE_1 can be used in neonates to maintain patency of the ductus arteriosis. Infants born with certain congenital heart abnormalities depend on a patent ductus to maintain adequate pulmonary blood flow. **PGE_1** is used to temporarily maintain the patency until surgery can be performed. **PGE_1**, because of its vasodilatory action, can be injected into the corpus cavernosum of the **penis to induce erection**. This use has been largely supplanted by the **phosphodiesterase V inhibitors such as sildenafil**. **PGE_1 analogs have also been used for cytoprotection of NSAID-induced gastric and peptic ulcers**. This is based on the protective action mediated by the reduction in acid and pepsin production and increased mucus production produced by PGE_1. PGE_1 and PGI_2 and their congeners PGE_2 and PGI_2 have also been used to treat peripheral occlusive vascular disease and have been used for treating Raynaud disease and arteriosclerosis obliterans. Because of its effect to inhibit platelet aggregation and its short half-life, PGI_2 can be used during dialysis instead of heparin. It has also been used to treat pulmonary arterial hypertension.

15-methyl-$PGF_{2\alpha}$ stimulates uterine contractions. It can be used to control persistent postpartum hemorrhage secondary to uterine atony that is unresponsive to other drugs. 15-methyl-$PGF_{2\alpha}$ can be used in the first and second trimester to induce abortion. PGE_2 congeners are used to facilitate cervical ripening and for the induction of labor. PGE_2 is combined with the antiprogestin RU-486 (mifepristone) to induce first-trimester abortion. Side effects are usually nausea and vomiting. It is contraindicated in asthmatics because of its bronchoconstrictive activities.

Structure

Prostaglandins are derived by metabolism of the 20-carbon fatty acid arachidonic acid.

Mechanism of Action

There are a number of specific membrane receptors that mediate the action of the prostaglandins. There are four prostaglandin E receptors (EP_1-EP_4), two prostaglandin F receptors (FPA and FPB), one prostaglandin H receptor (IP), and two thromboxane receptors (TP_α and TP_β) and 2 prostaglandin D receptors (DP and $CRTH_2$). These receptors are coupled to increases or decreases in cAMP, and increases in inositol-3 phosphate.

Administration

Most prostaglandins or their analogs are administered by local instillation (e. g., vaginal or cervical gels or suppositories) or continuous infusion. Misoprostol, a PGE_1 analog, is available for oral administration.

Pharmacokinetics

Prostaglandins are rapidly absorbed and inactivated in lung, liver, and kidney. Both the natural prostaglandins and their analogs have a very short half-life (typically minutes).

Comprehension Questions

[27. 1] Which of the following enzymes do leukotrienes require for their biosynthesis?

A. COX-1 B. COX-2 C. 5-lipoxygenase D. 8-lipoxygenase

[27. 2] PGI_2 can be used to

A. Cause peripheral vasoconstriction

B. Control bleeding from the uterine artery

C. Facilitate blood clotting

D. Treat occlusive vascular disease

[27. 3] A 38-year-old woman is taking ibuprofen for severe dysmenorrhea but develops epigastric pain. The physician prescribes a medication to prevent gastritis. Which of the following best describes the medication?

A. PGE_1 analog B. PGE_1 antagonist

C. PGE_2 analog D. PGE_2 antagonist

E. PGE_2 analog F. PGE_2 antagonist

G. PGI analog H. PGI antagonist

Answers

[27. 1] **C.** Production of leukotrienes requires 5-lipoxygenase

[27.2] **D.** PGE_2 and PGI_2 are vasodilators in all vascular beds.

[27.3] **A.** PGE_1 analog, misoprostol, is used to prevent NSAID-associated gastritis.

PHARMACOLOGY PEARLS

❖ PGE_1 and PGH_1 can be used to produce relatively local vasodilation.

❖ PGE_2 and $PGF_{2\alpha}$ have obstetric uses to control uterine bleeding and to hasten parturition.

❖ 15-methyl-$PGF_{2\alpha}$ stimulates uterine contractions. It can be used to control persistent postpartum hemorrhage.

❖ Thromboxane is a potent vasoconstrictor.

REFERENCES

Rayburn, WF. Prostaglandin E2 gel for cervical ripening and induction of labor: a critical analysis. Am J Obstet Gynecol 1989; 160: 529-34.

词汇

1. vaginal delivery[阴道分娩]
2. injection[注射]
3. methylergonovine[甲基麦角新碱,甲麦角新碱,美占飞]
4. postpartum bleeding[产后出血]
5. uterus[子宫]
6. firm[坚硬的,结实的]
7. boggy[潮湿的]
8. heart rate[心率]
9. tachycardic[心动过速]
10. blood pressure[血压]
11. IM injection[intramusculary injection,肌肉内注射]
12. carboprost tromethamine[甲基前列腺素 $F_2\alpha$ 缓血酸胺,甲基前列腺素 $F_2\alpha$ 三羟甲基氨基甲烷(子宫兴奋药)]
13. prostaglandin[前列腺素]
14. arteriolar[微小动脉]
15. eicosanorc[类花生酸,二十(烷)类]
16. vein[静脉]
17. prostanoid[类前列腺类]
18. thromboxane[血栓素]
19. peroxidase[过氧化物酶]

注 1

病人仍然有轻微的心动过速，血压有所上升，这是由于病人注射了甲基麦角新碱的原因。甲基麦角新碱应用时可产生高血压、头痛、恶心、呕吐等副反应，故临床应用时应加以注意。

注 2

病人应该立即注射甲基前列腺素 $F_2\alpha$ 缓血酸胺（子宫兴奋药）。该药物可引起子宫平滑肌的强烈收缩，故一般对于产后出血病人效果良好。

点评

正常情况下，胎盘娩出后子宫收缩，子宫底平脐或脐下一横指，呈球形，质软。子宫收缩乏力时，子宫底升高，子宫质软，袋状，阴道流血多。根据该病例情况，阴道分娩 90 分钟后，阴道持续出血，在注射甲基麦角新碱后仍然出血不止。阴道触诊感到子宫内潮湿有血。建议病人应该立即注射甲基前列腺素 $F_2\alpha$ 缓血酸胺。

魏敏杰

❖ CASE 28

A 16-year-old female comes to the office because of menstrual[①] cramps[②]. She had menarche[③] at age 13. Her menses[④] lasts for 4-5 days, and she has 28-day cycles. For the first 2-3 days of her menses she states that she has very bad cramping. The cramps have occurred since menarche and seem to have worsened in the past year. They have been so bad at times that she has missed school and has not been able to participate[⑤] in her after-school sports. She has been taking acetaminophen[⑥注1] and over-the-counter "menstrual cramp" pills without adequate[⑦] relief[⑧]. She has no significant[⑨] medical history, takes no medications regularly, and is not sexually active. Her examination is normal. You assess the problem as primary[⑩] dysmenorrhea[⑪] and prescribe naproxen[⑫注2] to be used on an as-needed basis.

◆ **What are the therapeutic effects of nonsteroidal antiinflammatory drugs (NSAIDs)?**

◆ **What is the mechanism of the antiinflammatory action of NSAIDs?**

ANSWERS TO CASE 28: Nonsteroidal Antiinflammatory Drugs

Summary: A 16-year-old female with dysmenorrhea is prescribed Naprosyn.

- **Effects of NSAIDs**: Antiinflammatory, analgesic, and antipyretic[13].
- **Mechanism of action**: Antiinflammatory effect primarily resulting from inhibition of prostaglandin H synthase (cyclooxygenase); may also involve interference with other mediators of inflammation, modulation of T-cell function, stabilization of lysosomal membranes, and inhibition of chemotaxis[14].

CLINICAL CORRELATION

Nonsteroidal antiinflammatory drugs (NSAIDs) are widely used for acute and chronic conditions that cause pain, injury, inflammation, or fever. They are available over-the-counter and by prescription. The antiinflammatory effect is a result of the inhibition of cyclooxygenase (COX), which converts arachidonic acid to prostaglandins. There are two major subtypes of the COX enzyme, with the COX-2 subtype primarily mediating the pain and inflammation responses in tissues throughout the body. COX-1 has significant activity in producing prostaglandins that appear to protect the gastrointestinal (GI) mucosal lining. **Aspirin irreversibly inactivates both COX-1 and COX-2**, whereas all other **NSAIDs are reversible inhibitors of one or both of these enzymes**. The analgesic effect of these medications is thought to be related to the peripheral[15] inhibition of prostaglandin production, but there may be a central inhibition of pain stimuli as well. The antipyretic effect is thought to involve inhibition of IL-1 and IL-6 induced production of prostaglandins in the hypothalamus affecting the thermoregulatory system, resulting in vasodilation and increased heat loss. NSAIDs are metabolized in the liver and excreted by the kidney. They exhibit cross-sensitivity with each other and with aspirin. All NSAIDs can cause non-dose-related episodes of acute renal failure and nephrotic syndrome. They should be used with caution in those with renal insufficiency or in patients taking other potentially nephrotoxic agents. Aspirin and NSAIDs that nonselectively inhibit both COX-1 and COX-2 commonly produce GI disturbances and ulceration. They are contraindicated in persons with known peptic ulcer disease. Newer agents with higher selectivity for COX-2 inhibition have fewer gastrointestinal side effects and may reduce the rate of NSAID-related gastric ulcers but have been linked to increased risk of cadiovascular disease.

Pharmacology of NSAIDS

Objectives

1. Know the mechanism of action of aspirin and other NSAIDs.

2. Know the therapeutic uses of NSAIDs.
3. Know the adverse effects, toxicities[16], and contraindications to NSAID use.

Definitions

Inflammation: A local response to cellular injury that is marked by capillary dilatation, leukocytic infiltration, redness, heat, pain, and swelling.

Familial adenomatous polyposis (FAP) is a genetic disorder leading to abnormal growths in the colon.

Discussion of Class

(See Case 27 on eicosanoids for a description of the biosynthesis of the prostaglandins and leukotrienes.)

NSAIDs are among the most widely used drugs and are available in various formulations both over-the-counter and by prescription. They are widely used for the relief of pain and fever and to reduce inflammation. There are more than 23 NSAIDs available, and they represent a number of structural classes. Table 28-1 summarizes this class of drugs. They are all small acidic compounds. All are orally active with some pharmacologic differences but they all share the following:

Analgesic activity. Effective against pain of low to moderate intensity. Lower maximal effects compared to opioids[17], but no central nervous system (CNS) liability.

Antiinflammatory activity, which is their chief clinical application. They provide symptomatic relief only.

Antipyretic activity.

Gastric and intestinal ulceration. Two mechanisms include local irritation caused by acidic[18] drug, and inhibition of prostaglandins, which exert a cytoprotective effect.

Table 28-1

CLASSES OF NSAIDS

CARBOXYLIC ACIDS			PYRAZOLONES	OXICAMS
Salicylates	Acetic acids	Proprionic acids	Phenylbutazone	Piroxicam
Acetylsalicyclic acid	Indomethacin	Ibuprofen	Apazone[19]	Meloxicam[20]
Salicyclic acid	Diclofenac	Naproxen		
	Sulindac Tolmetin	Ketoprofen Pranoprofen Miroprofen		

Carboxylic Acids

The salicylates, acetylsalicylic acid (ASA, aspirin) and sodium salicylate have been used for hundreds of years for their analgesic properties. **ASA acts to covalently and irreversibly inhibit both COX-1 and COX-2.** COX-1 becomes acetylated at a serine in the cyclooxygenase active site, rendering the enzyme inactive. COX-2 is also covalently modified but at a different serine residue. This also eliminates cyclooxygenase activity and alters COX-2 to produce 15-HETE. 15-HETE can be further metabolized to a potent antiinflammatory compound, 15-epilipoxin A_4. Some of the antiinflammatory activity of aspirin might be mediated by this metabolite. Inhibition of cyclooxygenase activity of both COX isoforms decreases prostaglandin and thromboxane production but does not effect the production of eicosanoids through the lipoxygenase pathway. Sodium and magnesium salicylate lack the acetyl group that modifies the COXs and are much weaker antiinflammatory agents. Their mechanism of action may be to reduce free radical production that is necessary to activate the cyclooxygenases.

Aspirin can be used to reduce pain, temperature, and inflammation. The antiinflammatory properties make it useful in rheumatoid arthritis, rheumatic fever, and other diseases that produce joint pain.

The **adverse effects of aspirin are dose related. At low doses**, most adverse effects are confined to the **gastrointestinal tract, commonly gastritis.** At **higher** doses patients suffer **"salicylism," tinnitus, vomiting, and vertigo.** Serious aspirin overdose effects the medulla directly and **depresses respiration.**

Acetic and Propionic Acids

Indomethacin, ibuprofen, and naproxen are other important NSAIDs. Although they reduce prostaglandin production by **inhibiting COX-1 and COX-2**, the mechanism of this inhibition is different from aspirin. These drugs are **reversible inhibitors** of the enzyme and appear to act by interfering with the **binding of arachidonate.** All have been approved for rheumatic disorders, osteoarthritis, localized musculoskeletal pain, dysmenorrhea, and headache. All are readily absorbed from the GI tract. Indomethacin is the most potent of these drugs in inhibiting cyclooxygenase. **Indomethacin also has the highest incidence (35%-50%) of adverse effects, most commonly gastrointestinal. Indomethacin** has been found to produce **ulceration of the upper gastrointestinal tract.** Naproxen and ibuprofen are also associated with frequent gastrointestinal adverse effects but are less severe and better tolerated. **All of the NSAIDs can produce renal toxicities including acute renal failure.**

Specific COX-2 Inhibitors

Considerable effort has gone into the development of agents that **specifically inhibit**

COX-2 compared to COX-1. In theory, such agents would be efficacious for **treating inflammatory states but have fewer adverse effects**, especially in the GI tract because COX-1 would still be able to provide cytoprotection. Two clinical trials support this notion but these drugs still produce adverse effects in the GI tract. Additional studies on total mortality and morbidity will be necessary. **These drugs—celecoxib, meloxicam, and valdecoxib—that are specific COX-2 inhibitors** are currently marketed in the United States. They are between 10 and 100 times more specific for COX-2 compared to COX-1 in vivo. A fourth drug, refecoxib, was removed from the US market in 2004 when studies suggested that the drug caused a significant increase in cardiovascular disease and stroke. It is unclear whether all members of this class are associated with this increase in cardiovascular risk. These drugs are useful in treating osteoarthritis, rheumatoid arthritis, dysmenorrhea, acute pain, and pain caused by migraine. **Celecoxib is approved for the treatment of familial adenomatous polyposis (FAP)**. Adverse effects are diminished with COX-2 specific inhibitors, but there are still significant side effects. Rare instances of serious stomach and intestinal bleeding have been reported. Hepatotoxicity and acute renal failure have also occurred. Less serious side effects include dyspepsia, diarrhea, peripheral edema, and dizziness.

Other Agents

Acetaminophen is a non-antiinflammatory analgesic agent. It is about as effective at reducing fever and as an analgesic as aspirin, but it lacks antiinflammatory activity and does not inhibit platelet aggregation. Its mechanism of action is thought to be **inhibition of a COX-1 variant named COX-3** that is expressed in brain and heart. This would account for the CNS effects and the lack of peripheral effects. The most important toxicity of acetaminophen is hepatotoxicity. This is caused by the metabolism of the drug to *N*-acetyl-pbenzoquinoneimine (NAPB), which is usually **eliminated by hepatic conjugation with glutathione**. Toxic levels of acetaminophen deplete glutathione and NAPB accumulates to toxic levels. Other adverse effects include skin rash and mild dyspepsia.

Comprehension Questions

[28.1] Which of the following is the most effective in reducing risk of myocardial infarction?

A. Acetaminophen B. Aspirin C. Celecoxib D. Ibuprofen

[28.2] The advantage of specific cyclooxygenase-2 (COX-2) inhibitors is

A. Decreased gastrointestinal side effects

B. Decreased vasoconstrictor activity

C. Increased antiinflammatory activity

D. Increased inhibition of platelet aggregation

[28. 3] A 26-year-old woman takes a "handful" of acetaminophen in a suicide attempt. At the emergency department, it is determined that she has taken enough to be potentially harmful. Which of the following is the best treatment for this patient?

A. Calcium gluconate B. IgG against acetaminophen

C. N-acetylcysteine D. Penicillamine

Answers

[28. 1] **A.** Aspirin. Because aspirin irreversibly inhibits cyclooxygenase, it effectively eliminates thromboxane production by platelets. It can do this at low doses that do not impair the production of beneficial PGI_2 by endothelial cells.

[28. 2] **A.** In theory, inhibition of COX-2 would reduce inflammation and pain while leaving the cytoprotective actions of COX-1 intact. However, the two enzymes appear to overlap in their functions to a considerable degree.

[28. 3] **C.** Excess acetaminophen is metabolized in the liver via the mixed function oxidase P450 system to a toxic metabolite, NAPB, which has an extremely short half-life and is rapidly conjugated with glutathione, a sulfhydryl donor, and removed from the system. Under conditions of excessive NAPB formation or reduced glutathione stores, NAPB is free to covalently bind to vital proteins and the lipid bilayer of hepatocytes; this results in hepatocellular death and subsequent centrilobular liver necrosis. The antidote for acetaminophen poisoning is *N*-acetyl-L-cysteine (NAC), which prevents the formation and accumulation of NAPB, increases glutathione stores, combines directly with NAPB as a glutathione substitute, and enhances sulfate conjugation.

PHARMACOLOGY PEARLS

- Aspirin is an irreversible inhibitor of both COX-1 and COX-f2.
- Acetaminophen does not have antiinflammatory activity.
- The COX-2 specific antiinflammatory agents may have fewer gastrointestinal side effects.

REFERENCES

Bombardier C, Laine L, Reicin, et al. Comparison of upper gastrointestinal toxicity of rofecoxib and naproxen in patients with rheumatoid arthritis. VIGOR study group. N Engl J Med 2000; 343: 1520-28.

Silverstein FE, Faich G, Goldstein JL, et al. Gastrointestinal toxicity with celecoxib vs nonsteroidal antiinflammatory drugs for osteoarthritis and rheumatoid arthritis: the CLASS study: a randomized controlled trial. Celecoxib long-term arthritis safety study. JAMA 2000; 284: 1247-55.

词汇

1. menstrual[月经的]
2. cramp[绞痛,痉挛]
3. menarche[月经初潮]
4. menses[月经]
5. participate[参加,参与]
6. acetaminophen[对乙酰氨基酚]
7. adequate[足够的]
8. relief[缓解]
9. significant[显著的]
10. primary[主要的]
11. dysmenorrhea[痛经]
12. naproxen[甲氧萘丙酸,萘普生]
13. antipyretic[解热药,退热药]
14. chemotaxis[趋化性的]
15. peripheral[周围的,外用的,末梢的]
16. toxicities[毒力,毒性]
17. opioids[类鸦片的]
18. acidic[酸性的]
19. apazone[阿扎丙宗]
20. meloxicam[美洛昔康]

注 1

对乙酰氨基酚又名扑热息痛，是非甾体抗炎药苯胺类，是非那西丁的体内代谢产物。在体内几乎无抗炎作用，临床上用来缓解发热、镇痛。

注 2

萘普生与布洛芬是同类药，是芳香丙酸类的解热镇痛抗炎药，特点：具有较好的抗炎，解热及镇痛作用，被广泛地应用于治疗风湿性关节炎和骨关节炎。其不良反应是胃肠道反应，但程度较轻，易于耐受。

点评

本病例患者是16岁年轻女性，13岁初潮，每次持续4~5天，月经周期28天，表明该女性生理正常，但月经前3天疼痛剧烈，以致影响正常的日常学习和生活，如不能正常上课和参加学校的体育活动。这时的痛经称为原发性痛经，如果妇科检查没有发现任何问题，就只能对症处理，常规镇痛药如阿托品、颠茄片等药物解痉。待其生育后会得到缓解。相反，如果并不是从初潮时就开始疼痛，而是后来才开始的，这时就称为继发性痛经，这时就有必要进行系统的妇科检查，明确是否有子宫内膜移位症或子宫腺瘤病。从而根据病情进行药物或手术治疗。

近年来的研究证明，子宫内膜与血内前列腺素含量的增高、游离钙离子增加、子宫肌纤维痉挛性收缩是原发性痛经发病的三个环节。那么抑制前列腺素的合成、阻止游离钙的增加、抑制子宫平滑肌过度收缩的药物都可以用于痛经的治疗。常用药物为：消炎痛，每次 25 毫克，每日 2 ~ 3 次口服；甲氯灭酸，每次 250 毫克，每日 3 次；乙酰水杨酸(阿司匹林)，每次 0.3 ~ 0.6 克，每日 3 次口服等。另外，一直沿用的止痛经药物还有阿托品、黄体酮等。上述药物可于疼痛开始时服用，疼痛缓解后可停药。抗前列腺素药物有胃肠道反应，严重时可引起消化道出血，故有溃疡病者慎用。

魏敏杰

CASE 29

A 58-year-old man presents for follow-up of gout. He has had multiple episodes[①] of gouty[②] arthritis[③], primarily in the great toe. Each episode has been successfully treated with oral antiinflammatory[④] medications[⑤]. He takes no medications regularly and has a normal examination today. [注1] Laboratory[⑥] studies following his last episode showed an elevated uric acid level and normal renal function. A 24-hour urine collection showed normal excretion of uric acid. [注2] You prescribe allopurinol to be taken daily in an effort to lower his uric acid level and prevent recurrent gout episodes. [注3]

- **Which medications are used for the treatment of acute gout?**
- **Which medications are used for the treatment of chronic gout?**
- **What is the mechanism of action of allopurinol?**

ANSWERS TO CASE 29: Medications Used for Gout

Summary: A 58-year-old man with hyperuricemia and recurrent gout is prescribed allopurinol.

- **Drugs for the treatment of acute gout**: nonsteroidal antiinflamatories (NSAIDs), colchicine, corticosteroids.
- **Drugs for the treatment of recurrent gout**: Probenecid, sulfinpyrazone, allopurinol.
- **Mechanism of action of allopurinol**[7]: Inhibition of xanthine[8] oxidase, an enzyme that converts hypoxanthine to xanthine and xanthine to uric acid.

CLINICAL CORRELATION

Allopurinol is the only medication used in clinical practice to **lower uric acid production**. Uric acid is the end product of purine metabolism. The **enzyme xanthine oxidase converts hypoxanthine to xanthine and xanthine to uric acid**. Allopurinol and its metabolite, alloxanthine, inhibit the synthesis of uric acid by inhibiting xanthine oxidase. Allopurinol may precipitate acute gout when therapy is initiated. Colchicine may be coadministered for the first week of allopurinol therapy to try to reduce the risk of an acute gout flare. Its primary side effects are gastrointestinal (GI) disturbance and rash. There is a very rare, but potentially life-threatening, hypersensitivity reaction that may cause fever, bone marrow[9] suppression, hepatic dysfunction, and renal failure.

Medications for Gout

Objectives

1. Know the primary drugs used for gout and their mechanisms of action.
2. Know the adverse effects and contraindications to their usage.

Definitions

Prophylactic: Prevention of a disease or adverse event.

Gout: Condition of painful deposits of urate crystals[10] in the joints and other parts of the body such as the ear pinna[11].

PHARMACOLOGY OF CLASS

Allopurinol is a prophylactic drug that reduces the biosynthesis of uric acid. In this manner, **serum uric acid levels are typically reduced**, and the formation of **inflammatory tophi within joints is reduced**. It is a useful **long-term therapy** for patients with chronic gouty arthritis. It is also indicated for the **treatment of hyperuricemia secondary to**

blood dyscrasias. Allopurinol can be used to **prevent the progression of uric acid nephropathy**, and for the prophylaxis of both uric acid and calcium oxalate renal stone formation that is typically associated with hyperuricemia. Allopurinol is useful in patients with **recurrent renal stones** or with renal impairment or those that do not respond to probenecid. Patients treated with allopurinol should have adequate renal secretion of uric acid. **Adverse effects include nausea, vomiting, and diarrhea and an allergic skin reaction is reported in 3 percent of patients**. On initial use of allopurinol, uric acid is mobilized from tissues and joints and this may **precipitate an acute gouty attack**.

Structure

Allopurinol is a structural analog of xanthine.

Mechanism of Action

Allopurinol inhibits xanthine oxidase (Figure 29-1) and reduces the biosynthesis of urate. Allopurinol is metabolized to alloxanthine by xanthine oxidase and this metabolite inhibits two steps in the conversion of purines to uric acid.

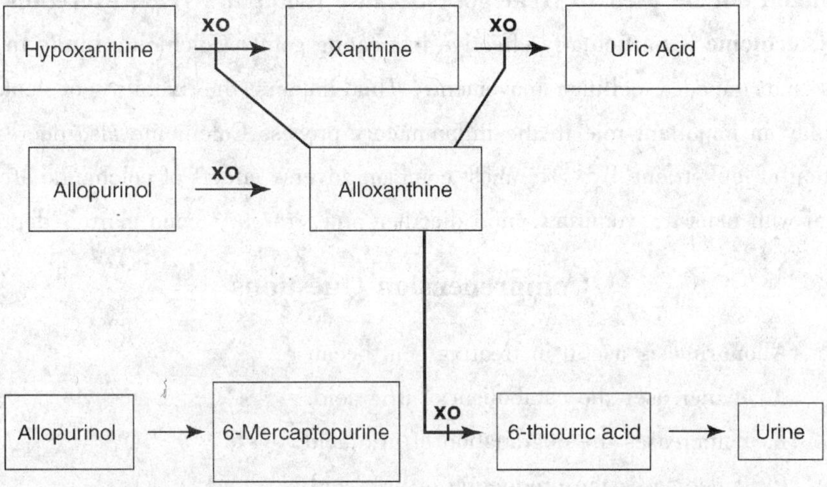

Figure 29-1. Uric acid pathway. XO = xanthine oxidase, which is blocked by alloxanthine, a metabolite of allopurinol.

Allopurinol also increases the reutilization of xanthine and hypoxanthine via hypoxanthine guanine phosphoribosyltransferase (HGPRT) to increase for nucleic acid and nucleotide synthesis. This causes a negative feedback that decreases de novo purine[12] biosynthesis. These actions decrease both serum and urine uric acid.

Administration

Allopurinol has good oral bioavailability and its half-life, 1-3 hours and the half-life of its active metabolite alloxanthine, 12-30 hours, permits once-a-day dosing.

Pharmacokinetics

A significant reduction on serum uric acid concentration usually requires 2-3 days, and the reduction of serum urate to normal levels may take 1-3 weeks. About 80 percent of allopurinol is eliminated by the kidney as alloxanthine and the remainder is eliminated in the feces.

Other Drugs Used to Treat Gout

Allopurinol is useful in managing gout in patients with normal levels of uric acid excretion. In those patients with gout secondary to impaired renal excretion of uric acid (see Case 8), **probenecid or sulfinpyrazone** is more effective. These **drugs block renal reabsorption of uric acid and thereby increase excretion.**

The pain associated with acute attacks of gout are typically treated with NSAIDs or **colchicine**. Virtually all NSAIDs have been used successfully to treat the pain associated with gout, but **indomethacin remains the most frequently used. Aspirin should not be used to treat gout because it impairs renal excretion of uric acid. Colchicine** is particularly effective in treating gout. Colchicine **binds to microtubules** and impedes cellular movement. This impairs the mobility of leukocytes, which play an important role in the inflammatory process Colchicine also decreases the production of leukotriene B_4. The most common adverse effects of colchicine are gastrointestinal with nausea, vomiting, and diarrhea and, rarely, bone marrow depression.

Comprehension Questions

[29.1] Allopurinol is useful in treating gout because

A. It increases the catabolism of uric acid.

B. It increases the degradation of uric acid.

C. It decreases the production of uric acid.

D. It increases renal excretion of uric acid.

[29.2] Colchicine is especially useful in treating an acute attack of gout because it

A. Decreases uric acid deposition

B. Is potent antiinflammatory agent

C. Impairs leukocyte migration

D. Increases the solubility of uric acid

[29.3] A 44-year-old man is suffering from recurrent gouty arthritis. His serum uric acid level is elevated, and you prescribe allopurinol. Within 1 week of the allopurinol, he develops a painful episode that "feels like gout." Which of the following is the best explanation?

A. The patient is resistant to the allopurinol and should be placed on another medication.

B. The patient likely has an arthritis syndrome produced by allopurinol and should have an antinuclear antibody(ANA)drawn.

C. The patient likely developed acute gout as a result of mobilization of the urate from joints and tissue.

D. This likely represents a drug-drug interaction, and so the allopurinol should be discontinued.

Answers

[29.1] **C.** The mechanism of action of allopurinol is to decrease the production of uric acid.

[29.2] **C.** Impairing leukocyte migration reduces the inflammation associated with a gouty attack.

[29.3] **C.** The patient likely developed an acute episode of gout as a result of the mobilization of urate from joints and tissue, a phenomenon commonly seen with initiation of allopurinol.

PHARMACOLOGY PEARLS

❖ Allopurinol can precipitate an acute gouty attack. Initial therapy should be combined with an NSAID or colchicine to avoid this effect.

❖ Uric acid is the end product of purine metabolism.

❖ Allopurinol lowers uric acid production, by inhibiting the enzyme xanthine oxidase which converts hypoxanthine to xanthine and xanthine to uric acid.

REFERENCES

Ettinger B, Tang A, Citron JT. Randomized trial of allopurinol in the prevention of calcium oxalate calculi. N Engl J Med 1986; 315: 1386-9.

Bomalaski JS, Clark MA. Serum uric acid-lowering therapies: where are we heading in management of hyperuricemia and the potential role of uricase. Curr Rheumatol Rep 2004; 6: 240-7.

词汇

1. episode[发作]
2. gout[痛风]
3. arthritis[关节炎]
4. antiinflammatory[抗炎药]

5. medication［药物治疗］
6. laboratory［实验室］
7. allopurinol［别嘌呤醇］
8. xantihine［黄嘌呤］
9. marrow［髓,骨髓］
10. crystals［晶体,结晶］
11. pinna［耳部,耳廓］
12. purine［嘌呤］

注 1

痛风是一种与生活密切相关的代谢性疾病，与饮食习惯有关，常因为高嘌呤食物的过量摄入，导致嘌呤代谢紊乱，是痛风发病的主要原因。

注 2

痛风患者的实验室检查包括有血尿酸、尿尿酸的检测，在受累关节 X 线摄片检查 ，必要时作肾 B 超探测，肾功能等检查。其中血和尿中的尿酸水平升高，是痛风的实验室诊断指标之一。

注 3

痛风的治疗临床上使用别嘌呤醇为首选治疗药物。别嘌呤醇能够降低血中尿酸浓度，纠正高尿酸血症，缓解关节疼痛。

点评

痛风是一种与生活密切相关的代谢性疾病，其发病原因是血液中尿酸浓度过高，形成尿酸结晶沉积在组织中。如沉积在关节就会引起关节炎，沉积在肾脏就会导致肾结石。本例中关节炎是主要临床表现。大多数痛风患者最早出现的症状是急性痛风性关节炎。急性痛风性关节炎大多发生于下肢小关节，特别是第一趾跖关节。而且，常在夜间突然发病，患处关节局部红肿、剧烈疼痛，对温度、触摸、震动极为敏感。痛风发病急骤，消退也快，可在一周左右自行缓解。由于这种关节炎不是由细菌感染引起，所以一般不伴有发烧，使用抗生素治疗无效。痛风易复发，反复发作后，可累及多个关节，并导致关节畸形，还可引起严重的肾功能损害。少数患者以肾结石起病，可有腰痛、血尿等症状。临床上实验室检查尿酸水平升高，是痛风的实验室指标之一，应用别嘌呤醇是治疗药物首选。

本病例痛风反复发作，尿酸水平升高，肾功能正常，临床上使用别嘌呤醇能够降低血中尿酸浓度，纠正高尿酸血症，缓解关节疼痛。另外，临床上还可以应用丙磺舒和秋水仙碱对痛风进行治疗。

魏敏杰

❖ CASE 30

A 40-year-old woman has had rheumatoid[1] arthritis[2] for 5 years. She has been on multiple[3] NSAIDs[4注1] with some symptomatic[5] relief[6]. On a few occasions she has taken corticosteroids[7] for severe exacerbations[8]. She feels that her disease is getting worse. She has more stiffness[9] and swelling[10] in her wrists and hands. She is currently taking the maximum recommended[11] dosage of ibuprofen[12], but admits to taking more than she should on bad days. On examination you note active synovitis[13] of both wrists and all of her metacarpo-phalangeal joints[14]. There is subtle[15] ulnar deviation[16注2] of all of her fingers. She has several firm, subcutaneous nodules[17] on her arms. You assess[18] her as having an acute exacerbation of rheumatoid arthritis, along with overall worsening of the disease. You prescribe[19] a short course of oral corticosteroids and start her on methotrexate[20].

◆ **What is the mechanism of immune suppression mediated by glucocorticoids?**

◆ **What is the mechanism of action of methotrexate?**

ANSWERS TO CASE 30: Agents Used to Treat Rheumatoid Arthritis

Summary: A 40-year-old woman with worsening rheumatoid arthritis(RA) is prescribed corticosteroids and methotrexate.

- **Mechanism of immune suppression by glucocorticoids**: Interference with cell cycle of activated lymphoid cells and activation of apoptosis in some lymphoid lines.
- **Mechanism of action of methotrexate**: Inhibition of deoxyribonucleic acid (DNA) synthesis by inhibition of dihydrofolate reductase. Inhibits replication and function of T cells and possibly B cells.

CLINICAL CORRELATION

Rheumatoid arthritis(RA) is an autoimmune disorder in which the body's immune system attacks its own synovium. This causes joint stiffness, swelling and, if unchecked, joint destruction and disfigurement. Several immunosuppressive agents have been used with success in the treatment of RA. Glucocorticoids are used both for their antiinflammatory effect and their immunosuppressive effects. They are thought to interfere with the cell cycle of activated lymphoid cells and may activate apoptosis in some lymphoid lines. Its long-term use is limited by multiple side effects and toxicities, including induction of a Cushingoid syndrome, glucose intolerance, and reduction in bone density. Methotrexate is a cancer chemotherapeutic agent that also has immunosuppressive effects. It is a folate analog that interferes with DNA synthesis by inhibition of the dihydrofolate reductase enzyme. Its immunosuppressive effect is mediated through its inhibition of the replication and function of T, and possibly B, lymphocytes. Methotrexate can cause hepatotoxicity[21], bone marrow suppression and severe gastrointestinal side effects.

Pharmacology of Agents Used in Rheumatoid Arthritis

Objectives

1. Know the agents used for RA and their mechanisms of action.
2. Know the toxicities and adverse effects of agents used for RA.

Definitions

Rheumatoid arthritis: Chronic disease that is characterized especially by pain, stiffness, inflammation, swelling, and sometimes destruction of joints.

Osteoarthritis[22]: Arthritis characterized by degenerative and sometimes hypertrophic changes in the bone and cartilage of one or more joints and a progressive wearing down of apposing joint surfaces with consequent distortion of joint position usually without bony stiffening.

Discussion of Class

Rheumatoid arthritis is caused by an **inappropriate immune response** that results in **chronic inflammation in and around joints**. The chronic inflammatory process includes the production of a number of **cytokines and inflammatory mediators** that cause **destruction of cartilage within the joint**. Pharmacologic treatment of rheumatoid arthritis includes **treatment of the acute pain**, **treatment of the inflammation**, **and inhibition of the immune system.**

Glucocorticoids such as prednisolone or cortisone are potent antiinflammatory agents and are also **immunosuppressive**. Glucocorticoids may be administered orally or injected into an affected area. Drugs with an **11-keto group** on the steroid nucleus (cortisone or prednisone) are converted to **11-hydroxyl group** in the liver (to give cortisol and prednisolone). Other synthetic corticosteroids include dexamethasone, betamethasone and triamcinolone. Various chemical substitutions within these drugs decrease first-pass inactivation by the liver, decrease binding to plasma proteins such as corticosteroidbinding globulin (CBG), and increase the affinity of the drug for its receptor. The actions of glucocorticoids are mediated by a **specific nuclear receptor**, **the glucocorticoid receptor** (**GR**). Receptor activation occurs on drug binding, which ultimately leads to increased or decreased transcription of specific genes. The **antiinflammatory action of the glucocorticoids** is a result, in part, of **induction of marocortin**, which is a **specific inhibitor of phospholipase A_2**. This **decreases the production of prostaglandins**. In addition, the production of a number of cytokines including IL-1, IL-2, IL-6, and TNF-α, are decreased by glucocorticoids. This is caused in part by the induction of apoptosis in lymphocytes and leukocytes. Thus the antiinflammatory and immunosuppressive actions of the glucocorticoids are closely linked. Glucocorticoids are potent inhibitors of cell-mediated immunity but have little effect on humoral immunity.

Glucocorticoids are useful in the management of inflammation in RA, bursitis, lupus erythematosus, nephrotic syndrome, and ulcerative colitis. Glucocorticoids are also used to treat hypersensitivity reactions and allergic reactions and to reduce organ or graft rejection.

The use of **glucocorticoids** is limited by a number of **adverse effects**. Most of these adverse effects are predicable as exaggerated physiological effects. **Suppression of the pituitary-adrenal axis**, **hyperglycemia**, **increased protein metabolism**, **altered fat metabolism**, **and increased salt retention** (**a mineralocorticoid effect**) are frequently seen. **Osteoporosis and peptic ulcers** can be induced by glucocorticoids, and increased susceptibility to **infections** and **poor wound healing** also occur.

Methotrexate is a **folate analog that inhibits dihydrofolate reductase**. This enzyme is responsible for the production of tetrahydrofolate cofactors necessary for purine and thymidylate biosynthesis. Inhibition of the enzyme leads to impaired DNA synthesis, which has the greatest impact on rapidly dividing cells. Methotrexate is **immunosuppressive**, and this activity has led to its use in rheumatoid arthritis, psoriasis, and other autoimmune disorders. Its use as an **anticancer agent** includes childhood acute lymphoblastic leukemia, lymphoma, and osteogenic sarcoma. Serious adverse effects associated with methotrexate include **myelosuppression**, producing severe leukopenia, bone marrow aplasia, and thrombocytopenia. **Gastrointestinal effects** are common with nausea and vomiting, as well as mouth sores or ulcers. Hepatotoxicity, including acute elevations in transaminase levels, fibrosis, and cirrhosis, has been reported. Pulmonary effects include a nonproductive cough and pneumonitis. Methotrexate is a teratogen and is contraindicated in pregnancy.

More disease-specific approaches in treating RA have led to the development of the **disease modifying agents for rheumatoid disease** (**DMARDs**).

Recent evidence supports a central role of **tumor necrosis factor alpha** (TNF-α) in the pathogenesis of rheumatoid arthritis. **TNF-α appears responsible for much of the tissue injury in the disease**. Based on these observations, two new classes of drugs have been developed that specifically target the TNF pathway. One class of drugs is **antibodies specific for human TNF-α**. These antibodies interact with TNF-α and block its ability to interact with TNF-α receptors. **Infliximab** is a chimeric antibody containing a human constant region and murine variable regions. It is administered by infusion approximately once every 8 weeks. Infliximab is also indicated in refractory luminal and fistulizing Crohn disease. **Adalimumab** is a similar, fully human anti-TNF-α antibody that is self-injected twice weekly. **Etanercept** is a fusion protein created by combining the ligand binding portion of the human TNF-α receptor with the Fc portion of IgG. The protein acts to bind TNF-α and blocks the association of TNF with its receptor. It is self-injected 4 times a week. These drugs have proven very effective in patients with RA, and disease progression has been markedly diminished and even reversed in some instances. TNF-α also plays an important role in the body's immune responses, especially to infectious agents.

One of the **most serious adverse effects seen with the anti-TNF antibody preparations are severe infections such as tuberculosis**. These drugs should not be administered to patients who have any sign of infection. An increased risk of malignancy has also been reported in patients treated with the anti-TNF antibodies. **Neurological problems** including dizziness, visual disturbances, and peripheral weakness have also been reported. The adverse effect profile of etanercept is similar with serious infections, neurological disturbances and a high frequency, 20-30 percent, of injection site reactions.

Other Agents Used to Treat Rheumatoid Arthritis

Azathioprine is a **cytotoxic agent that suppresses T-cell activity** to a greater extent than B-cell activity. It is an orally active agent that is metabolized to mercaptopurine, which is also **immunosuppressive**. It is used alone or in combination with corticosteroids in the treatment of rheumatoid arthritis and other autoimmune disorders such as lupus erythematosus. Adverse effects include bone marrow suppression, leukopenia, and, less frequently, anemia.

Cyclophosphamide is an alkylating agent developed as an anticancer drug. It **suppresses B-cell function** more than T-cell function. It has been used to treat a number of autoimmune disorders including Wegener's granulomatosis, RA, and nephrotic syndrome in children. Its anticancer uses include nonHodgkin's lymphoma and Burkitt lymphoma. Myelosuppression, nausea and vomiting, and alopecia are common adverse reactions.

Gold salts have been used to treat patients with progressive RA who have not obtained relief from NSAIDs. Use of gold salts has diminished with the introduction of the DMARDs discussed above. Gold has a **high affinity for sulfur**, and most preparations contain gold attached to a sulfur atom. Aurothioglucose, gold sodium thiomalate and auranofin all contain a gold atom attached to a sulfur moiety. Gold preparations are injected IM and reach peak concentrations in 2-6 hours. Gold accumulates in organs that are rich in phagocytes and in the lysosomes of synovial cells. **Gold salts decrease the migration and the activity of macrophages**, but its precise mechanism of action is unclear. Gold salts do not have antiinflammatory activity. The **most common adverse effect** of gold salts are **skin lesions and ulceration in mucus membranes**. Impaired **renal function** and **blood dyscrasias** are also seen in about 10 percent of patients treated with gold salts.

Comprehension Questions

[30.1] Infliximab is effective in rheumatoid arthritis because it

A. Binds to TNF-α and sequesters it from receptors

B. Is a TNF-α receptor agonist

C. Is a TNF-α receptor antagonist

D. Is a synovium-specific antiinflammatory agent

[30.2] The immunosuppressive effect of methotrexate is a result of its inhibition of

A. Dihydrofolate reductase B. Leukocyte migration
C. Microtubule function D. Phospholipase A_2

[30. 3] A 55-year-old woman is being treated for RA. Her disease has become much worse, and a new medication is added. After 6 months, she notes night sweats, weight loss, chronic cough, and a chest radiograph that indicates a cavitary lesion. Which of the following medications was most likely prescribed for the RA?

A. Gold salts B. Infliximab C. Methotrexate D. Naprosyn

Answers

[30. 1] **A.** The anti-TNF-α antibodies bind to TNF-α and prevent its association with receptors. They are not direct receptor antagonists.

[30. 2] **A.** Methotrexate inhibits dihydrofolate reductase, which impairs rapidly dividing cells such as lymphocytes and leukocytes.

[30. 3] **B.** The anti-TNF-α immunoglobulin agents are usually well tolerated and modify the disease process of RA; however, they tend to predispose patients to infections, particularly tuberculosis. The patient in the question has a typical clinical presentation of tuberculosis. Diagnosis would be confirmed by sputum culture and acid fast smear, and therapy started with multiple antituberculosis agents.

PHARMACOLOGY PEARLS

- ❖ DMARDS, specifically the anti-TNF-α agents, stop the progression of rheumatoid arthritis and may induce remission.
- ❖ Methotrexate is a folate analog that inhibits dihydrofolate reductase and acts as an immunosuppressive agent.
- ❖ Glucocorticoid agents act as immunosuppressive agents and antiinflammatory agents but have numerous adverse effects.

REFERENCES

Gossec L, Dougados M. Combination therapy in early rheumatoid arthritis. Clin Exp Rheumatol 2003; 21(5 suppl 31): S174-8.

Toussirot E, Wendling D. The use of TNF-alpha blocking agents in rheumatoid arthritis: an overview. Expert Opin Pharmacother 2004; 5: 581-94.

词汇

1. rheumatoid[风湿样的,患风湿症的,似风湿症的]
2. arthritis[关节炎]
3. multiple[多样的,复杂的]
4. nonsteroidal anti-inflammatory drugs(NSAIDs)[非甾体类抗炎药]
5. symptomatic[症状的,征兆的]
6. relief[减轻,缓解]
7. corticosteroid[(肾上腺)皮质类固醇]
8. exacerbation[加重,恶化]
9. stiffness[四肢强直,僵硬]
10. swelling[肿胀,增大]
11. recommended[介绍,推荐]
12. ibuprofen[布洛芬]
13. synovitis[滑膜炎,关节膜炎]
14. metacarpo-phalangeal joint[掌指关节]
15. subtle[微细的,精细的,敏锐的]
16. ulnar deviation[尺骨偏斜,尺侧偏差]
17. subcutaneous nodule[皮下小结]
18. assess[评价,估计]
19. prescribe[开药方,开处方]
20. methotrexate[甲氨蝶呤]
21. hepatotoxicity[肝毒性]
22. osteoarthritis[骨关节炎,骨性关节炎]

注 1

化学结构上没有甾体结构，其最大的作用是抗炎，能够缓解红肿热痛等炎性症状，改善某些肌肉骨骼关节功能。这类药物一经吸收入血，会很快发挥药效，对慢性疾病用数周即有作用，但停药将使原有症状迅速恶化。第二个作用是镇痛，适用于轻中度疼痛。第三个作用是退热，该药可以使过高的体温下降，对正常体温影响甚微。第四个作用是抑制血小板凝集。

注 2

由于关节滑囊的慢性炎症，导致血管翳的形成，进而侵犯关节软骨、软骨下骨、韧带和肌腱等，造成关节软骨、骨和关节囊破坏，最终导致关节畸形和功能丧失。最为常见的关节畸形是腕和肘关节强直、掌关节半脱位、手指向尺侧偏斜和呈“无鹅颈”样及钮孔花样表现。非甾体类抗炎药能够减轻该症状，但不能改变病程和预防关节破坏，需与肾上腺皮质激素类药物联用。

点评

本病例具有典型的类风湿性关节炎病史，患者目前出现十指尺侧偏斜，并且双上肢可触及数个坚硬的皮下结节，因此考虑该患属于类风湿性关节炎急性加重。患者有长期服用非甾体抗炎药物史。过度疲劳、营养不良、精神抑郁均可能是病情加重的原因。目前患者已经服用最大推荐剂量的布洛芬，甚至比此剂量更大，但并没有阻止病情恶化，因此再继续服用非甾体抗炎药已起不到治疗效果。对于该患者可先进行血象(有正细胞正色素性贫血，淋巴细胞及血小板增多为活动期表现,血沉加快,嗜酸性细胞增多是类风湿性关节炎伴严重全身性并发症的象征）、X 线检查（关节 X 线片可见到关节面模糊，有侵蚀性损害，在疾病早期近关节处骨质疏松，软组织肿胀，骨质有侵蚀现象，晚期关节软骨坏死，可使关节间隙变狭窄及纤维化）。然后根据患者的具体情况，可以先给予短期的激素（长期应用可导致严重副作用，因此不作为常规治疗，只有经 NSAIDs，青霉胺等治疗效果不好，症状重，影响日常生活，才可应用皮质类固醇，症状控制后逐步减量至最小维持量）治疗，待病情稳定后开始给予氨甲蝶呤（有免疫抑制与抗炎作用，可降血沉，改善骨侵蚀，每周 5 ~ 15mg 肌注或口服，3 个月为一疗程）治疗。

魏敏杰

❖ CASE 31

A 67-year-old woman is receiving chemotherapy for metastatic ovarian cancer[①]. She is on her fourth cycle of a multidrug regimen[②], including cisplatin[注1] and doxorubicin. She has developed nausea and vomiting,[注2] among other side effects. You decide to premedicate her with IV ondansetron prior to her next dose of chemotherapy and provide oral ondansetron for home use as well.

◆ **What is the mechanism of action of ondansetron?**

◆ **What are the common side effects associated with ondansetron?**

ANSWERS TO CASE 31: Antiemetics

Summary: A 67-year-old woman has chemotherapy-induced nausea and vomiting and is prescribed ondanestron.

◆ **Mechanism of action of ondansetron**: Serotonin ($5\text{-}HT_3$) receptor antagonist in the central nervous system (CNS) and gastrointestinal (GI) tract.

◆ **Side effects of ondansetron**: Headache, diarrhea, dizziness, agitation.

CLINICAL CORRELATION

Nausea and vomiting are frequent side effects of cancer chemotherapy. Control of these symptoms is an important adjunct to chemotherapy. Several agents with varied mechanisms of action are available. The serotonin ($5\text{-}HT_3$) receptor system in the CNS and GI tract is felt to be a major trigger of chemotherapyinduced nausea and vomiting. Ondansetron and granisetron are specific $5\text{-}HT_3$ receptor antagonists that are widely used for the treatment of this problem. Granisetron has a higher receptor affinity, is longer acting, and is more potent than ondansetron. Both drugs can be administered intravenously or orally. Metoclopramide[3], which is primarily a dopamine antagonist, will also antagonize the $5\text{-}HT_3$ receptor when given in high doses. Metoclopramide also blocks receptors in the chemoreceptor trigger zone in the brain that contribute to nausea. Metoclopramide sensitizes the GI tract to acetylcholine[4] activity, which increases GI motility and gastric emptying. It is somewhat less effective for chemotherapy-induced vomiting than ondansetron or granisetron and has the potential for extrapyramidal side effects[5] that are seen with dopamine antagonists.

Pharmacology of Antiemetic Agents

Objectives

1. List the therapeutic uses of antiemetic[6] medications.
2. Describe the mechanism of action of the antiemetic medications.
3. Describe the adverse effects of the antiemetic medications.

Definitions

Emesis: vomiting; a complex reflex that results in emptying of the contents of the small intestine and stomach.

Discussion of Class

Vomiting is a **complex reflex** controlled by the **vomiting center** in the **lateral reticu-**

lar formation of the medulla. The vomiting center has **five primary afferents** (see Figure 31-1):

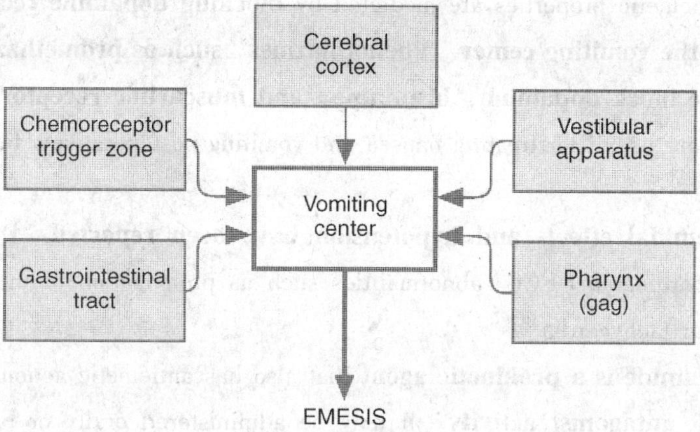

Figure 31-1. Primary afferent components to the vomiting center.

1. The **chemoreceptor trigger zone** (CTZ)[7] is located outside the blood-brain barrier and is exposed to blood-borne and cerebrospinal fluid emetogenic chemicals. Primary receptors associated with emesis are dopamine D_2, 5-HT_3, and opioid receptors.
2. The **vestibular apparatus**[8] is located in the inner ear, sending afferents pertaining to motion. Primary receptors are histamine H_1 and muscarinic cholinoreceptors[9].
3. The **pharynx** via the vagus nerve sends afferents of the gag reflex.
4. **Enteric affrents arise** from the gastrointestinal tract. 5-HT_3 receptors play an important role in these signals.
5. **Cerebral cortical afferents** with information such as stress, anticipation, psychiatric disorders[10].

Current antiemetic therapy blocks one or more of these afferents to reduce the activity in the vomiting center.

Serotonin 5-HT_3 Antagonists

Selective 5-HT_3 antagonists are potent antiemetic agents for emetogenic signals arising in the gastrointestinal tract and from the CTZ. These agents are especially useful for nausea from **chemotherapeutic agents and for postoperative or postradiation** induced vomiting. 5-HT_3 antagonists are not useful for motion sickness or nausea of vertigo[11]. Three agents are currently available: **ondansetron, granisetron, and dolasetron**. They are all administered either orally or intravenously, and are most effective if given 30 minutes prior to chemo-or radiotherapy. Oral agents may be administered once or twice daily.

Dopamine Antagonists

Droperidol is an **antipsychotic**[12] **butyrophenone** that has significant antiemetic actions. Its antiemetic properties are mediated by **blocking dopamine receptors in the CTZ and in the vomiting center**. **Phenothiazines**[13] **such as promethazine and prochlorperazine block dopamine, histamine, and muscarinic receptors** in the same regions. All are useful for treating nausea and vomiting postoperatively but are very sedating.

Extrapyramidal effects and hypotension have been reported. Droperidol may cause electrocardiogram (ECG) abnormalities such as prolongation of the Q-T interval and ventricular tachycardia[14].

Metoclopramide is a prokinetic agent that also has antiemetic actions based on its **dopaminergic antagonist activity**. It may be administered orally or parenterally for nausea following chemotherapy or for postoperative nausea. As with the other dopamine antagonists, side effects are rare but may include ex**trapyramidal**: **dystonias**[15] **and Parkinson syndrome** may appear days to months after treatment.

Corticosteroids

Glucocorticoids such as dexamethasone and prednisolone are used to treat nausea and vomiting associated with **chemotherapy**. They are most frequently used in combination with other antiemetics. The molecular basis for the antiemetic action of glucocorticoids is not understood.

Antihistamines

First-generation antihistamines such as cyclizine, diphenhydramine, and dimenhydrinate are useful to treat nausea associated with motion sickness and vertigo. They are **able to penetrate the blood-brain barrier** and their action is most likely to decrease afferents from the vestibular apparatus. The most common adverse effect of these agents is sedation.

Anticholinergic Agents

Scopolamine is the most effective agent for treating nausea associated with **motion sickness or vertigo**. It is **not effective for nausea of chemotherapy**. It is administered via a **transdermal patch** that delivers drug at a uniform rate for up to 72 hours. By avoiding the peak levels associated with oral administration, incidence of side effects is also reduced. **Scopolamine reduces afferents from the vestibular apparatus** and **decreases the excitability of the labyrinthine receptors**. Side effects, typical of antimuscarinic agents, include **dry mouth**, **blurred vision**, **and drowsiness**. It should **not be used in patients with glaucoma or prostatic hypertrophy**[16].

Other Agents Used for Antiemesis

Benzodiazepines such as lorazepam or diazepam may be used **prior to chemo-or radiotherapy** to reduce the frequency and severity of anticipatory vomiting that occurs in patients who undergo multiple rounds of anticancer therapy. **Dronabinol** is Δ^9-tetrahydrocannabinol, the major active ingredient in marijuana. It is an orally active agent that has been used to stimulate appetite and as an antiemetic. The mechanism of these activities is not known. It is frequently administered in conjunction with a phenothiazine, which reduces the adverse effects of both agents while producing a synergistic antiemetic effect. Adverse effects include euphoria, sedation, dry mouth, and hallucinations[17].

Comprehension Questions

[31.1] Droperidol is effective in reducing nausea because it

A. Blocks acetylcholine receptors in the periphery

B. Blocks dopamine receptors in the CTZ

C. Blocks glucocorticoid receptors in the vomiting center

D. Blocks 5-HT_2 receptors in the CTZ

[31.2] A patient undergoing chemotherapy with cisplatin has severe nausea. Which of the following would be the drug to use in this patient?

A. Cyclizine B. Naloxone C. Ondansetron D. Scopolamine

[31.3] A fisherman uses a transdermal scopdamine patch to assist with the nausea associated with being on a boat. What is the most likely side effect he will experience?

A. Acute dystonic reaction B. Euphoria

C. Sedation D. Tremor

Answers

[31.1] **B.** Droperidol is a dopamine receptor antagonist that diminishes the activity of the CTZ. It is effective in reducing nausea associated with chemotherapy or radiotherapy.

[31.2] **C.** Ondansetron is a serotonin 5HT_3 receptor antagonist with fewer side effects and greater effectiveness than the other agents in treating patients on chemotherapy.

[31.3] **C.** Sedation is the most common side effect associated with scopolamine patches as a result of stimulation of the muscarinic cholinoreceptor.

PHARMACOLOGY PEARLS

- ❖ The scopolamine patch is one of the most effective methods to treat motion-sickness.
- ❖ Dopaminergic agents such as droperidol and promethazine can lead to extrapyramidal side effects.
- ❖ The selective 5-HT_3 antagonists are potent antiemetic agents for chemotherapy but are not effective for motion sickness.

REFERENCES

Gralla, RJ. New agents, new treatment, and antiemetic therapy. Semin Oncol 2002; 29(suppl 2): 119-24.

Habib AS, Gan TJ. Evidence-based management of postoperative nausea and vomiting: a review. Can J Anaesth 2004; 51: 326-41.

词汇

1. metastatic ovarian cancer[转移性卵巢癌]
2. multidrug regimen[联合用药方案]
3. metoclopramide[甲氧氯普胺]
4. acetylcholine[乙酰胆碱]
5. extrapyramidal side effects[锥体外系副作用]
6. antiemetic[止吐药]
7. chemoreceptor trigger zone(CTZ)[化学受体激发区]
8. vestibular apparatus[前庭器官]
9. muscarinic cholinoreceptor[毒蕈碱受体]
10. psychiatric disorder[精神障碍]
11. vertigo[眩晕]
12. antipsychotic[抗精神病药物]
13. phenothiazine[吩噻嗪类]
14. ventricular tachycardia[室性心动过速]
15. dystonias[张力障碍]
16. prostatic hypertrophy[前列腺肥大]
17. hallucination[幻觉]

注 1

顺铂对多种实体肿瘤均有效，为当前联合化疗中常用药物之一。主要不良反应为胃肠道反应、骨髓抑制等。它能使小肠释放出 5-HT_3，后者作用于肠道神经原的 5-HT 受体，将神经冲动传入到脑干部，诱发呕吐。

注 2

呕吐的时间、性质、强度未做说明，昂丹司琼对延迟性呕吐的疗效有待进一步证实。

点评

本病例介绍了肿瘤化疗过程中常见不良反应——呕吐的发生机制并介绍了止吐药物的分类及作用机制。延脑的呕吐中枢，可接受来自催吐化学感受区（CTZ）、前庭器官、内脏等传入冲动而引发呕吐。已知 CTZ 含有丰富的多巴胺、组胺、胆碱受体，前庭器官有胆碱能、组胺能神经纤维与呕吐中枢相连。5-羟色胺的 5-HT_3 亚型受体通过外周、中枢部位如孤束核也与呕吐有关。各种止吐药物的作用机理即阻断其中一种或多种传入途径，以达到止吐的作用。

止吐药物主要有以下几类：(1)5-HT_3 受体阻断剂：选择性阻断中枢及迷走神经传入纤维 5-HT_3 受体，产生强大止吐作用。对抗肿瘤药顺铂、环磷酰胺、阿霉素等引起呕吐的止吐作用迅速强大，尤其适用于放化疗及术后呕吐的病人。(2)多巴胺受体拮抗剂：拮抗 CTZ 与呕吐中枢内的多巴胺受体，还可促进胃肠道平滑肌动力作用，止吐作用较轻。(3)皮质类固醇：止吐效果肯定，作用机制不明。常与其他止吐药联合应用。(4)抗组胺药：主要是第一代如赛克利嗪，常用于晕动病呕吐，不良反应有头晕、嗜睡、视力模糊和口干。(5)抗胆碱能药：主要是抑制中枢神经系统而产生镇静催眠作用，是防治晕动病的最有效药物之一，也能有效预防耳源性眩晕症(梅尼埃病)。对化疗所致呕吐无效。(6)其他止吐药：苯二氮䓬类有较强的镇静止吐作用，对晕动病和术后呕吐有效，对药物作用于 CTZ 引起的呕吐效果差。

应用止吐药需注意几个原则：首先明确引起呕吐的病因，尽可能去除病因和对因治疗；纠正可能存在的代谢和水、电解质紊乱；在没有其他治疗办法的前提下，权衡止吐药的利弊和不良反应而应用；各类药的作用机制和止吐效果不同，用药时应掌握各类药物的特点而选用；对晕动病、放射病和抗癌治疗引起的呕吐，预防性应用止吐药效果好。

王冠蕾

❖ CASE 32

A 58-year-old woman with a 20-year history of poorly controlled type II diabetes mellitus[①] comes in for routine follow-up. She has had multiple complications[②] from her diabetes, including retinopathy[③] and peripheral neuropathy[④]. She complains of having several months of feeling as if her stomach is full after eating very little. She is frequently nauseous and bloated[⑤]. She is on a combination of regular and neutral protamine Hagedorn (NPH)[⑥] insulin for her diabetes, an angiotensin-converting enzyme (ACE)[⑦]-inhibitor for her blood pressure, and an 3-hydroxy-3-methylglutaryl-coenzyme A (HMG-CoA)[⑧] reductase inhibitor for her lipids.[注1] Her examination today is unremarkable. A radiographic gastric emptying study shows a prolonged gastric emptying time. You diagnose her with diabetic gastroparesis[⑨][注2] and prescribe metoclopramide.

◆ **What is the mechanism of action of metoclopramide for gastroparesis?**

◆ **What are some common side effects of metoclopramide?**

ANSWERS TO CASE 32: Prokinetic Agents

Summary: A 58-year-old woman presents with diabetic gastroparesis and is prescribed metodopramide.

- **Mechanism of action of metoclopramide**: Dopamine D_2-receptor antagonist in the gastrointestinal (GI) tract.
- **Common side effects**: Sedation, extrapyramidal side effects, increased prolactin secretion.

CLINICAL CORRELATION

Metoclopramide, administered orally or parenterally, works as a prokinetic[10] agent in the gastrointestinal tract. In the GI tract, dopamine acts as an inhibitor, and acetylcholine (ACh) acts as a stimulator of gastrointestinal motility. As a dopamine D_2-receptor antagonist, metoclopramide allows for a greater stimulatory effect of ACh. It may also promote the release of ACh. The increased ACh effect at muscarinic receptors results in increases in lower esophageal sphincter[11] tone, rate of gastric emptying, and transit through the small intestine. Diabetic gastroparesis is an uncommon complication of poorly controlled diabetes, particularly in diabetics with peripheral neuropathy. In this setting, metoclopramide can promote emptying of the stomach and help to alleviate the symptoms. It is also used clinically in combination with antacids to treat gastroesophageal reflux disease (GERD)[12]. Metoclopramide also has central actions. Dopamine D_2-receptor blockade in the chemoreceptor trigger zone (CTZ)[13] in the CNS is the basis for clinical use of metoclopramide for treatment of nausea and vomiting. Restlessness[14], anxiety, and insomnia[15] are common adverse effects of metoclopramide and, like other dopamine D_2-receptor antagonists such as haloperidol and metoclopramide can cause extrapyramidal[16] side effects and tardive dyskinesia[17], and also increased prolactin[18] secretion that can result in galactorrhea[19], menstrual dysfunction, gynecomastia[20], and sexual dysfunction. Other prokinetic agents include cisapride (see Case 25) and domperidone, which is also a dopamine D_2-receptor antagonist, but one that acts only peripherally and, therefore, has few neural-related adverse effects.

Comprehension Questions

[32.1] Metoclopramide is a

A. β_1-adrenoceptor antagonist

B. Dopamine D_2-receptor antagonist

C. Muscarinic cholinoreceptor antagonist

D. Serotonin 5-HT_1 receptor antagonist

[32. 2] Which of the following is the most likely adverse effect of metoclopramide?

A. Hallucinations
B. Hyperactivity
C. Hyperthyroidism
D. Tardive dyskinesia

[32. 3] Metoclopramide

A. Decreases rate of gastric emptying
B. Decreases transit through the small intestine
C. Increases lower esophageal sphincter tone
D. Stimulates vomiting

Answers

[32. 1] **B**. Metoclopramide is a dopamine D_2-receptor antagonist.

[32. 2] **D**. Adverse effects of metoclopramide include insomnia, tardive dyskinesia and sexual dysfunction, as well as extrapyramidal side effects similar to haloperidol and endocrine effects related to increased prolactin secretion (galactorrhea, menstrual dysfunction, gynecomastia).

[32. 3] **C**. Metoclopramide increases lower esophageal sphincter tone. It also increases the rate of gastric emptying and transit through the small intestine and inhibits vomiting.

PHARMACOLOGY PEARLS

❖ Metoclopramide works as a prokinetic agent in the gastrointestinal tract, acting as a dopamine antagonist.

❖ Common side effects of metoclopramide are restlessness and anxiety. Also, like other dopamine D_2-receptor antagonists such as haloperidol, metoclopramide can cause extrapyramidal side effects and tardive dyskinesia.

❖ Metoclopramide increases prolactin secretion that can result in galactorrhea and menstrual irregularities.

REFERENCES

Booth CM, Heyland DK, Paterson WG. Gastrointestinal promotility drugs in the critical care setting: a systematic review of the evidence. Crit Care Med 2002; 30(7): 1429-35.

Smith DS, Ferris CD. Current concepts in diabetic gastroparesis. Drugs 2003; 63(13): 1339-58.

Tonini M，Cipollina L，Poluzzi E，et al. Review article：clinical implications of enteric and central D_2 receptor blockade by antidopaminergic gastrointestinal prokinetics. Aliment Pharmacol Ther 2004；19(4)：379-90.

词汇

1. diabetes mellitus[糖尿病]
2. complication[并发症]
3. retinopathy[视网膜病变]
4. peripheral neuropathy[周围神经病变]
5. bloated[发胀的]
6. neutral protamine hagedorn(NPH)[低精蛋白锌胰岛素]
7. angiotensin-converting enzyme(ACE)[血管紧张素转化酶]
8. 3-hydroxy-3-methylglutary-coenzyme a(HMG-CoA)[羟甲基戊二酰辅酶 a]
9. diabetic gastroparesis[糖尿病性胃轻瘫]
10. prokinetic[促动力药]
11. esophageal sphincter[食管括约肌]
12. gastroesophageal reflex disease(GRED)[胃食管反流病]
13. chemoreceptor trigger zone(CTZ)[化学促发带,在延髓呕吐中枢周围]
14. restlessness[烦乱不安]
15. insomnia[失眠]
16. extrapyramidal[锥体外系的]
17. tardive dyskinesia[迟发性运动障碍]
18. prolactin[催乳素]
19. galactorrhea[溢乳]
20. gynecomastia[男性乳腺发育]

注 1

该患者糖尿病病史长，因此有程度不同的并发症出现：视网膜病变和周围神经病变，并伴有血脂紊乱和高血压。因此该患者选用血管紧张素转化酶抑制剂降血压和 HMG-CoA 抑制剂控制高脂血症。

注 2

糖尿病性胃轻瘫属自主神经病变，在糖尿病病人中较常见并较早出现，伴有周围神经病变的病人更易出现胃轻瘫表现。治疗时应联合应用降糖药和促胃动力药。

点评

本病例糖尿病病史长，出现多种并发症，近来又有恶心、胀满等胃肠道症状，胃排空延迟，经胃动力检查，诊断为糖尿病性胃轻瘫，给予促动力药甲氧氯普胺治疗。

胃轻瘫是胃排空延缓的一种特殊类型，是指胃排空功能明显受损，但无机械性梗阻，主要表现为腹胀、恶心、呕吐和早饱，甚至在餐后几小时仍可呕出大量胃内容物。

甲氧氯普胺和多潘利酮是多巴胺 D_2 受体拮抗剂。它们对胃肠道多巴胺 D_2 受体有阻断作用，可引起从食道至近段小肠平滑肌运动，加速胃的正向排空(多巴胺使胃体平滑肌松弛，幽门肌收缩）和加速肠内容物从十二指肠向回盲部推进，发挥胃肠促动药作用。另外，甲氧氯普胺还阻断呕吐中枢 CTZ 的 D_2 受体，发挥止吐作用。

促胃动力药还包括抗胆碱药，5-HT_4 受体激动剂（如西沙必利）和胃动素受体激动剂。西沙必利和多潘利酮只对外周起作用，因此没有中枢相关副作用。

王冠蕾

❖ CASE 33

A 48-year-old woman presents for evaluation of abdominal pain. She reports that she gets right upper-abdominal pain after eating. It is worse if she eats fatty or fried food. She has tried over-the-counter antacids without relief. She has no significant medical history, has had no surgeries, and takes no medications on a regular basis. Both her mother and an older sister have had to have their gallbladders[①] removed. On examination, she is moderately obese,[注1] but her examination is otherwise normal. An abdominal x-ray is normal. An ultrasound of her abdomen reveals several small gallstones. You diagnose her with cholelithiasis[②] and recommend surgical evaluation.[注2] She is adamant in wanting to do anything to avoid surgery, so you prescribe ursodiol[③].

◆ **What is the mechanism of action of ursodiol?**

◆ **How long does it take to see full effect of this medication?**

◆ **What effect does ursodiol have on low-density lipoprotein (LDL)[④] cholesterol levels?**

ANSWERS TO CASE 33: Drugs Used to Dissolve Gallstones

Summary: A 48-year-old woman presents with cholelithiasis who does not desire surgery, and is prescribed ursodiol.

- **Mechanism of action of ursodiol**: Reduces cholesterol secretion into bile.
- **Length of time to see full effect**: Months to years.
- **Effect on LDL cholesterol levels**: No change.

CLINICAL CORRELATION

Gall stones are a common cause of abdominal pain. Gall stones often consist of a high proportion of cholesterol, which is excreted from the liver into bile. The bile is taken up in the gall bladder, where the cholesterol may precipitate into stones. Ursodiol is ursodeoxycholic acid, a bile acid. It reduces cholesterol secretion into bile with little change in the secretion of bile acid. It is used in an effort to dissolve cholesterol[⑤] gall stones in patients who either do not want surgery or are not surgical candidates. The full effect of this medication can take from several months to several years. It is also used as an adjunct[⑥] to shock wave lithotripsy[⑦] of gall stones. In this treatment, sound waves are used to break gall stones into small fragments. Ursodiol may then be used to attempt to dissolve the fragments. Radiopaque[⑧] gall stones, which contain calcium, are not effectively dissolved with ursodiol. It is administered orally, and its side effects[注3] are primarily gastrointestinal[⑨] (GI), with nausea and diarrhea being common. Ursodiol does not alter LDL cholesterol levels in the blood.

Pharmacology of Agents Used to Dissolve Gallstones

Objectives

1. Know the drugs used to dissolve gallstones and their mechanism of action.
2. Know the routes of administration and side effects of these drugs.

Definitions

Cholelithiasis[⑩]: The presence of stones in the gallbladder or common bile duct, or the process of formation of such stones.

Cholecystitis: Inflammation of the gallbladder.

Lithotripsy: Reduction of gallstones using sound waves to small particles that can be excreted from the gall bladder.

Discussion of Class

Gallstones are a major cause of morbidity and mortality, and surgical removal of the gallbladder is among the most common gastrointestinal surgeries. Although surgical removal is the preferred treatment, other treatments, including **ultrasound lithotripsy** or **pharmacologic dissolution**, are therapeutic options in patients who cannot have surgery. Gallstones can be transported into the duodenum⑪ and block the exit of the pancreatic duct, causing pancreatitis⑫. Gallstones can be radiotranslucent⑬, indicating a stone high in cholesterol content, or **radiopaque**, **indicating a stone with significant mineral**(usually **calcium**) content. **Ursodeoxycholic acid** (**ursodiol**) is a **naturally occurring bile acid that is a minor component of bile**. It has been used **successfully to treat** relatively **small**, **radiotranslucent stones**, especially those within the common bile duct. It decreases the synthesis of bile and reduces the concentration of cholesterol in bile. **Ursodiol solubilizes cholesterol by forming bile acid micelles** and disperses liquid crystals of cholesterol in an aqueous environment. These actions will **slowly cause the dissolution of the gallstone**. Complete dissolution occurs in about 30 percent of patients with stones less than 20 mm in diameter. It also decreases the biliary colic⑭ that is associated with gall stones in some patients. The prophylactic⑮ administration of ursodiol caused a marked reduction in the incidence of gallstones after cardiac surgery. Older approaches to pharmacologic dissolution of gallstones employed organic solvents such as methyl-*tert*-butyl ether (MTBE)⑯ or monoglycerides⑰ such as monooctanoin⑱. Although rapid dissolution of gallstones could be achieved, leakage of the solvent materials into the lumen of the bowel was associated with serious adverse effects, and these approaches have been largely discontinued. **Adverse effects of ursodiol are minor**, **typically GI upset and mild diarrhea**.

Structure

Ursodiol is derived from 7β-hydroxycholesterol⑲ and is a naturally occurring component in bile.

Administration

Ursodiol is administered orally, two to three times a day, and complete dissolution of stones may require a year. Treatment effectiveness should be monitored by diagnostic ultrasound.

Comprehension Questions

[33.1] Ursodiol reduces the size of common bile duct gallstones by

A. Chelating Ca^{2+} out of the stone

B. Decreasing the synthesis of bile

C. Increasing the cholesterol content in bile

D. Slowly dissolving cholesterol from the stone

[33.2] Complete dissolution of a gallstone by ursodiol typically requires

A. Several hours B. Weeks

C. Months to years D. Several years

[33.3] Ursodiol has been useful to treat

A. Cholestasis of pregnancy B. Cirrhosis

C. Diabetes mellitus D. Pancreatitis resulting from trauma

Answers

[33.1] **D**. Ursodiol is a detergent[20] that slowly causes dissolution of gallstones that are rich in cholesterol. It decreases the amount of cholesterol in bile as well as total bile acid synthesis.

[33.2] **C**. Ursodiol treatment typically takes months to a year for dissolution of a typical gallstone.

[33.3] **A**. Ursodeoxycholic acid has been used successfully to treat the symptoms of pruritus[21] associated with cholestasis of pregnancy, a disease thought to be caused by the accumulation of bile salts.

PHARMACOLOGY PEARLS

❖ Ursodiol is the best nonsurgical therapy for small, radiotranslucent gallstones in patients who are not candidates for surgery.

❖ Ursodeoxycholic acid has also been used to treat cholestasis of pregnancy.

REFERENCES

Ai T, Azemoto R, Saisho HJ. Prevention of gallstones by ursodeoxycholic acid after cardiac surgery Gastroenterol 2003; 38: 1071-6

Gonzalez-Koch A, Nervi F. Medical management of common bile duct stones. World J Surgery 1998; 22: 1145-50.

词汇

1. gallbladder[胆囊]
2. cholelithiasis[胆石症]
3. ursodiol[熊去氧胆酸]
4. low-density lipoprotein (LDL)[低密度脂蛋白]
5. cholesterol[胆固醇]
6. adjunct[辅助治疗]
7. shock wave lithotripsy[体外震波碎石术]

8. radiopaque[不透射线的]
9. gastrointestinal[胃肠道的]
10. cholecystitis[胆囊炎]
11. duodenum[十二指肠]
12. pancreatitis[胰腺炎]
13. radiotranslucent[透射线的]
14. biliary colic[胆绞痛]
15. prophylactic[预防性的]
16. methyl-tert-butyl ether(MTBE)[甲基叔丁醚];methyl-[甲基]
17. monoglyceride[单酸甘油酯]
18. monooctanoin[半合成甘油衍生物]
19. 7β-hydroxycholesterol[7β-羟胆固醇]
20. detergent[去污剂]
21. pruritus[瘙痒感]

注 1

胆结石根据含钙盐多少而分为不透X线结石与可透X线结石两类。10%~20%胆结石含钙较多,平片可以显示,称为不透X线结石;80%~90%胆结石含钙少,平片不能见到,是可透X线结石,需造影才能显示。患者腹部平片示可透X线结石,口服熊去氧胆酸对可透X线结石中的部分胆固醇结石有效。

注 2

胆囊结石可分为内科保守疗法及手术疗法两种。有下列情形应采取手术治疗:(1)凡胆囊结石病伴有明显症状和反复胆囊炎发作;(2)胆囊结石多颗、细小形,易落入胆总管导致胆管炎和胰腺炎;(3)结石过大,虽无症状但疑有胆囊癌变者。部分患者(如该患者)因怕手术而采用口服药物治疗,也有的人因合并高血压病、心脏病、糖尿病,或年老体弱,不具备手术条件,而采用内科治疗;或经溶石药物治疗一段时间为手术创造条件;或作为体外碎石治疗的辅助治疗手段。考虑该患者有胆结石的家族史,若药物溶石治疗效果不佳,仍应选择手术治疗。

注 3

溶石药物的不良反应:甲基叔丁醚等有机溶剂溶解胆石后,胆石碎屑进入肠道可以引起胆石性肠梗阻和胆源性胰腺炎等;另外,还可引起急性血管内溶血和急性肾衰。熊去氧胆酸对肝脏基本无损害,口服药物有胃肠道不适。轻度腹泻是由于胆汁酸抑制肠管内水和电解质的吸收而引起。

点评

本病例具有典型胆石症症状,进食后右上腹疼痛,进食油腻实物尤甚,服用抗酸药无效,超声提示胆结石。腹部平片提示为阴性结石(含胆固醇多而钙盐少的胆结石),有胆石症家族史。胆囊切除是胆结石治疗的首选方法。患者不愿手术并且其胆结石为含钙量较少的胆固醇结石,因此可先采用口服药物溶石疗法。胆固醇结石的形成,与胆汁中胆汁酸、磷脂浓度降低、胆固醇过饱和，即成石性胆汁的生成有关。此外，胆固醇结石患者加速胆固醇合成的HMG-CoA还原酶活性增强，而使胆固醇转化为胆汁酸的胆固醇7a羟基化酶活性降低。胆酸制剂可以抑制HMG-CoA还原酶的活性，使胆固醇的合成及分泌减少。但药物溶石效果有限，仅对30%患者有效，且需长期服药，有一定副作用，容易复发。考虑该患者有胆结石家族史，需对其进行手术评价，若药物溶石效果差，仍应主张手术治疗。

王冠蕾

❖ CASE 34

A 45-year-old woman presents with bloating① and "gas" after drinking milk. Her symptoms usually start about 2 hours after ingesting most dairy products②, although she has found that yogurt with active cultures doesn't bother her much. This has been worsening over the past several years. She has learned to avoid dairy products as much as possible but would like to be able to drink milk or eat ice cream occasionally. She has no significant medical history, takes no medications regularly, and has a normal examination. You diagnose her with lactose intolerance③ and suggest a trial of lactase④ when she plans to ingest dairy products. [注1]

◆ **What is the cause of lactose intolerance?**

◆ **What is the mechanism of action of lactase?**

ANSWERS TO CASE 34: Enzyme Replacements

Summary: A 45-year-old woman with lactose intolerance is prescribed lactase.

- **Cause of lactose intolerance**: Insufficient production of lactase by brush border cells of the small intestine.
- **Mechanism of action of lactase**: Hydrolyzes[⑤] lactose to glucose and galactose[⑥].

CLINICAL CORRELATION

Lactose intolerance is a very common digestive condition in which there is an underproduction of the natural enzyme lactase by the brush border of the small intestine. Lactase hydrolyzes lactose into the sugars glucose and galactose, which can then be transported from the lumen of the small intestine across cell membranes. A deficiency or absence of lactase results in lactose remaining within the intestinal lumen. The presence of this undigested disaccharide[⑦] will osmotically attract fluid into the intestinal lumen. As it passes further into the gastrointestinal (GI) tract, lactose will be metabolized by colonic bacteria, which produces bowel gas. The combination of increased amounts of fluid and gas in the intestine contributes to the symptoms of lactose intolerance. Most people with lactose intolerance learn to avoid lactose containing foods. The low levels of endogenous lactase production in these individuals can be supplemented by lactase given orally with meals containing dairy products. This often reduces, but not completely relieves, the symptoms of gas, bloating, and diarrhea that may occur.

Pharmacology of Enzyme Replacements

Objectives

1. Know the conditions for which digestive enzyme replacement can be used. [注2]
2. Know the specific digestive enzymes which can be replaced and the therapeutic effects of enzyme replacement.

Definitions

Pancreatin[⑧]: A preparation of principally amylase[⑨], lipase[⑩], and proteases[⑪].

Pancrelipase[⑫]: A preparation that is principally lipase that also contains amylase and proteases.

Discussion of Class

Digestive enzymes hydrolyze triglycerides[⑬] to fatty acids and glycerol[⑭], peptides and proteins to amino acids, and **carbohydrates into simple sugars.** Enzyme replacement is used in patients with a congenital[⑮] lack of enzyme activity as a result of mutation in specific enzymes, or secondary to other disorders that cause deficient pancreatic exocrine secretions such as in **cystic fibrosis**[16], **chronic pancreatitis**[17], **post-pancreatectomy**[18], **pancreatic ductal obstruction, and postgastrectomy**[19]. Greater than 90 percent of pancreatic function must be lost before clinically significant effects on digestion are apparent: steatorrhea[20] (from fat malabsorption) and protein malabsorption. **Sucrase**[21] is expressed on the brush border of the small intestine primarily in the distal duodenum and jejunum[22]. It converts sucrose into glucose and fructose[23]. **Isomaltase**[24] **and maltase**[25] hydrolyze isomaltose and maltose, respectively, into two molecules of glucose. **Lactase** (β-galactosidase) is normally expressed in villus enterocytes[26] in the small intestine. It breaks lactose into the monosaccharides[27] glucose and galactose.

Pancreatic Enzyme Preparations

There are **more than 35 preparations of pancreatin and pancrelipase** currently available. These are **all prepared from porcine pancreas**, but they are not bioequivalent and are not necessarily interchangeable. These agents can prevent malabsorption from the disorders mentioned above and palliation of pain in chronic pancreatitis. Pancreatic enzyme replacements are well tolerated, but can cause gastrointestinal disturbances such as nausea and diarrhea; allergic reactions to the porcine preparations have also been reported. Very high doses can cause hyperuricemia[28] and hyperuricosuria[29].

Pancreatic enzyme replacements are administered orally prior to a meal or snack. They are available in enteric-coated capsule or as noncoated capsules.

Small Intestine Enzyme Preparations

More than 15 percent of adults are lactose intolerant as a result of deficiency in the enzyme lactase. This deficiency leads to **lactose delivery to the colon**, where it osmotically **traps water and it is fermented**, producing **bloating sensations**, discomfort, and intestinal gas. Preparations of lactase for enzyme replacement are prepared from the yeast *Kluyveromyces lactis*[30]. **Lactase is administered orally**, typically taken just prior to ingestion of dairy products. The dosage may be increased until satisfactory results are obtained. Few adverse effects are reported beyond mild gastrointestinal upset.

Congenital sucrase-isomaltase deficiency (CSID)[31] **is a chronic autosomal**[32] **disease** with highly variable levels of enzyme activity. CSID is frequently characterized by nearly complete deficiency in sucrase activity, less severe reductions in isomaltase and maltase activity, and normal lactase activity. In the absence of sucrase activity, unhydrolyzed sucrose and starch are not absorbed from the small intestine, causing osmotic water retention, loose stools, and the typical manifestations of malabsorption.

Sacrosidase is derived from baker's yeast (*Saccharomyces cerevisiae*[33]). It is approved for use in CSID and is effective in improving carbohydrate absorption and alleviating the gastrointestinal sequelae[34]. It is administered orally just prior to eating food. Adverse effects are rare with one case of hypersensitivity reported to date.

Besides replacing enzymes in the digestive system, enzyme replacement has been useful to correct **genetic deficiencies in lysosomal[35] enzymes. Anderson-Fabry disease[36]** is an **X-linked lysosomal storage disease** that results from a deficiency in **α-galactosidase A[37]**. This enzyme hydrolyses globotriaosylceramide[38] to galactose and lactosylceramide[39]. In patients with the enzyme deficiency, globotriaosylceramide accumulates and is deposited in vascular endothelium, smooth muscle cells, renal glomerular and epithelial cells, myocardial cells and valvular fibrocytes, and neurons. This results in severe pain as a result of damage of small neurons, as well as cardiomyopathy and renal impairment and failure. The disease can be **treated with agalsidase alpha**, which is a **recombinant α-galactosidase A** produced in vitro in fibroblast cells. A similar replacement enzyme is agalsidase beta, which is a recombinant protein produced in a genetically engineered Chinese hamster ovary cell line. Both drugs are given intravenously biweekly, and both drugs reduce the globotriaosylceramide deposits and improve organ function. Both drugs are well tolerated.

Comprehension Questions

[34.1] A 17-year-old patient enters your office complaining that every time he drinks a glass of milk he gets gastrointestinal pain and cramping. Which of the following would be the best choice to treat his condition?

A. Aspirin B. Lactase C. Niacin D. Sucrase

[34.2] A 9-year-old patient whose main complaint is shooting pain in the arms and legs is seen in your hospital. After careful study you make the diagnosis of Anderson-Fabry disease. The best course of treatment for this patient would be

A. α-galactosidase A B. High-dose glucocorticoids

C. Indomethacin D. Sacrosidase

[34.3] A 45-year-old man has developed chronic pancreatitis as a result of alcohol abuse, and he has been noted to have pancreatic insufficiency. Which of the following circumstances contraindicates the use of pancreatic enzyme replacement in this patient?

A. Allergy to eggs B. Allergy to pork

C. Diabetes mellitus D. Pseudogout[40]

Answers

[34.1] **B**. This case of lactose intolerance would be treated with lactase before consumption of dairy products.

[34.2] **A**. Anderson-Fabry disease can be treated successfully with α-galactosidase A.

[34.3] **B**. All pancreatic enzyme replacements are porcine and so an allergy to pork products is a contraindication.

PHARMACOLOGY PEARLS

- ❖ Enzyme replacement therapy is effective in treating specific genetic enzyme deficiencies and acquired enzyme deficiencies and is associated with very few adverse effects.
- ❖ Lactose deficiency is a common problem and is addressed by avoidance of lactose-containing products or taking lactase orally prior to ingestion of lactose.
- ❖ All pancreatic enzyme preparations currently are prepared from porcine pancreas.

REFERENCES

Hauser AC, Lorenz M, Sunder-Plassmann G. The expanding clinical spectrum of Anderson-Fabry disease: a challenge to diagnosis in the novel era of enzyme replacement therapy. J Intern Med 2004; 255: 629-36.

Poisindex, from MICROMEDEX(R) Healthcare Series Vol. 119 expires 2004.

Sly WS. Enzyme replacement therapy for lysosomal storage disorders: successful transition from concept to clinical practice. Mo Med 2004; 101: 100-4.

Swagerty DL, Walling AD, Klein RM. Lactose intolerance. Am Fam Physician 2002; 65: 1845-50, 1855-6.

词汇

1. bloating[气胀]
2. dairy product[乳制品]
3. lactose intolerance[乳糖不耐受]
4. lactase[乳糖酶]
5. hydrolyze[水解]
6. galactose[半乳糖]
7. disaccharide[二糖]
8. pancreatin[胰酶]
9. amylase[淀粉酶]
10. lipase[脂肪酶]
11. protease[蛋白酶]
12. pancrelipase[胰脂酶]
13. triglyceride[甘油三酯]
14. glycerol[甘油]
15. congenital[先天性的]
16. cystic fibrosis[囊性纤维化]
17. pancreatitis[胰腺炎]
18. postpancreatectomy[胰切除术后]post-[后]
19. postgastrectomy[胃切除术后]
20. steatorrhea[脂肪泻]
21. sucrase[蔗糖酶]
22. jejunum[空肠]
23. fructose[果糖]

24. isomaltase[异麦芽糖酶]
25. maltase[麦芽糖酶类]
26. villus enterocyte[肠绒毛上皮细胞]
27. monosaccharide[单糖]; mono-[单]
28. hyperuricemia[高尿酸血症]
29. hyperuricosuria[高尿酸尿]
30. *Kluyveromyces lactis*[乳酸克鲁维酵母菌株]
31. congenital sucrase-isomaltase deficiency (CSID)[先天性蔗糖酶-异麦芽糖酶缺陷症]
32. autosomal[常染色体]
33. saccharomyces cerevisiae[酿酒酵母]
34. sequelae[后遗症]
35. lysosomal[溶酶体的]
36. Anderson-Fabry disease[安德森-法布里综合征,一种脂质贮积病]
37. α-galactosidase A[α-半乳糖苷酶 A]
38. globotriaosylceramide (Gb3)[神经酰胺已三糖苷]
39. lactosylceramide[乳糖酰鞘氨醇]
40. pseudogout[假痛风,软骨钙质沉着病]

注 1

该患者被诊断为乳糖不耐受症，此病症是由于体内乳糖酶的缺乏，乳糖不能完全被分解吸收，当未分解吸收的乳糖进入结肠后，被肠道内的细菌发酵成为小分子的有机酸和气体，引起肠鸣、腹胀、腹痛、排气、腹泻等症状。乳糖酶缺乏和乳糖不耐受影响着世界不同地区、不同种族的人们对乳制品的摄入。

注 2

机体可因先天性某些酶突变或某些疾病引起体内酶缺乏。如囊性纤维化，慢性胰腺炎等引起胰腺消化酶的减少，治疗上常给予各种外源性胰酶制剂(内含胰蛋白酶、胃蛋白酶、脂肪酶、糜蛋白酶等)作替代疗法，临床证明非常有效并且不良反应少。

点评

选择此病例是因为在我国，随着生活水平日益提高和乳制品摄入量的提高，乳糖不耐受这一问题应引起人们的重视。乳糖不耐受的长期危害在儿童表现为钙吸收不良、腹泻、软骨病、体重低下及生长发育迟缓，尤其先天性和继发性乳糖酶缺乏可导致婴幼儿难治性腹泻和慢性腹泻，在老年人尤其老年妇女易表现为骨质疏松等症状。

该患者为继发性乳糖不耐受。近几年出现对乳糖不耐受的典型症状：如服用乳制品后 2 小时内发生腹胀，嗳气等症状，并逐渐加重。患者为中年女性，考虑应摄取适量乳制品以避免出现骨质疏松等症状。服用乳制品时补充外源性乳糖酶可以提高乳糖消化和吸收，并预防和减缓不适症状，这属于酶替代疗法。还可采取的措施包括饮用发酵乳制品和含乳糖酶的奶粉。

王冠蕾

❖ CASE 35

A 48-year-old man presents for evaluation of heartburn. He reports a burning feeling in his chest after eating. It is worse when he eats spicy foods or tomato sauce. He sometimes is awakened at night with symptoms. He has tried over-thecounter antacids and histamine H_2-blockers with partial relief. He is on no medications regularly. His examination today is normal. An upper gastrointestinal (GI) x-ray series reveals gastroesophageal reflux.[注1] Along with appropriate diet and lifestyle modification recommendations, you prescribe omeprazole.[注2]

◆ **What is the mechanism of action of omeprazole?**

◆ **What is the mechanism of action of antacid medications?**

◆ **What is the mechanism of action of histamine H_2-receptor antagonists?**

ANSWERS TO CASE 35: Agents for Upper GI Disorders

Summary: A 48-year-old man with gastroesophageal reflux disease (GERD)[1] is prescribed omeprazole.

- **Mechanism of action of omeprazole**: Irreversible inhibition of the H^+, K^+-ATPase proton pump in parietal cells, reducing transport of acid from the cell into the lumen.
- **Mechanism of action of antacids**: Weak bases that directly neutralize gastric acid and reduce pepsin[2] activity.
- **Mechanism of action of histamine H_2-receptor antagonists**: Competitive antagonists of histamine at the histamine H_2-receptor; the receptor activation mediates cyclic adenosine monophosphate (cAMP)-dependent stimulation of acid release from gastric parietal cells[3].

CLINICAL CORRELATION

Gastroesophageal reflux disease (GERD), a common cause of recurrent heartburn and dyspepsia, is caused by gastric acid irritating the lining of the esophagus. It can be treated by numerous medications. Antacid medications, widely available without a prescription, usually contain aluminum hydroxide, magnesium hydroxide, calcium carbonate, or combinations thereof. They are weak bases that partially neutralize gastric acid. Histamine H_2-receptor antagonists, available over-the-counter or by prescription, competitively antagonize the effect of histamine (released from nearby gastric mucosa enterochromaffin-like [ECL] cells)[4], at the histamine H_2-receptor in gastric parietal cells. Histamine stimulates gastric acid secretion via a cAMP mediated stimulation of the H^+, K^+-adenosine triphosphatase (ATPase) proton pump, which transports H^+ from gastric parietal cells into the lumen of the stomach. Omeprazole was the first medication in a class known as proton pump inhibitors (PPIs)[5]. PPIs directly and irreversibly inhibit the action of the H^+, K^+-ATPase, reducing both the basal and stimulated release of gastric acid. PPIs are used for the treatment of refractory GERD, hypersecretory conditions such as Zollinger-Ellison syndrome[6], for peptic ulcer disease, and as a part of the treatment regimen (in combination with antibiotics) for *Helicobacter pylori*[7] infections. *H. pylori* is the most common cause of non-drug-induced peptic ulcer disease.

Pharmacology of Agents for Upper GI Disorders

Objectives

1. List the antacid agents and describe their mechanisms of action, therapeutic uses, and adverse effects.
2. List the histamine H_2-receptor antagonists and PPIs that inhibit gastric acid production and describe their mechanisms of action, therapeutic uses and adverse effects.
3. List the drugs used therapeutically to promote the defense of the gastrointestinal tract from the effects of acid, and describe their mechanisms of action, therapeutic uses, and adverse effects.

Definitions

Prodrugs[8]: Inactive compounds that are metabolized in the body to therapeutically active agents.

Discussion of Class

Drugs used to **treat acid-peptic diseases** (Table 35-1) either **reduce gastric acidity** (antacids, histamine H_2-receptor antagonists, and proton pump inhibitors) or **promote the defense of the GI mucosa** (sucralfate[9], bismuth subsalicylate[10], and the prostaglandin analog, misoprostol[11]).

Available **antacid preparations** are used primarily to treat heartburn and dyspepsia[12]. When given concomitantly with other drugs, antacids may reduce their absorption through direct binding or, as a result of an increase in gastric pH, by altering their dissolution or solubility.

Available **histamine H_2-receptor antagonists** are used to treat dyspepsia, GERD, peptic ulcer disease, and stress-induced gastritis[13].

Proton pump inhibitors are generally considered the first-line drugs for treating acid-peptic disease as a result of their superior efficacy and safety profile. Available PPIs are also used to **treat dyspepsia, GERD, peptic ulcer disease, and stress-induced gastritis, as well as gastrinomas**[14]. For treating peptic ulcer disease caused by ***H. pylori***, **PPIs** are used in a multidrug regimen that includes the antibiotics **clarithromycin and amoxicillin or metronidazole.**

Sucralfate use has for the most part been supplanted by other agents for the treatment of upper GI disorders. It is still used clinically to treat stress-related gastritis.

Misoprostol is a **prostaglandin E_1 analog** used primarily to **treat nonsteroidal anti-inflammatory drug (NSAID)-induced peptic ulcer disease.**

Bismuth subsalicylate (Pepto Bismol) is available as a nonprescription agent and is used to treat **dyspepsia**, **acute diarrhea**, and, as a second line agent in a multidrug combination, ***H. pylori* infection** where it is thought to inhibit growth of the organism.

Structure

Proton pump inhibitors (PPIs) are substituted benzimidazoles. They resemble histamine H_2-receptor antagonists but have a different mechanism of action. Sucralfate is a complex salt of sucrose sulfate and aluminum hydroxide. Misoprostol is a prostaglandin analog of prostaglandin E_1 (PGE_1). Bismuth subsalicylate is a combination of bismuth and salicylate.

Table 35-1

MEDICATIONS FOR PEPTIC ULCERS

ANTACIDS	ADVERSE EFFECTS
Sodium bicarbonate	Bloating[15], belching[16], metabolic acidosis as a result of absorbed unreacted alkali at high doses, and fluid retention caused by absorption of sodium chloride that may compromise patients with heart failure and hypertension. Hypercalcemia[17] at high doses when administered with dairy products containing calcium.
Calcium carbonate	Bloating, belching, metabolic acidosis, hypercalcemia.
Magnesium hydroxide	Osmotic diarrhea from unabsorbed magnesium.
Aluminum hydroxide	Constipation[18] from unabsorbed aluminum.
HISTAMINE H_2-RECEPTOR ANTAGONIST	**ADVERSE EFFECTS**
Cimetidine (prototype) *Ranitidine* *Famotidine* *Nizatidine*	Mild diarrhea or constipation, headache, myalgia[19]. Confusion, hallucinations[20], and excitement, particularly cimetidine, when administered IV to elderly or patients with renal or liver disease.
PROTON PUMP INHIBITORS	**ADVERSE EFFECTS**
Omeprazole (prototype) *Esomeprazole* *Lansoprazole* *Pantoprazole* *Rabeprazole*	Small increase in incidence of diarrhea and headache. Otherwise, no significant adverse effects documented in humans, although there are theoretical concerns with long-term therapy regarding the development of certain cancers and enteric[21] infections.
GI PROTECTIVE AGENTS	**ADVERSE EFFECTS**
Sucralfate	Constipation as a consequence of the aluminum salt. It may bind other drugs to limit their absorption (phenytoin[22], quinoline[23] antibodies).

续表

GI PROTECTIVE AGENTS	ADVERSE EFFECTS
Bismuth Subsalicylate	Black stools and darkening of the tongue.
PROSTAGLANDIN analogs *Misoprostol*	Diarrhea and abdominal discomfort. Contraindicated[24] in women unless proved negative for pregnancy.

Mechanism of Action

Antacids are weak bases that directly neutralize gastric hydrochloric acid to form a salt and water and to reduce pepsin activity. They may also stimulate the production of prostaglandins and thus increase the defense of the GI mucosa.

Histamine H_2-receptor antagonists are highly specific and selective competitive antagonists of histamine binding to gastric parietal cell histamine H_2-receptors, thus preventing activation of adenylyl cyclase and accumulation of cAMP, which mediate acid release into the gastric lumen. Parietal cell acid secretion induced by the secretagogues[25] gastrin and acetylcholine, which act synergistically with histamine, is also inhibited by histamine H_2-receptor antagonists, albeit indirectly.

PPIs irreversibly inhibit the H^+, K^+-ATPase proton pump in parietal cells, thus reducing transport of acid from the cell into the lumen of the stomach.

Sucralfate in its viscous form may bind to positively charged proteins to coat epithelial cells and to form a physical barrier in the gastrointestinal tract that protects the luminal surface and any already formed ulcers from the deleterious effects of gastric acid and pepsin.

Misoprostol stimulates bicarbonate and mucus secretion and mucosal blood flow, resulting in enhanced neutralization and action of secreted acid. It also binds to parietal cell prostaglandin receptors to modestly inhibit secretagogueinduced acid secretion.

Bismuth subsalicylate, like sucralfate, coats epithelial cells to form a physical barrier in the gastrointestinal tract and protect it from the deleterious[26] effects of gastric acid and pepsin. It may also stimulate bicarbonate and prostaglandin E_2 secretion.

Administration

All antacids, histamine H_2-receptor antagonists, PPIs, sucralfate, misoprostol, and bismuth subsalicylate can be given orally. The proton pump inhibitor pantoprazole and the histamine H_2-receptor antagonists (cimetidine, famotidine, and ranitidine) are available for parenteral[27] use.

Proton pump inhibitors are inactive, acid-labile, prodrugs that are administered in acid-resistant, enteric-coated preparations to protect them from destruction in the stomach.

In the acidic environment of the stomach, sucralfate forms a viscous gel.

Pharmacokinetics

The acid neutralizing capacity of available antacid preparations varies considerably, being highly influenced by their rate of dissolution, their solubility in water, and the rate of gastric emptying among other factors. Sodium bicarbonate and calcium carbonate react more rapidly with HCl to produce CO_2 and water than do magnesium or aluminum hydroxide and, therefore, may cause bloating and belching. As over-the-counter preparations, magnesium hydroxide, which can cause diarrhea, and aluminum hydroxide, which can cause constipation, are usually administered in combination to balance their effects on the GI tract.

Histamine H_2-receptor antagonists are absorbed rapidly; however, cimetidine, ranitidine and famotidine have a bioavailability of only 50 percent. Their clearances can be reduced in the elderly and by renal and hepatic dysfunction. Cimetidine inhibits the activity of several hepatic cytochrome P450 enzymes that can prolong the duration of action of a number of other drugs.

PPI bioavailability is decreased significantly by food. Because maximal inhibition of H^+, K^+-ATPase occurs when proton pumps are actively secreting acid, PPIs are best administered within an hour or so of meals. After dissolution of the enteric-coated PPI capsule in the intestine, the lipophilic[28] prodrug diffuses into the acidic environment of the parietal cell where it becomes protonated and highly concentrated, and where it is then converted to a reactive sulfonamide[29] cation[30] that irreversibly binds to and inactivates parietal cell H^+, K^+-ATPase through a covalent[31] disulfide[32] linkage. Although their serum halflife is short, PPI inhibition of the proton pump lasts up to 24 hours while synthesis of new H^+, K^+-ATPase occurs. PPIs are metabolized by hepatic P450 microsomal enzymes; however, no clinically significant drug-drug interactions have been documented.

Sucralfate is very insoluble, and therefore it **acts locally** with little systemic absorption from the gastrointestinal tract.

Misoprostol is absorbed rapidly and is metabolized to an active agent that has a very short serum half-life and short duration of action and therefore must be administered three to four times daily.

Bismuth subsalicylate is rapidly dissociated in the stomach into bismuth, which is eliminated in the stool, and salicylate[33], which is absorbed systemically.

Comprehension Questions

[35.1] The most common adverse effect of omeprazole is

A. Black stools B. Constipation

C. Headache D. Vomiting

[35.2] Ranitidine inhibits

A. Gastrin binding to parietal cells

B. Histamine binding to parietal cells

C. H^+, K^+-ATPase

D. Parietal cell prostaglandin receptors

[35.3] Cimetidine

A. Is a prostaglandin analog of PGE_1

B. Is a prodrug

C. Is associated with confusion and hallucinations in elderly patients

D. Reduces the duration of action of other drugs

Answers

[35.1] **C.** The most common adverse effect of omeprazole is headache. Diarrhea, not constipation, is another common adverse effect. Black stools are associated with use of bismuth subsalicylate. Vomiting is not a typical effect.

[35.2] **B.** Ranitidine is a histamine H_2-receptor antagonist that inhibits histamine binding to parietal cells and reduces acid secretion. It indirectly inhibits the synergistic[34] acid secretion stimulated by gastrin binding to parietal cell gastrin receptors. Proton pump inhibitors inhibit parietal cell H^+, K^+-ATPase.

[35.3] **C.** Cimetidine, a histamine H_2-receptor antagonist, uniquely causes confusion and hallucinations, particularly in elderly patients. It also inhibits hepatic microsomal enzymes to increase, not decrease, the duration of action of other drugs. PPIs are prodrugs.

PHARMACOLOGY PEARLS

- Histamine H_2-receptor antagonists cross the blood-brain barrier and placenta, are secreted into breast milk, and therefore should be used judiciously during pregnancy and in nursing mothers.
- Three to four days of PPI administration are necessary to achieve maximal inhibition of acid secretion (up to 98%). Likewise, 3-4 days are needed for acid secretion to return to normal after discontinuation of therapy.
- PPIs are considered first-line agents for peptic ulcer disease and GERD.

REFERENCES

Aihara T, Nakamura K, Amagase K, et al. Pharmacological control of gastric acid secretion for the treatment of acid-related peptic disease: past, present and future. Pharmacol Ther 2003; 98(1): 109-27.

Chan FK, Leung WK. Peptic-ulcer disease. Lancet 2002; 360(9337): 933-41.

Suerbaum S, Michetti P. Heliobacter pylori infection. N Engl J Med 2002; 347(15): 1175-86.

词汇

1. gastroesophageal reflux disease (GRED)[胃食管反流性疾病]
2. pepsin[胃蛋白酶]
3. parietal cell[胃黏膜壁细胞]
4. enterochromaffin-like (ECL) cells[肠嗜铬样细胞]
5. proton pump inhibitors (PPIs)[质子泵抑制剂]
6. Zollinger-Ellison syndrome[卓-艾综合征，即胃泌素瘤]
7. *Helicobacter pylori*[幽门螺杆菌]
8. prodrug[前体药]
9. sucralfate[硫糖铝]
10. bismuth subsalicylate[碱式水杨酸铋]
11. misoprostol[米索前列醇]
12. dyspepsia[消化不良]
13. gastritis[胃炎]
14. gastrinoma[胃泌素瘤]
15. bloat[胃气胀]
16. belch[嗳气]
17. hypercalcemia[高钙血症]
18. constipation[便秘]
19. myalgia[肌痛]
20. hallucination[幻觉]
21. enteric[肠道的]
22. phenytoin[苯妥英]
23. quinoline[喹啉]
24. contraindicated[禁用的]
25. secretagogue[促分泌素]
26. deleterious[有害于，有毒的]
27. parental[非肠道的，如皮下、肌肉、静脉内注射]
28. lipophilic[亲脂的]
29. sulfonamide[磺胺]
30. cation[阳离子]
31. covalent[共价]
32. disulfide[二硫化物]
33. salicylate[水杨酸盐]
34. synergistic[相互促进的]

注 1

胃食管反流病(GERD)发病机制是抗反流防御机制下降和反流物对食管黏膜攻击作用的综合结果。其治疗中的基础药物是质子泵抑制剂(PPI)。这是因为：1. PPI 抑制胃酸分泌作用强大，可有效缓解症状；2. PPI 促进损伤的食管粘膜快速愈合，治愈潜在的食管炎，预防和治疗 GRED 并发症。

注 2

奥美拉唑(Omeprazole)是 PPI 中第一个获准应用于临床的药物。PPI 的机制是通过抑制 H^+，K^+-ATP 酶，使其不可逆的失活，抑制壁细胞内 H^+ 进入胃腔中而抑制胃酸分泌。PPI 是目前已知抑酸作用最强的药物，是治疗 GRED 的最佳选择。

点评

该患者男性，年龄 48 岁，有典型的餐后烧心症状，可于夜间发生，上消化道 X 线检查也显示胃食管反流，故诊断胃食管反流疾病基本确立。该病治疗的主要措施是在改变生活方式的基础上应用 PPI，以完全(充分)缓解烧心和其他症状，治愈潜在的食管炎，维持症状缓解和胃镜检查上的缓解，治疗或预防并发症。以下药物也可用于控制胃食管反流疾病的症状：(1) H_2受体拮抗剂：竞争性拮抗 H_2 受体，能抑制组胺引起的胃酸分泌，但不能有效抑制进食刺激的胃酸分泌；(2)促胃肠动力药：改善食管蠕动，促进胃排空，从而达到减少胃内容物食管反流及减少其在食管的暴露时间；(3) 抗酸药：中和胃酸，缓解症状。以上药物对 GRED 的疗效均远不及 PPI。本病常见的并发症有上消化道出血，食管狭窄和食管炎；可有少数 GRED 随时间进展为 Barret 食管，Barret 食管大大增加发生食管腺癌的危险性，故应积极治疗基础病，预防并发症的发生和发展。

王冠蕾

❖ CASE 36

A 22-year-old man presents for the evaluation of abdominal pain and diarrhea. He states that for about a month he has had progressively worsening cramping pains. He has had watery diarrhea and, from time to time, has noted blood mixed in with his stool. He has lost about 5 pounds. He has tried over-the-counter antidiarrheal medications without relief. He is on no medication regularly and has no significant medical history. Examination of his abdomen reveals it to be distended① and to have hyperactive bowel sounds. It is diffusely tender with no palpable masses. Rectal② examination is very painful and reveals heme positive watery stool. A blood count shows that he has iron deficiency anemia and an erythrocyte sedimentation rate③ that is markedly elevated. An office sigmoidoscopy④ reveals changes consistent with ulcerative colitis⑤.[注1] You start him on a short course of corticosteroids⑥ and plan to place him on long-term sulfasalazine⑦.[注2]

◆ **What is the mechanism of action of sulfasalazine**?

◆ **Sulfasalazine cannot be used by persons allergic to which class of antibiotics**?

ANSWERS TO CASE 36: Agents for Lower Gastrointestinal (GI) Disorders

Summary: A 22-year-old man with ulcerative colitis is started on a short course of corticosteroids and long-term sulfasalazine.

- **Mechanism of action of sulfasalazine**: 5-aminosalicylic acid (5-ASA) component of sulfasalazine inhibits leukotriene and prostaglandin production in the colon.
- **Sulfasalazine cannot be used by persons allergic to**: Sulfonamides.

CLINICAL CORRELATION

Sulfasalazine is used to achieve and maintain remission in persons with inflammatory bowel disease (IBD: ulcerative colitis and Crohn disease). It is composed of two constituents—5-ASA bound by an AZO bond (N = N) to sulfapyridine. The AZO bond limits the gastrointestinal (GI) absorption of the inactive, parent compound. However, in the terminal ileum⑧ and colon, bacteria break down sulfasalazine into its two components. 5-ASA⑨ is the active antiinflammatory component. Its mechanism of action, while not entirely known, is thought to involve inhibition of the production of inflammatory leukotrienes and prostaglandins in the colon. Its activity is terminated by hepatic acetylation⑩. Sulfapyridine⑪, which is also acetylated, does not appear to play an active role in the reduction of inflammation in the colon. Sulfapyridine mediates the allergic cross reaction with sulfonamide drugs. 5-ASA can also be administered as mesalamine, balsalazide, and olsalazine, which do not have a sulfa component. Sulfasalazine, balsalazide, and olsalazine are administered orally. Mesalamine has oral, suppository⑫, and enema⑬ formulations. The many adverse effects of sulfasalazine, attributable primarily to the systemic actions of sulfapyridine, which for many patients is not tolerated, and which is more common in slow acetylators than fast acetylators, includes severe GI discomfort with nausea, headache, myalgia⑭, bone marrow suppression, possible oligospermia⑮ that is reversible, and a hypersensitivity with numerous attendant serious sequelae.

Pharmacology of Agents That Act on the Lower GI Tract

Objectives

1. List drugs used as antidiarrheal agents and describe their mechanisms of action, therapeutic uses, and adverse effects.
2. List drugs used as laxatives⑯ and describe their mechanisms of action and adverse effects.
3. List drugs used to treat irritable bowel syndrome (IBS)⑰ and inflammatory bowel

disease(IBD).

Discussion of Class

The agents used for **acute treatment of diarrhea of mild to moderate severity**(Table 36-1) may also be used for control of **chronic diarrhea** resulting from **inflammatory bowel disease(IBD) and irritable bowel syndrome(IBS)**(Table 36-2).

Octreotide is used primarily to treat diarrhea stemming from **gastrointestinal tumors, AIDS, short-bowel syndrome, vagotomy**[18]**, and dumping syndrome**[19]. At low doses(50 mcg subcutaneously), octreotide is used to stimulate intestinal motility in patients with conditions that lead to intestinal obstruction or bacterial overgrowth.

Opioids

Prolonged use of high doses of **diphenoxylate can result in opioid dependence**.

Table 36-1

ANTIDIARRHEAL AGENTS

SELECTED ANTIDIARRHEAL AGENTS	SELECTED LAXATIVES
Opioid agonists	*Bulk-forming laxatives*
Loperamide	Psyllium
Diphenoxylate	Methylcellulose
	Polycarbophil
Kaolin	*Osmotic laxatives*
	Magnesium citrate
	Sodium phosphate
	Magnesium oxide
	Sorbitol
	Lactulose
	Polyethylene glycol(PEG)
Pectin	*Stool softeners*
	Docusate
	Glycerin
	Mineral oil
Methylcellulose resins	*Stimulant laxatives*
Cholestyramine	(infrequently used)
Colestipol	Aloe, senna, cascara, cator oil
Bismuth subsalicylate	

Table 36-2

DRUGS USED TO TREAT BOWEL DISORDERS

DRUGS USED TO TREAT IBS	DRUGS USED TO TREAT IBD
Alostetron Tegaserod	*Aminosalicylates* Sulfasalazine Balsalazide Olsalazine Mesalamine
	Glucocorticoids
	Purine analogs Azathioprine 6-Mercaptopurine
	Methotrexate
	Anti-TNF-Alpha agents Infliximab

IBS = irritable bowel syndrome; IBD = inflammatory bowel disease.

Kaolin-Pectin

When administered concomitantly (within 2 hours of one another) **kaolins and pectins may bind other drugs in the gastrointestinal tract and reduce their absorption.**

Methylcellulose Resins

Cholestyramine and colestipol may cause **bloating and constipation** and in some patients may result in insufficient absorption of fat. Like kaolin-pectin, the use of **octreotide** may result in constipation and abdominal pain. The formation of gallstones resulting from reduced gallbladder contractility, and the development of hyperglycemia[20], and sometime hypoglycemia, as a consequence of an imbalance in the secretions of insulin, glucagons[21], and growth hormone may also occur with octreotide therapy. **Reduced pancreatic secretions may result in steatorrhea[22] and deficiency of fat-soluble vitamins.**

Bulk-Forming and Osmotic Laxatives

Bulk-forming and osmotic laxatives (except polyethylene glycol [PEG])[23] can cause flatulence and bloating. Osmotic laxatives can result in electrolyte imbalance and should be used cautiously in patients with renal insufficiency or cardiac dysfunction. PEG is used to cleanse the colon prior to endoscopy[24]. If aspirated, mineral oil can cause severe lipid pneumonia and when used chronically can result in decreased fat-soluble vitamin absorption.

Structure

Kaolin is a natural occurring hydrated magnesium aluminum silicate, whereas pectin is derived from apples.

Octreotide is a more stable, biologically active octapeptide analog of the 14-amino acid regulatory peptide, somatostatin[25].

PEG is an osmotically active sugar.

Mechanism of Action

Kaolin and **pectin absorb fluids as well as bacteria** and other toxic agents in the gastrointestinal tract.

The **opioids loperamide**[26] **and diphenoxylate inhibit** the **release of acetylcholine** from cholinergic nerves in the submucosa and myenteric complex to disrupt coordinated colonic motility and to increase water absorption and transit time through the gastrointestinal tract.

Cholestyramine and colestipol bind excess diarrhea-causing bile salts[27] that may accumulate in Crohn disease or from resection of the terminal ileum where bile salts are normally absorbed.

Octreotide, like somatostatin, **inhibits the release of numerous GI hormones**(e.g., gastrin, cholecystokinin, serotonin) that results in decreased intestinal fluid secretion and, depending on the subcutaneous dose, increased(50 mcg) or decreased(100-250 mcg) motility among many other effects, including reduced pancreatic secretions.

Bulk-forming laxatives, which are not absorbed from the GI tract, absorb water to form a gel or increase the fluidity of the stools that distends the colon and induces peristalsis[28]. Osmotic laxatives, which are also not absorbed from the GI tract, increase the fluidity of stools. Stool softeners increase the penetration of water and lipids into compacted fecal material(docusate, glycerin) or coat it(mineral oil) to prevent the loss of water.

Administration

Loperamide, administered orally, is a nonprescription opioid agonist. Diphenoxylate is administered orally in combination with low doses of atropine(which also may contribute to the antidiarrheal activity of the preparation) to preclude its self-administration as a drug of abuse[29].

Octreotide can be administered intravenously or subcutaneously and in a subcutaneous depot formulation.

All laxatives are administered orally except glycerin, which is administered rectally as a suppository.

Polyethylene glycol is administered with an isotonic balanced salt solution to prevent the development of intravascular fluid or electrolyte imbalance.

Pharmacokinetics

Commercial preparations of kaolin and pectin are not absorbed from the gastrointestinal tract.

Loperamide does not cross the blood-brain barrier and therefore has no analgesic[30] activity or, importantly, potential for abuse that limits the use of other opioids as antidiarrheal agents.

Diphenoxylate, although very insoluble, does penetrate the central nervous system (CNS), and therefore its continuous use can result in opioid dependence.

Octreotide has a serum half-life of 90 minutes, compared with somatostatin, which has a serum half-life of approximately 3 minutes. Its duration of action can be extended up to 12 hours by subcutaneous administration and up to a month by using a depot formulation.

Sorbitol and lactulose are metabolized by colonic bacteria.

Comprehension Questions

[36.1] Which of the following drugs best crosses the blood-brain barrier?

A. Diphenoxylate
B. Kaolin
C. Loperamide
D. Methylcellulose

[36.2] Which of the following drugs inhibits the release of acetylcholine from cholinergic nerves in the submucosa and myenteric complex?

A. Cholestyramine
B. Docusate
C. Loperamide
D. Pectin

[36.3] Which of the following drugs shows an allergic cross reaction with an antibiotic?

A. Diphenoxylate
B. Octreotide
C. Psyllium
D. Sulfasalazine

Answers

[36.1] **A.** Diphenoxylate can cross the blood-brain barrier and cause dependence. Methylcellulose and kaolin are not absorbed from the GI tract. Loperamide does not cross the blood-brain barrier.

[36.2] **C.** The opioid loperamide inhibits release of acetylcholine from cholinergic nerves in the submucosa and myenteric complex to disrupt coordinated colonic motility and to increase water absorption and transit time through the GI tract. Pectin absorbs fluids in the gastrointestinal tract. Stool softeners like docusate[31] increase the penetration of water and lipids into compacted fecal material.

[36.3] **D.** Sulfasalazine is composed of 5-ASA and sulfapyridine. Sulfapyridine, which does not appear to play an active role in the reduction of inflammation in the colon, mediates an allergic cross reaction with sulfonamide drugs.

PHARMACOLOGY PEARLS

- ❖ Antidiarrheal agents should not be used be used to treat patients experiencing bloody stools or high fever because of the increased risk of aggravating the underlying condition.
- ❖ Cholestyramine and colestipol bind excess diarrhea-causing bile salts.
- ❖ Many laxatives are commonly overused by the lay public.

REFERENCES

Borum ML. Irritable bowel syndrome. Prim Care 2001; 28(3): 523-38.

Schiller LR. Review article: the therapy of constipation. Aliment Pharmacol Ther 2001; 15(6): 749-63.

Stein RB. Medical therapy for inflammatory bowel disease. Gastroenterol Clin North Am 1999; 28(2): 297-321.

Wald A. Constipation. Med Clin North Am 2000; 84(5): 1231-46.

Wingate D, Phillips SF, Lewis SJ, et al. Guidelines for adults on self-medication for the treatment of acute diarrhea. Aliment Pharmacol Ther 2001; 15(6): 773-82.

词汇

1. distended[膨胀的]
2. rectal[直肠的]
3. erythrocyte sedimentation rate (ESR)[红细胞沉降速率]
4. sigmoidoscopy[乙状结肠镜检查]
5. ulcerative colitis (UC)[溃疡性结肠炎]
6. corticosteroid[皮质类甾醇]
7. sulfasalazine[柳氮磺吡啶(简称 SASP)]
8. ileum[回肠]
9. 5-aminosalicylic acid (5-ASA)[5-氨基水杨酸]
10. acetylation[乙酰化作用]
11. sulfapyradine[磺胺吡啶]
12. suppository[栓剂]
13. enema[灌肠剂]
14. myalgia[肌肉痛]
15. oligospermia[少精液症]
16. laxative[轻泻药]
17. irritable bowel syndrome (IBS)[肠易激综合征]
18. vagotomy[迷走神经切断术]
19. dumping syndrome[倾倒综合征]
20. hyperglycemia[高血糖]
21. glucagon[胰高血糖素]

22. steatorrhea[脂肪痢]
23. polyethylene glycol (PEG)[聚乙烯二醇]
24. endoscopy[内镜检查]
25. somatostatin[促生长抑素]
26. loperamide[洛哌丁胺，一种阿片样镇痛药]
27. bile salt[胆盐]
28. peristalsis[蠕动]
29. abuse[滥用]
30. analgesic[镇痛的]
31. docusate (sodium)[多库酯钠，粪便软化剂]

注 1

溃疡性结肠炎是一种原因不明的慢性结肠炎，一般而言，症状严重性和结肠受侵范围与炎症程度相关。病变主要限于结肠的黏膜，表现为炎症或溃疡，由于发病机理目前还不十分清楚，临床药物治疗主要采用抗炎和调节免疫反应以对症治疗。国内近年有关溃疡性结肠炎的报道明显增加，对此疾病应引起重视。

注 2

皮质甾醇类药物是治疗溃疡言结肠炎的经典药物，主要机制包括：广泛的抗炎作用，对细胞因子、致炎因子产生和作用的抑制。常用于临床溃疡性结肠炎急性期控制症状。柳氮磺吡啶(SASP)是用以长期控制溃疡性结肠炎症状并缓解疾病的常用药。该药经口服后在肠道被肠菌分解为5-氨基水杨酸与磺胺吡啶，前者是主要有效成分，滞留在结肠内与肠上皮接触而发挥抗炎作用。但因为同时产生磺胺吡啶，因此对磺胺过敏者禁用。

点评

该患者有典型腹痛、腹泻症状，且症状逐渐加重，出现稀水样血便，体重下降，实验室检查显示缺铁性贫血及血沉明显升高，乙状结肠镜检查显示溃疡性结肠炎改变，故诊断为溃疡性结肠炎基本成立。该病除了进行一般治疗，强调加强休息、营养和饮食外，主要有三大类药物治疗：①氨基水杨酸制剂　柳氮磺吡啶，是磺胺吡啶和5-氨基水杨酸(5-ASA)的偶氮配位化合物，有抗炎和抗菌的双重作用。作用机制为抑制前列腺素合成，清除氧自由基而减轻炎症反应，抑制免疫细胞的免疫反应。长期应用时应注意其不良反应，包括过敏反应，中性粒细胞减少或缺乏症、血小板减少症及再生障碍性贫血；溶血性贫血及血红蛋白尿；和肝肾损害等，因此长期用药需定期检查全血象，尿液和肝肾功能。②糖皮质激素　对急性期有较好疗效，属于非特异性抗炎抗免疫。适用于对氨基水杨酸制剂疗效不佳的轻、中型患者，特别适用于重型活动期患者及暴发型患者。③免疫抑制剂　可试用于糖皮质激素治疗效果不佳或对糖皮质激素依赖的慢性活动性病例，加用这类药物后可逐渐减少糖皮质激素用量甚至停用。当出现严重并发症时，还有可能要进行手术治疗。本病活动期治疗方案的选择主要根据病情和病变部位，结合治疗反应来决定。缓解期主要以氨基水杨酸制剂作维持治疗。

王冠蕾

❖ CASE 37

An 8-year-old boy is brought to your office because of a chronic cough. His mother says that he coughs frequently throughout the day and will have symptoms 2 or 3 nights a month as well. This has been a problem on and off for about a year, but seems to be worse in the spring and fall. He also coughs more when he is riding his bike or playing soccer. He has been treated twice in the past year for "bronchitis" with antibiotics and cough suppressants but he never seems to clear up completely.[注1] His examination is normal except for his lungs, which reveal expiratory wheezing. Your diagnose him with asthma and prescribe an albuterol inhaler.[注2]

◆ **What is the mechanism of action of the albuterol?**

◆ **What are the most common side effects of the albuterol?**

◆ **What medications can be used to provide long-term control of the asthma symptoms?**

ANSWERS TO CASE 37: Agents Used to Treat Asthma

Summary: An 8-year-old boy with asthma is prescribed an albuterol inhaler.

- **Mechanism of action of albuterol**: β_2-adrenoceptor agonist in bronchial smooth muscle causing smooth muscle relaxation, also inhibits the release of mediators from mast cells and stimulates mucociliary clearance.
- **Most common side effects of albuterol**: Skeletal muscle tremor, tachycardia, and cough.
- **Medications for the long term-control of asthma**: Inhaled corticosteroids, long-acting β_2-adrenoceptor agonist, cromolyn, or nedocromil; second line agents include oral theophylline, leukotriene inhibitors, or corticosteroids.

CLINICAL CORRELATION

Asthma is a disease of chronic airway inflammation. This inflammation can cause episodes of wheezing, coughing, and breathlessness, which are reversible either spontaneously or with treatment. The inflammation can also increase bronchial reactivity to certain stimuli, such as allergens, infectious agents, or exercise, which may trigger bronchospasm and symptoms. Inhaled β_2-adrenoceptor agonists(β-agonists) are widely used to treat the acute bronchospastic episodes. They work to relax bronchial smooth muscle via a cyclic adenosine monophosphate(cAMP)-mediated reduction in intracellular calcium concentrations, resulting in relaxation. The increase in cAMP also reduces the release of mediators from mast cells in the airways. Frequent use of these agents can result in a tachyphylaxis. Patients who require frequent dosing with inhaled β-agonists should also be treated with medications to reduce the frequency of bronchospastic events. These include inhaled corticosteroids, long-acting β-agonists, cromolyn, or nedocromil and oral methylxanthines, corticosteroids, or leukotriene modifiers. Inhaled β-agonists commonly cause tremor, tachycardia, and cough.

Pharmacology of Drugs Used to Treat Asthma

Objectives

1. Understand the medications used in the treatment of asthma, their mechanisms of action, and adverse effects.
2. Know the difference between short-acting symptomatic treatments and long-acting preventive therapies.
3. List the mediators of airway inflammation involved in asthma.

Definitions

Bronchoconstriction[①]: Constriction of the bronchial air passages, as a result of increased tone in airway smooth muscle cells.

Discussion of Class

Asthma[②] is characterized by **acute episodes of bronchoconstriction** caused by **underlying airway inflammation**[③]. A common finding in asthmatics is **an increased responsiveness** of the **bronchi and trachea** to **exogenous or endogenous stimuli** that results in **inappropriate contraction of smooth muscle in the airway**, and production of **thick viscid mucus** and **mucosal thickening from edema and cellular infiltration**. Asthma typically occurs with both an **early-phase response** lasting about 1-2 hours that is triggered by autocoids and inflammatory mediators such as **histamine, leukotrienes, and prostaglandins**. Immunoglobulin E (IgE) sensitized mast cells play a key role in the early-phase response. The late-phase response that occurs 2-8 hours later is mediated by cytokines from T-helper type 2 (Th2) lymphocytes including granulocyte-macrophage colony-stimulating factor (GM-CSF), and interleukins 4, 5, 9 and 13. These mediators attract and activate eosinophiles and increase IgE production by B cells. This leads to the chronic bronchoconstriction, continued mucus production, and cellular infiltration that typify the underlying inflammation in asthma.

There are currently **six classes of drugs** used to treat asthma: **β-adrenoreceptor agonists**, **acetylcholine antagonists**, **glucocorticoids**, **leukotriene modifiers**, **chromones**, and **anti-IgE monoclonal antibodies.** The National Asthma Education and Prevention Program has revised its 1997 guidelines on the treatment of asthma as illustrated in Table 37-1.

Table 37-1

RECOMMENDATIONS FOR PHARMACOLOGIC MANAGEMENT OF ASTHMA IN ADULTS AND CHILDREN OLDER THAN 5

ASTHMA SEVERITY	SYMPTOM FREQUENCY	MEDICATIONS
Mild intermittent	< 2days/wk, < 2nights/mo	None; course of systemic glucocorticoids for occasional, severe exacerbations
Mild persistent	> 2/week but < once/day > 2nights/month	Low-dose inhaled glucocorticoids. Alternate: cromolyn, nedocromil, leukotriene modifier, OR sustained release theophylline

续表

ASTHMA SEVERITY	SYMPTOM FREQUENCY	MEDICATIONS
Moderate persistent	Daily, > 1night week	Low- to medium-dose glucocorticoids and long-acting inhaled β_2-agonists. Alternate: leukotriene modifier or theophylline
Severe persistent	Continual during day Frequent at night	High-dose glucocorticoids AND long acting inhaled β_2-agonist AND (if needed) systemic glucocorticoids

The recommendation for quick relief in all patients regardless of severity is two to four puffs of a **short-acting inhaled β_2-agonist**[4] **one to three times per occurrence**. Use of short-acting β_2-agonists more than two times a week may indicate the need to initiate long-term therapy. Short-acting β_2 selective drugs for use in asthma include albuterol, terbutaline, metaproterenol, and pirbuterol. These agents bind specifically to the β_2-adrenergic receptor and avoid the cardiovascular effects of β_1 activation. Activation of β_2-receptors causes bronchodilation. Onset of action occurs in minutes and lasts for 4-6hours. Albuterol[5] and terbutaline[6] can be administered orally; terbutaline is available for subcutaneous injection for emergency treatment. Few side effects of short-term use of β_2-agonist have been reported. Excessive use or the oral preparations may result in cardiovascular effects such as tachycardia.

Long-acting inhaled β_2-agonists[7] such as salmeterol[8] and formoterol[9], have a much longer half-life (up to 12 hours). These agents are available in metereddose inhalers that produce fewer side effects than systemic administration. Use of long-acting agents produces the same relaxation in airway smooth muscles and also appears to decrease the release of mediators from mast cells and lymphocytes. The long-acting agents should not be used to reverse an acute attack.

Glucocorticoids[10] are an important treatment for **mild persistent and more severe asthma**. Glucocorticoids are **potent antiinflammatory agents** and reduce the production of inflammatory mediators and cause apoptosis of leukocytes and decrease vascular permeability. They **do not cause relaxation of bronchial smooth muscle**. The glucocorticoids are used for the prophylactic treatment of asthma; they have no appreciable effect on an acute event. Glucocorticoids administered by **inhalation** provide a high concentration of drug where needed and **minimizes the amount in the systemic circulation**. However, some drug is swallowed during inhalation and some drug is absorbed into the systemic circulation through the lung. Adverse effects are attributable to local effects of the glucocorticoids or the drug entering the systemic circulation. These include **oral candidiasis, increase loss of calcium from bone**, and rarely, **suppression** of the

hypothalamic-pituitary-adrenal axis[11]. **Systemic use of glucocorticoids** is recommended in patients with **severe persistent asthma** (see Table 37-1).

Leukotrienes B_4, C_4, and D_4 play an important role in the pathogenesis of asthma. LCB_4 is a potent neutrophile chemoattractant, and LTC_4 and LTD_4 are involved in bronchoconstriction and overproduction of airway mucus. These mediators are derived from arachidonic acid via the enzyme 5-lipoxygenase. Two classes of drugs have been developed that interfere with leukotrienes. **Zileuton** is an **inhibitor of 5-lipoxygenase** and thereby **decreases the biosynthesis of leukotrienes. Zafirlukast** and **montelukast** are **specific, competitive, Cys-LT1 receptor antagonists**[12]. The **Cys-LT1** receptor is responsible for **mediating the bronchoconstrictor activity of all leukotrienes**. The two classes of drugs are equally **effective in the treatment of mild to moderate persistent asthma** and appear to be about **as effective as low-dose inhaled glucocorticoids**. All of the leukotriene modifiers are administered orally; the receptor antagonists may be taken once or twice a day, zileuton is taken four times a day. **Zileuton**[13] has been associated with **liver toxicity**, and **monitoring liver enzymes is recommended**.

The **methylxanthines**[14] include theophylline, theobromine, and caffeine; theophylline is used as a **second-line agent to treat asthma**. Theophylline is thought to act by **inhibiting cyclic nucleotide phosphodiesterases**, thereby **increasing intracellular cAMP and cyclic guanosine monophosphate (cGMP)**. Theophylline is also an **antagonist of adenosine receptors**[15], and this mechanism of action might be especially important in asthma because **activation of pulmonary adenosine receptors results in bronchoconstriction**. Theophylline[16] produces **bronchodilation** and improves long-term control of asthma. Theophylline is available for oral administration, as a suppository, and for parenteral use. Plasma levels of theophylline show considerable variability between patients, and the drug has a **narrow therapeutic window**; blood levels need to be monitored. Infants and neonates have the slowest rates of clearance.

The **chromones**[17], **cromolyn**[18] **and nedocromil**[19], are unique drugs used for the **prophylaxis** of **mild to moderate persistent asthma**. A variety of mechanisms of action have been proposed for these agents including inhibition of mediator release from mast cells and suppression of activation of leukocytes. These various effects are now thought to be mediated by **inhibition of various chloride channels**[20] **that are responsible for secretion and cellular activation**. They have **no effect on airway smooth muscle tone** and are **ineffective in reversing bronchospasm**; thus they are truly for prevention. Both agents are administered by inhalation and are effective in reducing both antigen and exercise-induced asthma. They are poorly absorbed into the systemic circulation and have mild adverse effects including throat irritation, cough, and nasal congestion. More serious adverse reactions including anaphylaxis, anemia, and pulmonary infiltration are rare.

Inhaled acetylcholine muscarinic cholinoreceptor antagonists[21] have a use in treatment of asthma, but they have been somewhat superseded by other agents. Muscarinic antagonists can effectively block the bronchoconstriction, and the increase in mucus secretion that occurs in response to vagal discharge. **Ipratropium bromide**[22] is a **quaternary ammonium derivative of atropine** that can be administered by inhalation and that is **poorly absorbed into the systemic circulation**. Ipratropium bromide causes variable degrees of **bronchodilation** in patients; this may reflect the variable degree that parasympathetic stimulation contributes to asthma in individual patients. Ipratropium bromide is useful in patients that are unresponsive or cannot tolerate β_2-receptor agonists. In addition, ipratropium bromide increases the bronchodilator activity of albuterol in the treatment of severe acute attacks.

IgE bound to mast cells plays an important role in antigen induced asthma. A newly developed **monoclonal antibody**[23] **that targets circulating IgE** and prevents its interaction with mast cells has recently been approved for the treatment of asthma. By decreasing the amount of IgE antibodies available to bind mast cells, IgE cross-linking is less likely and subsequently, the mast cell release of those mediators is decreased. In clinical trials **omalizumab significantly reduced IgE levels** and reduced the magnitude of both the early and late phase responses to antigen. **Omalizumab is indicated for adults and children older than 12 years with moderate-to-severe persistent asthma** who have a **positive skin test or in vitro reactivity to a perennial aeroallergen** and whose **symptoms are inadequately controlled with inhaled corticosteroids**. The **most frequent adverse events included injection site reaction, viral infections, upper respiratory tract infection (20%), sinusitis**[24]**, headache, and pharyngitis**[25]. These events were observed at similar rates in omalizumab treated patients and control patients. More serious adverse effects include malignancy (0.5%) and anaphylaxis.

Comprehension Questions

[37.1] Zileuton is effective in treating asthma because it

A. Antagonizes leukotriene receptors

B. Inhibits cyclooxygenase

C. Inhibits 5-lipoxygenase

D. Inhibits mast cell degranulation

[37.2] Which of the following drugs would be best for treatment of an acute attack of asthma?

A. Inhaled albuterol

B. Oral albuterol

C. Oral dexamethasone

D. Oral salmeterol

Match the following agents (A-H) to the described clinical situation [37.3-37.5].

A. Anticholinergic inhaler
B. β-agonist inhaler
C. Chromone agent
D. Glucocorticoid inhaler
E. IgE inhibitor
F. Leukotriene receptor antagonist
G. Lipoxygenase inhibitor
H. Methylxanthines

[37.3] A 21-year-old woman with moderately severe asthma on three-drug treatment has elevated liver function tests thought to be caused by one of her medications.

[37.4] A 25-year-old man has bronchospasm that is exercise induced, particularly in the cold weather. He takes his medication 15 minutes prior to anticipated exercise, which will help to prevent the asthmatic attack but does not produce bronchodilation.

[37.5] A 16-year-old female is placed on multiple medications. She has been taking her medications as instructed, but one of the medications is causing her to have tachycardia, nausea, and jitteriness. She has been informed of the need to measure serum levels of this medication.

Answers

[37.1] **C**. Zileuton diminishes the production of leukotrienes by inhibiting 5-lipoxygenase.

[37.2] **A**. Inhaled albuterol would provide the fastest acting and most localized therapy for an acute attack.

[37.3] **G. Zileuton** is an inhibitor of 5-lipoxygenase, thereby decreases the biosynthesis of leukotrienes; it is associated with liver toxicity.

[37.4] **C**. Chromones are prophylactic agents, useful especially for exercise or cold induced bronchospasm.

[37.5] **H**. The methylxanthine agents have a low therapeutic index and often can cause adverse effects.

PHARMACOLOGY PEARLS

❖ Inhaled corticosteroids are the treatment of choice for the long-term management of persistent asthma.

❖ Use of short-acting β_2-agonists more than twice weekly indicates inadequate control, and examination of long-term treatment should be considered.

REFERENCES

Lim KG. Management of persistent symptoms in patients with asthma. Mayo Clin Proc 2002; 77: 1333-8.

Ressel GW, Centers for Disease Control and Prevention, National Asthma Education and Prevention Program. NAEPP updates guidelines for the diagnosis and management of asthma. Am Fam Physician 2003; 68: 169-70.

词汇

1. bronchoconstriction[支气管收缩]
2. asthma[哮喘]
3. airway inflammation[气道炎症]
4. short-acting inhaled β-agonist[短效吸入 β-激动药]
5. albuterol[沙丁胺醇]
6. terbutaline[特布他林]
7. long-acting inhaled β-agonist[长效吸入 β-激动药]
8. salmeterol[沙美特罗]
9. formoterol[福莫特罗]
10. glucocorticoid[糖皮质类固醇]
11. hypothalamic-pituitary-adrenal axis[下丘脑-垂体-肾上腺轴]
12. cys-LT1 receptor antagonists[半胱氨酰白三烯受体拮抗药]
13. Zileuton[齐留通]
14. methylxanthines[甲基黄嘌呤类]
15. adenosine receptor[腺苷受体]
16. theophylline[茶碱]
17. chromones[色甘酸类]
18. cromolyn[色甘酸钠]
19. nedocromil[奈多罗米]
20. chloride channel[氯通道]
21. inhaled acetylcholine muscarinic cholinoreceptor antagonists[吸入 M-胆碱受体拮抗剂]
22. ipratropium bromide[异丙托溴铵]
23. monoclonal antibody[单克隆抗体]
24. sinusitis[(鼻)窦炎]
25. pharyngitis[咽炎]

注 1

哮喘往往被误诊为“支气管炎”，故仅用抗生素和镇咳药不能奏效。

注 2

沙丁胺醇系短效 β_2 受体激动剂，对支气管平滑肌细胞上的 β_2 受体有选择性激动作用，对心脏的 β_1 受体作用弱，故在松弛支气管平滑肌的同时较少产生心动过速等副作用。可口服或吸入给药。

点评

本病例为8岁患儿，有持续1年的慢性咳嗽症状，且于春秋季节加重。运动亦可使症状加重。曾按“支气管炎”治疗效不佳。这提示患儿为过敏性哮喘，并为肺中有严重喘鸣所证实。如能检查IgE或作过敏原皮试可有助于临床诊断。此例确诊后，采用沙丁胺醇(albuterol)气雾剂吸入治疗。儿童使用此类气雾剂需在医师和父母指导下用药，以免用药不当。由于哮喘患者常有呼吸道过敏性炎症，肾上腺皮质激素局部或全身用药均可发挥抗炎作用，并因此降低患者的支气管高反应性、避免内源性或外源性刺激诱发的哮喘发作。此患儿如吸入β-激动剂仍不能完全控制时，可考虑并用吸入皮质激素类药物，如丙酸倍氯米松气雾剂(becotide)。吸入肾上腺皮质激素类气雾剂通过其局部抗炎作用产生疗效，并较少全身不良反应。目前，主张用长效β_2受体激动剂与强效皮质激素类组成的复方制剂吸入治疗哮喘，如沙美特罗与氟替卡松组成的复方粉雾剂，一日仅吸入1～2次。吸入M-胆碱受体拮抗剂与β_2受体激动剂组成的复方气雾剂治疗哮喘亦是一种选择。

林志彬

❖ CASE 38

A 32-year-old woman comes to your office during the height of the spring pollen season complaining of sneezing and congestion. She gets these symptoms every year. Her nose runs constantly, her eyes water and itch, and she sneezes. She is only getting partial relief from oral antihistamines. She asks if there is anything else that she can do for her allergies. On examination she has red, irritated conjunctiva with clear eye drainage and periorbital discoloration ("allergic shiners"). Her nasal mucosa is boggy and appears congested. You agree with her diagnosis of seasonal allergic rhinitis and prescribe a corticosteroid nasal spray[注1] to be used along with her oral antihistamine.[注2]

◆ **How long does it take to see the full effect of nasal steroids?**

◆ **What are the common side effects of nasal steroids?**

ANSWERS TO CASE 38: Rhinitis and Cough Medications

Summary: A 32-year-old woman with seasonal allergic rhinitis is prescribed nasal steroid medication to take together with her antihistamine.

- **Length of time until maximal effect of nasal steroids**: 1-2 weeks.
- **Common side effects**: Nasal burning, throat irritation, nose bleeds.

CLINICAL CORRELATION

The mechanism of action of nasal steroids for allergic rhinitis is not entirely known. Corticosteroids have a wide range of activity on many inflammatory mediators, including histamine, cytokines and leukotrienes, and cell types such as mast cells, eosinophils, and macrophages, which are involved in allergic symptoms. Nasal steroids are effective at reducing the congestion, rhinitis, and sneezing associated with seasonal and environmental allergies. They require treatment for up to 2 weeks before maximal benefit is seen. For that reason it is recommended that they be used on a daily, not an as needed, basis. The adverse effects of nasal steroids are primarily a result of local effects, because they are not largely systemically absorbed. These include nasal burning and bleeding and throat irritation. Histamine (H_1-receptor) antagonists are also widely used for allergic rhinitis and may be used in combination with nasal steroid medications. H_1-receptors are membrane bound and coupled to G-proteins. Their activation leads to increased phospholipase C activity, with increases in diacylglycerol and intracellular Ca^{2+}. The net effect of this in blood vessels is vasodilation and increased permeability, which clinically contributes to the mucosal swelling and congestion seen in allergic rhinitis.

Pharmacology of Drugs Used to Treat Rhinitis and Cough

Objectives

1. Understand the characteristics of rhinitis and cough.
2. List the drugs used for rhinitis, their mechanisms of action, and adverse effects.
3. Know the agents used to treat cough, their mechanisms of action, and adverse effects.

Definitions

Rhinitis①: Inflammation of the mucus membranes of the nose.

Allergic conjunctivitis②: An inflammatory condition of the conjunctiva secondary to an allergic stimulus. Common symptoms include itchy, red, and tearing eyes.

Discussion of Class

Rhinitis is caused by **increased mucus production**, **vasodilation**, **and increased flu-**

id accumulation in mucosal spaces. Inflammatory mediators[3] including **histamine**, **leukotrienes**, **interleukins**, **prostaglandins**, **and kinins** are responsible for these effects. Increased production of these mediators can be provoked by an allergic response, or a bacterial or viral infection.

Allergic rhinitis affects 20 percent of the adult population and up to 40 percent of children. **The hallmark of allergic rhinitis is an immunoglobulin E(IgE)-mediated inflammatory response**. Antihistamines, anticholinergics, intranasal corticosteroids, and chromones have proven to be useful in treating allergic rhinitis.

Both **first-and second-generation histamine H_1-receptor blockers**[4] (see Case 24) are useful in treating **acute allergic rhinitis**[5], but their long-term benefits are questionable. First-generation agents, including diphenhydramine[6], cyclizine[7], and chlorpheniramine[8], have been shown to reduce sneezing, nasal congestion, and nasal itching. Second-generation agents, including fexofenadine[9], cetirizine[10], and loratadine[11], have comparable efficacy and significantly fewer adverse effects such as sedation and dry mouth. Second-generation antihistamines effectively reduce all seasonal allergic rhinitis symptoms in children, but dosages must be appropriately reduced. Following oral administration effects are seen with antihistamines in 1-2hours. The most common adverse effect seen with the second-generation agents are headache, back pain, and cough.

Inhaled nasal corticosteroids[12] such as beclomethasone, budesonide, flunisolide, fluticasone and triamcinolone acetonide are **useful for long-term management of allergic rhinitis.** This **route of administration reduces the frequent adverse effects associated with systemic administration of corticosteroids**. Corticosteroids are potent antiinflammatory agents and reduce both the production of inflammatory mediators (cytokines, leukotrienes, and prostaglandins) and cellular components (mast cells, eosinophils, basophils, lymphocytes, macrophages, and neutrophils). The major adverse effects seen with inhaled corticosteroids is **pharyngitis and an increased risk of upper respiratory tract infections**.

The **chromones**[13], cromolyn and nedocromil, have also been used to treat allergic rhinitis. These agents are administered by inhalation and are poorly absorbed into the systemic circulation. Their major action is to reduce the activity of a number of chloride channels that are important in the release of mediators such as histamine. The major adverse effects of these agents are bronchospasm, cough, and nasal congestion (which can be severe); less frequent adverse effects include anaphylaxis, dizziness, and anemia.

Nasal decongestants[14] are α-adrenoreceptor agonists that **reduce the discomfort** of allergic rhinitis, and to a lesser extent congestion associated with the common cold or flu, by decreasing the volume of nasal mucosa and **causing vasoconstriction of capaci-**

tance vessels in the nasal passages. The most common α-adrenergic agent[15] used as a decongestant is **pseudoephedrine**[16] (a stereoisomer of ephedrine), which acts directly on **α_1-adrenoreceptors**. Ephedrine[17] has largely been discontinued as a decongestant because it has significant central nervous system (CNS) effects. A major limitation in the use of these agents is rebound hyperemia and worsening of symptoms that often occurs with chronic use or after discontinuation. Nasal decongestants should be used with caution in patients with hypertension.

Cough and Antitussives[18]

Cough is produced by the cough reflex, which is integrated in the cough center in the medulla. The initial stimulus for cough arises in the bronchi where irritation causes bronchoconstriction. Stretch receptors in the trachea and bronchial tree monitor the state of this bronchoconstriction and send vagal afferents to the cough center that trigger the cough reflex. Agents that have antitussive activity act either to relieve the bronchoconstriction or reduce the activity of the cough center.

Codeine[19] **and hydrocodone are opioid congeners** that are used as antitussives. Cough suppression occurs at lower doses than required for analgesia. The exact mechanism of the antitussive activity of the opioids is unclear because isomers devoid of binding to classic receptors still display antitussive activity. Both codeine and hydrocodone are available as syrups for oral administration.

Dextromethorphan[20] **is the d-isomer of the codeine analog methorphan**. It has no analgesic or addictive properties and does not act through the classic opioid receptors. Binding sites for dextromethorphan have been identified in membrane preparations from various parts of the brain, but it is still unclear whether they mediate the antitussive actions of the drug.

β-adrenergic agonists have been shown to reduce cough without having any significant central effects. This **action is likely mediated within the bronchi** and reduces vagal afferent signals to the cough center.

Comprehension Questions

[38.1] Pseudoephedrine is used to treat nasal congestion because it

A. Is an α_1-adrenergic agonist
B. Is an α_2-adrenergic agonist
C. Inhibits leukotrienes
D. Inhibits the production of IgE

[38.2] Which of the following would be the best for long-term management of a patient with allergic rhinitis?

A. Diphenhydramine
B. Inhaled glucocorticoids
C. Oral glucocorticoids
D. Oral pseudoephedrine

[38.3] A 24-year-old man is taking two medications to help with the symptoms of allergic rhinitis. He is noted to have a blood pressure of 150/70 mmHg. The clinician notes that one of the medications may be responsible for the new-onset hypertension. The most likely etiology is

A. Inhaled chromone
B. Inhaled glucocorticoids
C. Oral diphenhydramine
D. Oral pseudoephedrine

Answers

[38.1] **A.** Pseudoephedrine is the most common agent used today as a decongestant. It is a directly acting α_1 sympathomimetic agent.

[38.2] **B.** Systemic glucocorticoids cause too many adverse effects; pseudoephedrine acts primarily only on nasal congestion; diphenhydramine is not useful for long-term management.

[38.3] **D.** Pseudoephedrine has activity on the α_1-adrenergic receptor, causing vasoconstriction to the nasal mucosa. Hypertension may also be seen at times.

PHARMACOLOGY PEARLS

- ❖ The hallmark of allergic rhinitis is an IgE mediated inflammatory response.
- ❖ Antihistamines are useful for treating symptoms of acute rhinitis but their long-term benefit is questionable.
- ❖ Pseudoephedrine has activity on the α_1-adrenergic receptor, causing vasoconstriction to the nasal mucosa.

REFERENCES

Ressel GW, Agency for Healthcare Research and Quality. AHRQ (agency for healthcare research and quality) releases review of treatments for allergic and nonallergic rhinitis. Am Fam Physician 2002; 66: 2164, 2167.

词汇

1. rhinitis[鼻炎]
2. allergic conjunctivitis[过敏性结膜炎]
3. mediators[炎症介质]
4. histamine H_1-receptor blockers[组胺 H_1-受体阻断药]
5. acute allergic rhinitis[急性过敏性鼻炎]
6. diphenhydramine[苯海拉明]
7. cyclizine[赛克利嗪]
8. chlorpheniramine[氯苯那敏]
9. fexofenadine[非索非那定]
10. cetirizine[西替利嗪]
11. loratadine[氯雷他定]

12. inhaled nasal corticosteroids[鼻吸入皮质类固醇]
13. chromones[对氧萘酮类]
14. nasal decongestants[解除鼻充血药]
15. α-adrenergic agent[α 肾上腺素能药]
16. pseudoephedrine[伪麻黄碱]
17. ephedrine[麻黄碱]
18. antitussives[镇咳药]
19. codeine[可待因]
20. dextromethorpha[右美沙芬]

注 1

肾上腺皮质激素鼻气雾剂如丙酸倍氯米松鼻气雾剂可通过其抗炎及抗过敏作用抑制鼻黏膜过敏性炎症，减轻症状。

注 2

口服抗组胺药即组胺 H_1 受体拮抗剂，可抑制组胺引起的鼻黏膜炎症反应，减轻过敏性鼻炎患者的鼻结膜充血、痒、流涕等症状。

点评

本病例为典型季节性过敏性鼻炎合并结膜炎患者，单用抗组胺药仅能部分缓解，故加用局部喷鼻给药的肾上腺皮激素类药物，以消除过敏性炎症，减轻症状。鼻腔喷入皮质激素类药物可显著减少全身给药的不良反应，但也要警惕其对粘膜局部的不良反应。此外，局部应用能减轻鼻粘膜充血水肿的α-肾上腺素受体激动药如伪麻黄碱等就有助于迅速缓解症状，但不宜久用，以避免由于产生快速耐受性，而降低疗效。如能明确致敏原可采取脱敏疗法，有时可达到根除疾病的目的。

林志彬

❖ CASE 39

A 67-year-old man complains of pain in his right hip for the past few weeks. He has had no injury to the area and describes the pain as a "bone ache" that does not radiate. Review of systems is positive only for some weakness of urinary stream and having to get up twice a night to go to the bathroom. His general physical examination is normal. His hip exam is normal with a full range of motion and no tenderness. Examination of his prostate reveals it to be firm, enlarged, and nodular. Blood tests show a markedly elevated prostate specific antigen (PSA), and biopsy of the prostate shows carcinoma.[注1] A bone scan confirms the presence of metastatic disease in the right hip. Along with other adjuvant therapies, a decision is made to start depot leuprolide acetate.[注2]

◆ **Leuprolide acetate is an analog of which hypothalamic hormone?**

◆ **What is the mechanism of action of leuprolide acetate?**

◆ **Which pituitary hormones are affected by leuprolide acetate, and how are they affected?**

ANSWERS TO CASE 39: Drugs Active on the Hypothalamus and Pituitary Gland

Summary: A 67-year-old man with metastatic prostate cancer is to receive depot leuprolide acetate.

- **Leuprolide acetate is an analog of which hypothalamic hormone**: Gonadotropin-releasing hormone (GnRH).
- **Mechanism of action of leuprolide acetate**: Chronic administration GnRH analog results in the reduction of the number of GnRH receptors in the pituitary (down-regulation), with resultant decreases in pituitary gonadotropin production.
- **Pituitary hormones affected**: Leuteinizing hormone (LH) and follicle-stimulating hormone (FSH) production is reduced.

CLINICAL CORRELATION

The hypothalamic-pituitary-gonadal axis is a classic example of a hormonal stimulation-feedback system. The hypothalamus produces GnRH, which binds to specific receptors on pituitary gonadotropic cells. These cells then produce LH and FSH, which act on the gonadal organs. LH and FSH regulate the female menstrual cycle by their effects on the ovarian production of estrogen and progesterone. In males, LH and FSH regulate the production of testosterone in the testes. Estrogen, progesterone, and testosterone then function as feedback signals for the hypothalamic production of GnRH. Leuprolide acetate is a synthetic 9-amino acid analog of GnRH. When initially administered, leuprolide acetate results in increases in LH, FSH, and gonadal steroid production because of its action as a GnRH agonist. However, with chronic administration, there is a reduction in the number of GnRH receptors in the pituitary gonadotropic cells. This causes a reduction in FSH or LH and a resultant reduction in gonadal hormone production. In women this effect may be beneficial in conditions such as endometriosis, where estrogen stimulates the growth, and activity of the ectopic endometrial tissue, which causes symptoms. The effect in men is to lower the production of testosterone to near castrate levels. Because prostate cancer is often testosterone-dependent, leuprolide acetate can be used as a treatment for prostate cancer in those who are not surgical candidates, do not desire surgery, or have metastatic disease. Leuprolide acetate must be administered parenterally, and it has a depot form, which is active for up to 3 months. It commonly causes "menopausal" side effects, such as hot flashes, as a result of the reduction in gonadal hormone production.

Pharmacology of Neuroendocrine Drugs

Objectives

1. Understand the receptors and second messengers involved in the endocrine system.
2. Understand the hypothalamic-pituitary axis and its feedback system.
3. Know the drugs used as agonists and antagonists on the hypothalamicpituitary axis, their therapeutic uses, mechanisms of action, and adverse effects.

Definitions

Prostate cancer[1]: Common malignancy in men which may be confined to the prostate gland or metastasize to pelvic lymph nodes or bone.

Hormonal therapy[2]: Various malignancies are sensitive to hormones, and thus medications that act as agonists or antagonists are used for therapy.

Discussion of Class of Agents

The **hypothalamic-hypophyseal-end organ system**[3] is a classic negative feedback pathway (Fig. 39-1). The multiple steps in this regulatory pathway, and both positive and negative regulation, provide several targets for pharmacologic intervention. The **hypothalamus**[4] secretes a number of **releasing factors**[5], including **GnRH**, **corticotropin-releasing hormone (CRH)**, **thyroid-releasing hormone (TRH)**, **and growth hormone-releasing hormone (GHRH)**[6], that are of clinical significance.

These neuroendocrine factors are secreted by the hypothalamus into the hypothalamic-hypophyseal portal circulation, and they act on cognate cell types within the pituitary and cause an increase in the secretion of specific pituitary hormones. For example, **GnRH** produces an increase in the synthesis and release of both **gonadotropins, LH and FSH**[7]. This action is mediated by a specific **seven-transmembrane G-protein coupled receptor**[8] that binds GnRH in cells called gonadotrophs.

FSH acts on the **ovary**[9] to cause **follicular development and maturation**[10]; **LH** causes an increase in the production of **estradiol**[11] and is required for maintenance of the **corpus luteum**[12]. The **LH surge**[13] at midmenstrual cycle triggers **ovulation**[14]. In men, **FSH is required for spermatogenesis**[15], **and LH causes an increase in testosterone**[16] **production**. The actions of the two gonadotropins are also mediated by specific G-protein coupled receptors in the ovary and testis.

Estradiol and testosterone are released into the circulation, and these sex hormones have effects in many tissues. Predominantly **estradiol in women**, and **testosterone and estradiol in men** (produced by peripheral conversion of testosterone to estradiol), act on the hypothalamus and pituitary to decrease the production of the releasing hormone and the gonadotropins, respectively. This closes the negative feedback loop. As in all target tissues, the estrogen and testosterone receptors in the pituitary and hypothalamus are nuclear receptors that modulate the transcription of target genes.

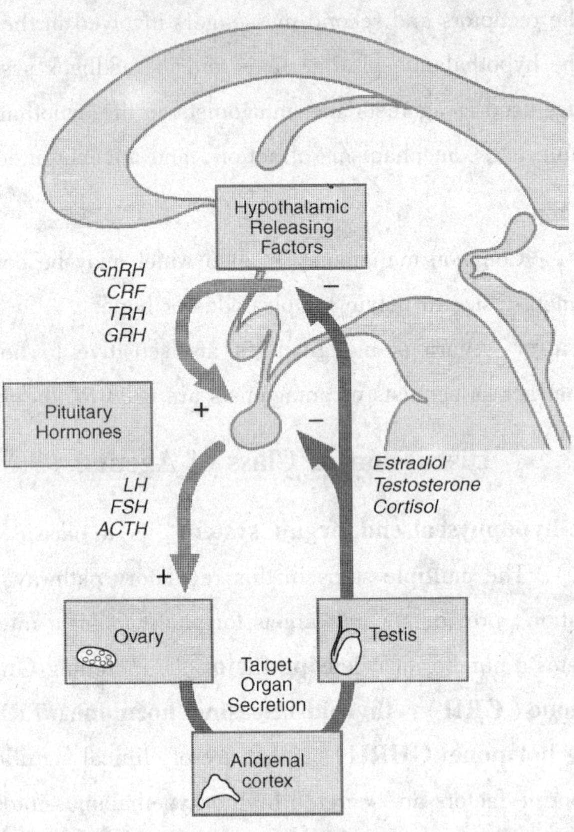

Figure 39-1. Interaction among the hypothalamus, pituitary, and gonad. GnRH = gonadotropic-releasing hormone; CRH = corticotropin-releasing hormone; TRH = thyrotropin-releasing hormone; GHRH = growth hormone-releasing hormone; LH = luteinizing hormone; FSH = follicular stimulating hormone; ACTH = adrenocorticotropic hormone.

The **adrenal cortex**[17] is regulated in a similar manner. **Corticotropin-releasing factor (CRF)**[18] is released **from the hypothalamus**, and it elicits the synthesis and release of **adrenocorticotropic hormone (ACTH)**[19] from the **pituitary**[20]. **ACTH acts on the adrenal cortex** and causes an increase in the synthesis of **cortisol from the zona fasciculata**[21] and **adrenal androgens from the zona reticularis**[22].

The secretion of **growth hormone by the pituitary** is regulated in a different manner. Growth hormone secretion is stimulated by the **hypothalamic hormone GHRH** and is **inhibited by somatostatin**[23]. Somatostatin acts in a number of tissues besides the pituitary; it inhibits the release of glucagon and insulin from the pancreas and inhibits the secretion of a number of gut peptides. **Prolactin**[24] secretion from the pituitary is also controlled by **positive and negative regulatory factors**[25]. The most important pharmacologically is the **prolactin inhibitory factor(PIF) activity of dopamine agonists.**

Pharmacologic Uses of Hypothalamic Peptides and Analogs

Leuprolide acetate and gonadorelin acetate[26] **are synthetic peptide GnRH analogs** that are administered either by subcutaneous injection, as a long-acting implant, or by IV infusion. Nafarelin acetate is a comparable peptide analog that can be administered by nasal spray. The frequency of administration is critical to the therapeutic goal. **Acute or pulsatile administration of GnRH analogs increases** production of **LH and FSH** by the pituitary. Used in this manner, GnRH analogs are useful to **stimulate spermatogenesis and testosterone production in men, and to induce ovulation or treat primary hypothalamic amenorrhea**[27] **in women. Chronic administration**, for example, daily injections or use of depot preparations, **decreases** the production of FSH and LH by the pituitary. This is caused by a **depression in the number of GnRH receptors on gonadotrophs**[28]. **Chronic leuprolide administration** can be used to achieve maximum androgen blockade(MAB), which **reduces testosterone production by the testis**[29] that is **therapeutically equivalent to orchiectomy**[30]. In men this is useful to control androgen-dependent hyperproliferation as in **advanced prostate cancer and prostatic hyperplasia**[31]. In women, chronic leuprolide leads to markedly diminished estrogen production which is useful in treating a number of estrogen-dependent hyperproliferative diseases. These include **endometriosis, polycystic ovarian disease, and uterine myomas**[32]. Chronic leuprolide has also been used to treat hirsutism in women. The major adverse effect in women is a chemical menopause with vasomotor symptoms and the potential for osteoporosis. In men, leuprolide has been associated with the flare phenomenon, increased cancer growth as a result of transient increase in testosterone production on initiation of therapy. Other adverse effects in men include hot flashes, gynecomastia, and testicular atrophy.

Somatostatin is unique among the hypothalamic peptides because of its widespread inhibitory activity on secretion and cellular proliferation. **Octreotide**[33] is an 8-amino acid cyclopeptide with potent somatostatin agonist activity. Its action to decrease secretion makes it useful to treat hypersecretory states such as VIPomas and chronic pancreatitis. Its antiproliferative uses include colorectal cancer and leukemia, and it is in clinical trials for additional malignancies. It has also been used to treat acute portal hypertension. Adverse effects include nausea, cramps and increased gallstone formation.

Other hypothalamic peptides are used primarily as diagnostic agents. **GHRH** is a 40 amino-acid peptide that can be administered IV for the diagnostic evaluation of idiopathic growth hormone deficiency. Similarly, IV administration of **TRH** is useful in the differential diagnosis of thyroid diseases. **CRF** is a 41-amino acid polypeptide found in the hypothalamus and the gut. CRH is used in cases of ACTH deficiency to distinguish between hypothalamic-pituitary or primary adrenal disease.

The **PIF**[34] activity of **bromocriptine**[35] or **levodopa**[36] can be used to treat states of prolactin excess as in some cases of amenorrhea, galactorrhea, and prolactin-secreting tumors.

Comprehension Questions

[39.1] Which of the following best describes the action of somatostatin?

A. Inhibition of growth hormone release

B. Inhibition of prolactin release

C. Stimulation of insulin release

D. Stimulation of LH release

[39.2] In the first 2 weeks following a single injection of leuprolide, one would be expected which of the following?

A. Decreased LH production

B. Decreased testosterone production

C. Increased LH receptors

D. Increased testosterone production

[39.3] A 22-year-old woman has severe endometriosis with dysmenorrhea. She is treated with depot leuprolide acetate. One week after her first injection, she notes a marked increase in the dysmenorrhea. What is the explanation?

A. Direct effect of leuprolide on the endometrial implants

B. Likely flare with increased gonadotropin effect prior to downregulation of receptors

C. Probable placebo effect

D. Resistance of her endometriosis to the leuprolide and probable need for another agent

Answers

[39.1] **A.** Somatostatin is a major regulator of growth hormone, and its effect is inhibitory of growth hormone release.

[39.2] **D.** Acute leuprolide will increase FSH/LH and sex steroid production and have little effect on receptor numbers.

[39.3] **B.** The initial response to gonadotropin releasing hormone analog is an increase in FSH and estrogen, leading to an exacerbation of the endometriosis.

Thereafter, there is a downregulation of GnRH receptors of the pituitary, leading to a decrease in FSH and estrogen.

PHARMACOLOGY PEARLS

- ❖ The frequency of administration of leuprolide determines its effect: Acute administration will increase FSH/LH and sex steroids, chronic administration will decrease FSH/LH and sex steroids.
- ❖ Chronic leuprolide administration leads to androgen blockade in men, which is useful in treating hormone-dependent cancers such as prostatic carcinoma.

REFERENCES

Holzbeierlein JM, Castle EP, Thrasher JB. Complications of androgen-deprivation therapy for prostate cancer. Clin Prostate Cancer 2003; 2: 147-52.

Valle RF, Sciarra JJ. Endometriosis: treatment strategies. Ann N Y Acad Sci 2003; 97: 229-39.

词汇

1. prostate cancer[前列腺癌]
2. hormonal therapy[激素疗法]
3. hypothalamic-hypophyseal-end organ system[下丘脑-垂体-靶器官系统]
4. hypothalamus[下丘脑]
5. releasing factor[释放因子]
6. GnRH, CRH, TRH, GHRH[促性腺释放激素,促肾上腺皮质激素释放激素,促甲状腺激素释放激素,生长素释放激素]
7. gonadotropins, LH and FSH[促性腺激素,黄体生成素,促卵泡激素]
8. G-protein coupled receptor[G 蛋白偶联受体]
9. ovary[卵巢]
10. follicular development and maturation[卵泡的发育和成熟]
11. estradiol[雌二醇]
12. corpus luteum[黄体]
13. LH surge[LH 峰]
14. ovulation[排卵]
15. spermatogenesis[精子生成]
16. testosterone[睾酮]
17. adrenal cortex[肾上腺皮质]
18. CRF[促肾上腺皮质激素释放因子]
19. ACTH[促肾上腺皮质激素]
20. pituitary[垂体]
21. zona fasciculata[束状带(肾上腺皮质)]
22. zona reticularis[网状带(肾上腺皮质)]
23. somatostatin[生长抑素]
24. prolactin[催乳素]
25. positive and negative regulatory factors[正性和负性调节因子]
26. leuprolide acetate and gonadorelin acetate[醋酸亮丙瑞林和醋酸高纳瑞林]
27. primary hypothalamic amenorrhea[原发性下丘脑性闭经]
28. gonadotrophs[促性腺细胞]
29. testis[睾丸]
30. orchiectomy[睾丸切除术]
31. prostatic hyperplasia[前列腺增生]

32. endometriosis, polycystic ovarian disease, and uterine myomas[子宫内膜异位症,多囊卵巢病,子宫肌瘤]
33. octreotide[奥曲肽]
34. PIF[催乳素抑制因子]
35. bromocriptine[溴隐亭]
36. levodopa[左旋多巴]

注 1

PSA 称为前列腺特异性抗原，自前列腺上皮分泌后，以高浓度储存于导管腔内，极少部分通过组织屏障进入血循环，成为血清 PSA。检验血清 PSA 是一项敏感而简便的前列腺癌的检查手段，在判断前列腺癌体积时要优于前列腺酸性磷酸酶(PAP)，目前已被广泛应用于临床。由于 PSA 是前列腺癌特异性的肿瘤标志物，利用 PSA 既具有肿瘤定位特异性，又具有丝氨酸蛋白酶水解活性的特性，设计合成能被 PSA 特异性识别并水解的抗肿瘤前体药物已成为前列腺癌靶向治疗中极具前景的策略，为高效、低毒、特异的治疗前列腺癌提供了新的思路，具有广阔的应用前景。

注 2

醋酸亮丙瑞林(LE)是一种促性腺激素释放增效剂，可刺激垂体分泌促性腺激素，诱发生殖器官生成类固醇，长期使用会抑制促性腺激素及性腺甾体生成。1998 年在法国批准上市，1992 年获得我国进口药品许可证。目前主要应用于临床治疗子宫内膜异位症、子宫肌瘤、前列腺癌等疾病。

对于前列腺癌患者，醋酸亮丙瑞林可调节垂体促性腺激素的合成以及释放，能有效降低睾丸激素水平，从而抑制肿瘤细胞的增殖。醋酸亮丙瑞林的适应证是进展期前列腺癌的姑息治疗，FDA 推荐在醋酸亮丙瑞林治疗期间要定期监测睾酮和 PSA 水平，特别是那些没有获得期望的生化或临床缓解的患者。

点评

本病例患者有典型的疼痛史，尿频且有排尿障碍，但其他各项一般检查正常。患者的前列腺检查显示前列腺坚硬、增大且有小结，血液检查显示 PSA 水平显著增高，活检提示前列腺癌。血清前列腺特异抗原浓度升高是提示前列腺癌的敏感监测指标，目前在临床上广泛用于前列腺癌的辅助诊断，但由于前列腺癌不是造成血前列腺特异抗原浓度升高的唯一原因，因此不能作为确诊指标。前列腺特异抗原(PSA)有总前列腺特异抗原(tPSA)、结合前列腺特异抗原(cPSA)、游离前列腺特异抗原(fPSA)之分，tPSA = cPSA + fPSA。f PSA /t PSA 比值对于鉴别前列腺癌与良性前列腺增生比 tPSA 精确。此外前列腺特异抗原密度(PSAD)，即血前列腺特异抗原浓度除以前列腺体积，有助前列腺癌相与良性前列腺增生症鉴别。由于良性前列腺增生是前列腺实质细胞数量增多而造成前列腺体积的增大，引起不同程度的血前列腺特异抗原(PSA)浓度升高。

治疗中采用醋酸亮丙瑞林，商品名抑那通。醋酸亮丙瑞林是高活性的促黄体生成释放激素(LH-RH)衍生物，由于它对蛋白分解酶的抵抗力和对LH-RH受体的亲和力都比LH-RH强，所以能有效地抑制垂体-性腺系统的功能。重复给予大剂量的醋酸亮丙瑞林，在首次给药后能立即产生一过性的垂体-性腺系统兴奋作用(急性作用)，然后抑制垂体生成和释放促性腺激素。它还进一步抑制卵巢和睾丸对促性腺激素的反应，从而降低雌二醇和睾丸酮的生成(慢性作用)。醋酸亮丙瑞林的促黄体生成激素(LH)释放活性约为LH-RH的100倍，它的抑制垂体-性腺系统功能的作用也强于LH-RH。此外，醋酸亮丙瑞林又是一种缓释制剂，它恒定地向血液中释放醋酸亮丙瑞林，故能有效地降低卵巢和睾丸的反应，产生高度有利的垂体-性腺系统的抑制作用。

对前列腺癌患者皮下注射醋酸亮丙瑞林，每4周1次，使血清睾丸酮浓度降至去势水平之下，表明本品有药理学的去势作用。醋酸亮丙瑞林在与其他LH-RH促进剂合用时可能在初期导致血清睾酮水平升高，这可能会引起在治疗最初几周短暂的前列腺癌进展或症状加重。暂时性骨痛也可能会加重，应该给予对症治疗。还曾发现过个别因输尿管梗阻和脊髓受压的伴或不伴严重并发症的麻痹。FDA禁止醋酸亮丙瑞林注射液在对促性腺激素释放激素(GnRH)、GnRH促进剂类似物或其组成成分过敏的患者中使用。

王毅群　姚明辉

❖ CASE 40

A 28-year-old woman presents for an evaluation of infertility. She and her husband have been attempting to conceive unsuccessfully for a year. She has never been pregnant. She has a history of irregular menstrual cycles, which were treated with oral contraceptive pills for 5 years. She has not taken contraceptives in the past 3 years. [注1] She has no other medical history, she takes no medications, and there is no family history of infertility. She does not smoke cigarettes or drink alcohol. Her routine physical and gynecologic examinations are normal. Blood tests were also normal. Basal body temperature charts that she brings in with her show no midcycle temperature elevation, and home urine ovulation prediction tests have all been negative. Her husband has already seen his physician, had a normal examination, and has had a normal semen analysis. She is diagnosed with infertility secondary to anovulation and started on clomiphene citrate. [注2]

◆ **What is the mechanism of action of clomiphene**?

◆ **How does clomiphene induce ovulation**?

ANSWERS TO CASE 40: Drugs Active on the Gonadal and Reproductive System

Summary: A 28-year-old woman with infertility and anovulation is treated with clomiphene citrate.

- **Mechanism of action of clomiphene**: Competitive antagonist of estrogen receptor.
- **Mechanism of induction of ovulation**: Inhibition of estrogen feedback on hypothalamus and pituitary with resultant increase in folliclestimulating hormone (FSH), which induces follicle production in the ovaries and ovulation.

CLINICAL CORRELATION

The menstrual cycle is regulated by the hypothalamic-pituitary-ovarian axis. Gonadotropin-releasing hormone (GnRH) produced in the hypothalamus stimulates the pituitary hormones FSH and luteinizing hormone (LH), which induce the maturation of follicles and release of ova from the ovaries. Estrogen and progesterone produced in the ovaries create a feedback loop on the hypothalamus and pituitary. Clomiphene is a competitive antagonist of the estrogen receptor. It is used for the treatment of infertility in women who have anovulatory menstrual cycles. By antagonizing estrogen receptors in the pituitary gland, clomiphene disrupts the normal negative feedback on the release of FSH. The elevated levels of FSH then help to induce the development of follicles in the ovaries. Potential risks of the use of clomiphene include the stimulation of multiple follicles and release of multiple eggs, with a resultant multiple gestation. It may also cause ovarian enlargement. The antiestrogen effect may precipitate hot flashes and abnormal uterine bleeding.

Pharmacology of Gonadal Steroids and Their Antagonists

Objectives

1. Understand the structures, mechanism of action, and effects of natural gonadal hormones.
2. Know the therapeutic uses and adverse effects of estrogens, progestins, and androgens.
3. List the types, uses, and adverse effects of hormonal contraceptives.
4. Describe the drugs used as antiestrogens, antiprogestins, and antiandrogens, their therapeutic uses, mechanisms of action, and adverse effects.

Definitions

Nuclear receptor[①]: A superfamily of receptor molecules that are activated by steroid hormones, fatty acid derivatives, or products of metabolism such as bile acids. They act by altering the rate of transcription of specific target genes.

ERE[2]: Estrogen-response element. A DNA sequence motif that binds estrogen receptors. The consensus sequence is GGTCANNNTGACC.

SERM[3]: Selective estrogen receptor modulator. A group of drugs that display tissue-specific estrogen agonist or antagonist activity.

Discussion of Class

Estrogens and Progestins[4]

The **gonadotropins**[5] **and sex steroids** comprise a collection of drugs that have a number of uses including **infertility**, **contraception**, **hormone replacement**, **osteoporosis**[6], **and cancer. Antagonists** acting within the system also have uses in treating **hormone-dependent cancers and as abortifacients**[7].

The **menstrual cycle**[8] is controlled by a complex feedback system between the hypothalamus, pituitary, and ovaries (see Case 39). LH and FSH are released from the pituitary on stimulation by GnRH released from the hypothalamus. **GnRH is released from the hypothalamus in a pulsatile manner under the control of the "pulse generator" in neurons in the arcuate nucleus**. In the proliferative phase of the menstrual cycle, the pulse generator causes release of GnRH at a rate of about one pulse per hour, and consequently **release of LH and FSH**[9] from the pituitary is also **pulsatile**. The **intermittent release of GnRH is key in controlling the menstrual cycle** because continuous infusion of GnRH results in cessation of release of the pituitary gonadotropins, estrogen and progesterone, and produces amenorrhea. FSH acts on the Graafian follicle to cause maturation of ova and to secrete estrogen. As estrogen levels rise, LH and FSH production is inhibited because of negative feedback that diminishes the *amplitude* of the GnRH pulse; release of FSH is also diminished by inhibin that is released by the ovary. At midcycle, alterations in the responsiveness of the pituitary to gonadotropins occur, and the negative feedback pattern is replaced by a period of positive feedback when estradiol causes an increase in the release of LH and FSH. This change in pituitary responsiveness requires levels of serum estradiol above 150 pg/ml for 36 hours. The positive feedback elicits the midcycle surge of LH and FSH that causes ovulation. After ovulation, the corpus luteum is able to secrete progesterone for its lifetime of 14 days if pregnancy does not occur. Progesterone decreases the frequency of the hypothalamic pulse-generator and inhibits LH and FSH release from the pituitary. A frequent cause of infertility is a disruption in the complex feedback regulatory patterns that results in anovulation.

The **ovary produces a number of estrogens**, the most important are **17β estradiol and estrone**[10]. 17β-estradiol and estrone are classical steroid hormones containing a four-ring structure and 18 carbon atoms. **Progesterone**[11] is also a classical steroid composed of **21 carbon atoms.**

The effects of estrogen and progesterone are mediated by **hormone-specific nuclear receptors**. There are **two types of estrogen receptors**, termed ER_α and ER_β. Most tissues express more ER_α, but the relative amounts of the two receptors is tissue and cell dependent. The precise role that each of these receptors plays in the mediating the various effects of the estrogens is unclear. 17β-estradiol has the highest affinity for the ERs; estrone binds to both receptors with a lower affinity. ER_α and ER_β are nuclear receptors that reside within the nucleus bound to the promoters of target genes at estrogen response elements even in the absence of ligand. On binding an estrogen, a conformational change occurs in the receptor such that additional proteins are recruited to the receptor. These proteins, called coactivators, are able to increase the transcription rate of estrogen-dependent target genes. There also are two forms of the progesterone receptor called PRA and PRB. These two isoforms are derived from a single gene by differential use of two promoters within the progesterone receptor gene. Human PRB contains an additional 164 amino acids on the amino terminus of the mature protein, the rest of the PRB is identical to PRA. Both receptors reside within the nucleus bound to PREs and activate gene expression in a fashion similar to ERs, but the target genes are different as a result of differences in the sequence of ERE compared to PRE. In most circumstances PRA inhibits the action of PRB (and of some other nuclear receptors such as ER_α and ER_β as well). Thus the amplitude of the effects elicited by progesterone depends on the ratio of the two isoforms.

Estrogens and progesterone have a variety of pharmacological uses including oral contraception, hormone replacement therapy (HRT) in postmenopausal women, treatment of osteoporosis, and for failure of ovarian development.

Oral Contraceptives[12]

Oral combination contraceptives contain **synthetic estrogens**, most commonly **ethinyl estradiol**[13], and a **progestin** (for example norethindrone or norgestrel). Over the past several years the doses of estrogen in combination oral contraceptives have diminished, and the ratio of estrogen to progestin has evolved from a fixed ratio (monophasic) to biphasic and triphasic regimens with varying ratios that attempt to more closely mimic the ratio during the normal menstrual cycle. **The primary mechanism of action of oral contraceptives is prevention of ovulation**[14]. The midcycle LH surge is absent, and endogenous estrogen levels are reduced. Oral contraceptives also alter transport of the ovum down the fallopian tube; increase the viscosity of mucus produced by the cervix, which impairs sperm entry; and create an endometrial environment less favorable to implantation.

Progestin-only contraceptives may be administered as a daily oral dose, a **depot injection** (medroxyprogesterone acetate), or as a **progestin** (L-norgestrel) **implant**. Their effectiveness approaches combination oral contraceptives, and both the depot injection and the implants have the advantage of a long duration of action (14 weeks for the injection, 5 years for the implants). Progestins alone inhibit ovulation about 70 percent of the time, but their effectiveness is increased by effects on the endometrium and cervical mucus production.

Several emergency ("morning-after") contraceptive regimens have been used effectively to prevent pregnancy if used within 72 hours of coitus. The most common regimen consists of two combination oral contraceptive pills containing 50 mcg of ethinyl estradiol and 500 mcg of norgestrel immediately and 2 at 12 hours. Alternative schedules include 2 doses of 750 mcg of Lnorgestrel over 1 day.

Hormone Replacement Therapy

The decline in the production of estrogens that occurs at and following menopause is associated with **increased rates of bone loss** that can result in frank **osteoporosis**, **vasomotor symptoms**⑮ such as hot-flashes and night sweats, vaginal dryness and thinning, and genital atrophy. All of these symptoms can be **alleviated by estrogens**, but careful assessment of the risk-benefit ratio for a given patient is essential. The most commonly prescribed oral estrogen preparation for postmenopausal therapy is a complex mixture of natural estrogens (conjugated equine estrogen, Premarin), by mass mostly estrone sulphate and equiline estrogens, and this is usually combined with medroxyprogesterone acetate to avoid unopposed estrogenic stimulation of the endometrium. Other HRT or estrogen replacement therapy (ERT) regimens include oral esterified estrogens, micronized estradiol, and transdermal delivery of estradiol.

Other Uses of Estrogens and Progestins

Estrogens can be used to treat circumstances of inadequate hormone production as in **primary hypogonadism**⑯. This treatment is usually begun early (ages 11-13) to facilitate the development of the secondary sexual organs and to stimulate maximal growth.

Estrogens are also useful in the treatment of **intractable dysmenorrhea**⑰ where inhibition of ovulation may be of therapeutic value. Relatively high doses of estrogens have been used to suppress ovarian production of androgens. Both of these therapeutic approaches depend on estrogen-mediated negative feedback inhibition of gonadotropin release.

Adverse Effects of Estrogens and Progestins

Most of the adverse effects associated with estrogens and progestins are extensions of their physiologic actions. **Uterine bleeding**[18] is the most common adverse effect associated with use of estradiol. The **increased risk of cancer** caused by estrogen and progesterone use remains a significant concern. **Unopposed estrogen treatment** has been well documented to cause about a threefold increase in the risk of **endometrial cancer**[19]. Addition of a progestin to a treatment regimen essentially eliminates this increased risk. Several recent very large clinical trials examining use of estrogens to treat postmenopausal women have indicated that there is an **increased risk of breast cancer with estrogen** plus progesterone treatment, and further studies suggest that it is the progestin that is likely responsible for this effect. The absolute number of breast cancers that might be attributable to the HRT was very low. These studies do also show that estrogens *decrease* the risk of endometrial, ovarian, and colon cancer. The net effect of estrogens and progestins on cancer remains unresolved.

Despite their action to improve serum lipid levels (decreasing low-density lipoprotein [LDL] cholesterol and increase high-density lipoprotein [HDL] cholesterol), and despite a history of anecdotal evidence, data are accumulating that the **most common HRT (Premarin**[20] **or Prempro), does not reduce the risk of cardiovascular disease**. Indeed, the data indicate there is an increased risk of myocardial infarction and stroke, especially in the first years of treatment. The underlying mechanism for this increased risk is unclear, but may involve the increased coagulability that is associated with estrogen treatment. Estrogens increase the synthesis of fibrin and coagulation factors II, VII, VIII, IX, and X, and decrease the concentration of antithrombin III. In addition, plasminogen activator inhibitor activity is increased. These changes all contribute to a heightened tendency to form blood clots. This mechanism may also participate in the increased risk of dementia in postmenopausal women treated with estrogens. It must be noted that these serious adverse effects have been documented only with Premarin or Premarin plus progesterone at a fixed dosage, and it is not certain if other dosing regimens or other estrogen preparations cause similar untoward effects.

Less serious adverse effects of estrogens include nausea and vomiting and peripheral edema. Some women complain of severe migraine when taking estrogens.

Antiestrogens and SERMS

Two compounds, **clomiphene and fulvestrant are pure antiestrogens**[21] that **antagonize** the action of estrogen in all tissues examined. Clomiphene is a triphenylethylene consisting of two isomers, cis-clomiphene and trans-clomiphene. Cis-clomiphene is a weak estrogen agonist, whereas trans-clomiphene a potent estrogen antagonist. **Clomi-**

phene[22] binds to both ER_α and ER_β, and block estrogen activation of these receptors. The major pharmacologic action of clomiphene is to **block estrogen-mediated negative feedback in the pituitary**. This increases the amplitude of LH and FSH pulses and induces ovulation in women with amenorrhea, Stein-Leventhal syndrome, and dysfunctional bleeding with anovulatory cycles. It does increase the number of ova released, thereby increasing the chances of twinning.

Fulvestrant[23] is a 7α-alkylamide derivative of estradiol that binds to both **ER_α and ER_β**. It is administered as a depot injection. The predominant action of fulvestrant is to increase the degradation of ER_α while having little effect on ER_β. This alteration in the ratio of ER_α/ER_β may explain its usefulness in women with tamoxifen-resistant breast cancer. **Adverse effects of the antiestrogens include hot flashes, ovarian enlargement, and nausea[24].**

The **SERMS**, tamoxifen, raloxifene, and toremifene are a new class of compounds that display a range of agonist to antagonist activities in a tissue specific manner. For example, tamoxifen is an estrogen receptor antagonist in the breast but is a weak estrogen agonist in the endometrium. The basis for this tissue specificity is a combination of drug-induced conformational changes in the receptor, the complement of coactivators expressed in a given cell type. As noted above, when estradiol binds to an ER, a conformational change occurs that facilitates an interaction between coactivator proteins and ER. The SERMs also bind to ER, but they induce a conformation that is different from that caused by estradiol. The configuration of the receptor dictates which coactivator can bind to the receptor; if a cell does not express a coactivator that can bind to the receptor, then the effect of drug binding will be antagonism in that cell type. If the cell does express a coactivator that recognizes a particular configuration, then the drug will have agonist (or partial agonist) activity.

Tamoxifen[25] is a triphenylethylene, is structurally related to diethylstilbestrol, and binds to both ER_α and ER_β. It acts as an **estrogen antagonist in the breast and in the brain**, but it has **weak estrogen agonist activity in the uterus and in bone**. It has mixed action in the liver, decreasing total cholesterol and LDL cholesterol but with no effect on triglycerides. **Tamoxifen is highly efficacious in the treatment of breast cancer**. Tamoxifen has been shown consistently to increase disease-free survival and overall survival; treatment for 5 years has reduced cancer recurrence by about 50 percent and death by nearly 30 percent. It is approved for primary prevention of breast cancer in women at high risk, where it causes a 50 percent decrease in the incidence of invasive breast cancer and a 50 percent reduction of noninvasive breast cancer. Because of the development of drug-resistant tumors, treatment should last for no more than 5 years. Adverse effects of tamoxifen include hot flashes, nausea, and vaginal bleeding.

Toremifene[26] also is a triphenylethylene with a chlorine substitution. It is also used for the treatment and prophylaxis of breast cancer.

Raloxifene[27] is a polyhydroxylated nonsteroidal compound with a benzothiophene core. Raloxifene binds with high affinity for both ER_α and ER_β. Raloxifene is an **estrogen agonist in bone**, where it exerts an antiresorptive effect. It reduces total cholesterol and LDL cholesterol. Raloxifene **does not have agonist activity in the uterus**. Its **primary use is the prevention of osteoporosis** in postmenopausal women. Adverse effects include **hot flashes**, **deep vein thrombosis**[28], and cramps in the lower extremities.

Antiprogestins

Mifepristone[29] (RU-486) is a 19-nor steroid that has both antiprogestational and antiglucocorticoid effects. It is used most commonly as an **abortifacient in the first trimester** of pregnancy. A single oral dose of mifepristone combined with a vaginal suppository containing prostaglandin E_1 is effective in terminating pregnancy in about 95 percent of cases if used in the first 7 weeks of gestation. Adverse effects include nausea, vomiting, and abdominal cramping.

Androgens and Antiandrogens

Testosterone[30] produced by the testes is the major androgen in humans. In many peripheral tissues, testosterone is converted to dihydrotestosterone by the enzyme 5_α-reductase. Most circulating testosterone is bound in the plasma to sex-steroid binding globulin (SSBG). Testicular production of testosterone is regulated by LH released from the pituitary in a manner similar to that of estrogen as previously described. Testosterone has two physiological actions. As an anabolic agent it promotes linear bone growth, development of internal genitalia and increases muscle mass. As an androgenic agent, it is responsible for the development of male secondary sexual characteristics. **Dihydrotestosterone**[31] is responsible for the development of external genitalia and hair follicle growth during puberty. Testosterone or dihydrotestosterone bind with high affinity to the androgen receptor (AR), another member of the nuclear receptor family of transcription factors.

There are two distinct chemical classes of androgens: **testosterone and its esters**[32] and the **17-alkyl androgens**[33]. Testosterone esters include testosterone enanthate, testosterone cypionate, and testosterone undecenoate. The 17-alkyl androgens include methyltestosterone, oxandrolone, danazol, and stanozolol. Testosterone and its esters are administered either as depot injections via transdermal patch, or as a gel. The 17-alkyl androgens are orally active.

The **major use of the androgens are the treatment of male hypogonadism**[34], both in adults and in prepubertal boys that produce low amounts of testosterone. Use in adults has been reported to increase libido, reduce senescence, and reduce the rate of bone resorption. The **major adverse effects of testosterone** and its esters are caused by the **androgenic actions**, which are especially apparent in women and prepubertal children. In women these adverse effects include hirsutism, acne, amenorrhea, and a thickening of the vocal chords. In **children, androgens can cause premature closure of the epiphyses**[35]. In men, androgens can produce azoospermia, decreased testicle size, and prostatic hyperplasia. The major adverse effect of the 17-alkyl androgens include masculinization and also serious hepatotoxicity. A cholestatic jaundice that is reversible on discontinuation of drug may occur.

Antiandrogens

Abnormal growth of the prostate is usually dependent on androgenic stimulation. This hormonal stimulation can be reduced by orchidectomy[36] or high doses of estrogens, but either of these treatments may be undesirable. **Chemical orchidectomy** can be accomplished with an inhibitor of GnRH synthesis such as **leuprolide**[37] or with **antiandrogens**.

Finasteride[38] **is a steroid derivative that competitively inhibits 5_{α}-reductase type Ⅱ**. Because **prostate growth is dependent on DHT rather than testosterone**, blockade of the enzyme can reduce stimulation of the gland. In clinical trials, finasteride decreased the incidence of prostate cancers but may have led to more aggressive tumors. **Bicalutamide and nilutamide**[39] **are moderately potent antiandrogens** that antagonize AR. These drugs are usually combined with a GnRH analog such as leuprolide to decrease LH and subsequently testosterone production. **Flutamide**[40] **is an AR antagonists** that blocks the action of testosterone in target organs. It has been used in the treatment of prostatic carcinoma.

Comprehension Questions

[40.1] Clomiphene acts to induce ovulation by

A. Diminishing ER mediated negative feedback at the pituitary

B. Increasing the action of ER_{α} in the hypothalamus

C. Increasing the action of ER_{α} in the ovary

D. Increasing the amount of estrogen receptor alpha

[40.2] Progesterone is added to estrogens in HRT to

A. Decrease the estrogen action on the breast

B. Decrease the occurrence of endometrial cancers

C. Increase the effectiveness of the estrogens

D. Inhibit bone resorption

[40.3] A 55-year-old woman is noted to be taking tamoxifen to help with breast cancer. She also complains of vaginal bleeding. She asks why she is having vaginal bleeding if the medication blocks estrogen effect in the body. Which of the following is the best explanation?

A. It has estrogen agonist effect of the breast and uterus, thereby leading to endometrial hyperplasia.

B. It is an estrogen antagonist in the breast and uterus, leading to loss of endometrial cells

C. It has an antagonist effect on the breast but an agonist effect on the uterus.

D. It has no effect on the uterus, and the vaginal bleeding is caused by something else.

Answers

[40.1] **A.** Clomiphene decreases estradiol's negative feedback in the pituitary, and this increases the amplitude of the LH pulse that is responsible for ovulation.

[40.2] **B.** Progestins are added to HRT regimens to decrease the risk of endometrial cancer.

[40.3] **C.** Tamoxifen has an estrogen antagonist effect on the breast but a weak agonist effect on the uterus, leading to endometrial hyperplasia in some women. Endometrial cancer is seen in some patients.

PHARMACOLOGY PEARLS

- ❖ Clomiphene is the agent of choice for treatment of infertility as a result of anovulation in women with an intact hypothalamicpituitary-ovarian axis.
- ❖ SERMs are tissue-specific estrogen antagonists that have uses in the treatment of breast cancer and osteoporosis.
- ❖ Antiandrogens are used to treat androgen dependent cancers such as prostate carcinoma.

REFERENCES

Burkman R, Schlesselman JJ, Zieman M. Safety concerns and health benefits associated with oral contraception. Am J Obstet Gynecol 2004 Apr; 190(suppl 4): S5-22.

Writitng Group for the Women's Health Initiative Investigators. Risks and benefits of estrogen plus progesterone in healthy postmenopausal women. JAMA 2002; 288: 321-333.

词汇

1. nuclear receptor[核受体]
2. ERE[雌激素反应元件]
3. SERM[选择性雌激素受体调节剂]
4. estrogens and progestins[雌激素和孕激素]
5. gonadotropins[促性腺激素]
6. osteoporosis[骨质疏松症]
7. abortifacients[堕胎药]
8. menstrual cycle[月经周期]
9. LH and FSH[黄体生成素和卵泡刺激素]
10. 17β estradiol and estrone[17β 雌二醇和雌酮]
11. progesterone[孕酮]
12. oral contraceptives[口服避孕药]
13. ethinyl estradiol[乙炔雌二醇]
14. ovulation[排卵]
15. vasomotor symptoms[血管收缩的症状]
16. primary hypogonadism[原发性性腺功能减退]
17. intractable dysmenorrheal[难治性痛经]
18. uterine bleeding[子宫出血]
19. endometrial cancer[子宫内膜癌]
20. premarin[结合型雌激素]
21. antiestrogens[抗雌激素药]
22. clomiphene[克罗米酚]
23. fulvestrant[氟维司群]
24. hot flashes, ovarian enlargement, nausea[潮红,卵巢增大,恶心]
25. tamoxifen[他莫西芬]
26. toremifene[托瑞米芬]
27. raloxifene[雷洛昔芬]
28. deep vein thrombosis[深静脉血栓]
29. mifepristone[米非司酮]
30. testosterone[睾酮]
31. dihydrotestosterone[二氢睾酮]
32. testosterrone and its esters[睾酮及其酯类]
33. 17-alkyl androgens[17-羟基雄激素]
34. male hypogonadism[男性性腺机能减退]
35. premature closure of the epiphyses[骨骺提前闭合]
36. orchidectomy[睾丸切除术]
37. leuprolide[醋酸亮丙瑞林]
38. finasteride[非那雄胺]
39. bicalutamide and nilutamide[比卡鲁胺和尼鲁米特]
40. flutamide[氟他胺]

注 1

月经不调有时可使用避孕药来调节。如孕激素、雌激素以及其他药物可调节下丘脑-垂体-卵巢轴，促使促性腺激素释放激素恢复正常节律，从而使月经周期恢复正常。要注意的是，避孕药也可引起月经不调。

注 2

枸橼酸氯米芬为非甾类抗雌激素药，能与雌激素竞争结合靶细胞的雌激素受体，对雌激素有弱的激动与强的拮抗双重作用。临床常用于治疗无排卵的女性不育症，但仅适用于体内有一定雌激素水平者。此外还可用于治疗黄体功能不足；测试卵巢功能；探测男性下丘脑-垂体-性腺轴的功能异常；治疗因精子过少的男性不育等。

点评

本病例患者曾有月经不调的病史，且使用避孕药5年，以治疗月经不调，但最近三年患者已没有服用避孕药。且家族中也没有任何不孕病史，无吸烟，酗酒等，各项常规及妇科检查也正常，但患者的基础体温变化及排卵实验的结果均提示患者排卵功能异常，表明患者不孕是由排卵异常引起的。

由于患者体内的雌激素还是有一定水平的，故选用抗雌激素药枸橼酸氯米芬。氯米芬是抗雌激素药，同时又有弱的拟雌激素作用。该药刺激排卵的机制尚不完全明了。由于本品对雌激素有弱的激动与强的拮抗双重作用，刺激排卵可能是在下丘脑部位，首先拮抗占优势，通过竞争性占据下丘脑雌激素受体，干扰着内源性雌激素的负反馈，促使黄体生成激素与促卵泡生成激素的分泌增加，继之刺激卵泡生长，卵泡成熟后，雌激素的释放量增加，通过正反馈激发排卵前促性腺激素的释放达峰值，于是排卵，治疗男性不育可能与FSH和LH升高以及促进精子生成有关。可以通过对抗内源性雌激素的负反馈作用，以增加促性腺激素的分泌达峰值，并最终达到刺激排卵的作用。

临床用药时，口服每日50mg，共5日。自月经周期的第5天开始服药。若患者系闭经，则应先用黄体酮撤退性出血的第5天始服用。患者在治疗后有排卵但未受孕可重复原治疗的疗程，直到受孕，或重复3~4个疗程。若患者在治疗后无排卵，在下一次的疗程中剂量可增加到每日100mg，共5日。个别患者药量可达每天150mg时，才能排卵。

王毅群　姚明辉

❖ CASE 41

A 45-year-old man presents for the evaluation of weight gain. He has noticed a 20-lb weight gain in the past few months without any change in his diet or activity level. He has started developing "stretch marks" on his abdomen as well. His wife has noted that even his face seems to be "growing fatter." Review of systems is significant for complaints of fatigue, multiple recent upper respiratory infections, and the development of facial acne. He has no significant medical history and takes no medications. There is a family history of diabetes and hypertension. On examination, his blood pressure is elevated at 165/95 mmHg, but his other vital signs are normal. His face is plethoric, and he has a small fatty hump developing on his upper back. His abdomen is obese but soft and nontender without masses or fluid. Skin exam is notable for moderate facial acne and multiple violaceous striae on the abdomen. Blood tests show an elevated glucose level of 150 mg/dL, normal electrolytes, and renal function. His thyroid function tests are normal. You suspect idiopathic Cushing disease[注1] and order a dexamethasone suppression test[注2] to assist with confirming the diagnosis.

◆ **Which pituitary hormone stimulates the release of adrenocortical steroids?**

◆ **What is the major glucocorticoid produced in the adrenal glands?**

◆ **What is the major mineralocorticoid produced in the adrenal glands?**

◆ **What is the major effect of mineralocorticoids?**

ANSWERS TO CASE 41: The Adrenal Cortex

Summary: A 45-year-old man has Cushing disease.

- **Pituitary hormonal stimulus of adrenocortical steroid production**: Adrenocorticotropic hormone (ACTH).
- **Primary adrenal glucocorticoid**: Cortisol.
- **Primary adrenal mineralocorticoid**: Aldosterone.
- **Major mineralocorticoid effects**: Regulation of salt and water balance in the kidney, promote sodium retention, and potassium loss.

CLINICAL CORRELATION

Cushing disease is caused by ACTH-secreting tumors in the pituitary gland. The continuous production of ACTH disrupts the normal circadian production of ACTH and overrides the feedback of adrenal steroids on the hypothalamus and pituitary, resulting in excessive adrenocortical steroid production. Glucocorticoids affect most organs and tissues in the body. Their effects are mediated by specific intracellular glucocorticoid receptors that modulate the transcription rates of specific genes and results in increases or decreases of specific proteins. The major glucocorticoid produced in the adrenal glands is cortisol (hydrocortisone). Glucocorticoids have numerous physiologic effects, including the stimulation of gluconeogenesis, increasing lipolysis, decreasing glucose uptake into fat cells, and redistributing body fat. These effects cause some of the symptoms and signs of Cushing disease, which include glucose intolerance or overt diabetes, weight gain, and increasing truncal obesity. Glucocorticoids also have antiimmune effects, which include decreasing circulating lymphocytes, monocytes, eosinophils, and basophils, increases in circulating neutrophils and atrophy of lymphoid tissue. The excess production of glucocorticoids can therefore lead to immune system suppression and recurrent infections. Under normal physiologic conditions, adrenocortical steroids will exert a negative feedback of ACTH release from the pituitary gland. ACTH release, and subsequent cortisol production, can be suppressed even more by the administration of synthetic steroids such as dexamethasone. ACTH, which is continuously produced by a tumor, will not be suppressed by a feedback mechanism. This formulates the basis for the dexamethasone suppression test, in which a dose of dexamethasone is administered and subsequent cortisol production is measured. Normally this would cause a reduction of circulating cortisol. In Cushing disease the measurement of cortisol will remain at normal, or even elevated, levels.

Pharmacology of the Glucocorticoids

Objectives

1. Understand the physiologic regulation of the hypothalamic-pituitaryadrenal axis.
2. List the natural and synthetic adrenocortical steroids, their actions, therapeutic uses, and adverse effects.
3. Know the glucocorticoid and mineralocorticoid effects of adrenocortical steroids.
4. Understand the adrenocortical antagonists, their mechanism of action, uses, and adverse effects.

Definitions

Glucocorticoids①: In humans the most important glucocorticoid is cortisol. These hormones regulate carbohydrate, protein, and lipid metabolism.

Mineralocorticoids②: In humans, aldosterone is the most important mineralocorticoid.

Aldosterone③ regulates Na^+ and K^+ homeostasis.

Discussion of Class

Control of the secretion of glucocorticoids by the adrenal gland is regulated by a classic negative feedback pathway that includes the hypothalamus, pituitary and the adrenal cortex (see Case 39). The **neuropeptide CRH (corticotropinreleasing hormone)**④ **is a 41-amino acid peptide produced in the hypothalamus** that is **secreted with a circadian rhythm**⑤. Secretion can also be increased by physiological or psychological stress. **CRH acts on the pituitary to stimulate the release of ACTH**(adrenocorticotropic hormone). ACTH released from the pituitary is transported in the systemic circulation to the **adrenal cortex**⑥, where it acts to stimulate the **zona fasciculata and reticularis**⑦ **to increase the biosynthesis of cortisol and weak androgens** such as **androstenedione**⑧ respectively. It also acts on the **zona glomerulosa**⑨ to slightly stimulate the production of **aldosterone**. ACTH is a true trophic hormone: It is necessary for the survival of cells of the adrenal cortex, although this effect is somewhat less pronounced in the zona glomerulosa. Cortisol secreted by the adrenal cortex is bound extensively to cortisol-binding globulin (CBG) in the plasma.

Glucocorticoids

Natural and synthetic glucocorticoids play a diverse role in **metabolism, catabolism, and immunity**⑩. Both cortisol, the natural glucocorticoid, and many synthetic glucocorticoids are used therapeutically (Table 41-1). The synthetic glucocorticoids have reduced mineralocorticoid activity and in general increased potency compared to cortisol. Glucocorticoids have a myriad of therapeutic uses. They are potent **antiinflammatory agents**⑪ because they **inhibit prostaglandin**⑫ **production by inhibiting phospholipase A**, the enzyme that yields arachidonic acid from plasma membrane phospholipids. Unlike NSAIDs, they also **inhibit leukocytes and macrophages**⑬ **that contribute heavily to inflammation**. Glucocorticoids are used to treat joint and bone inflammation, inflammatory bowel disease, bronchial asthma and dermatitis. Systemic inflammations such as in lupus erythematosus, rheumatoid arthritis, and acute respiratory distress syndrome are also treated with glucocorticoids. Glucocorticoids are potent immunosuppressive agents and are used either alone or in conjunction with other immunosuppressive agents to suppress organ rejection following transplant, and to reduce the severity of allergic reactions including contact dermatitis, serum sickness and allergic rhinitis. Other uses include prevention of respiratory distress syndrome in infants (by induction of surfactant), nephrotic syndrome, and at high doses to reduce cerebral edema. Adrenal insufficiency either acute or congenital is treated with glucocorticoids. Finally glucocorticoids are useful diagnostically as in the dexamethasone suppression test described above.

Table 41-1

COMMONLY USED ADRENOCORTICAL AGENTS

AGENT	EQUIVALENT DOSE (mg)	GLUCOCORTICOID POTENCY	MINERALOCORTICOID POTENCY	ANTIINFLAMMATORY POTENCY
Cortisol	20	100	1	1
Prednisone	5	100	0.4	4
Methylprednisolone	4	100	0.1	4
Triamcinolone	4	100	0.1	5
Dexamethasone	0.75	100	0.05	30
Fludrocortisone	2	100	250	10

Although they are highly efficacious agents, the **adverse effect profile** of glucocorticoids limits their use typically to short (approximately 2 weeks) periods. **Chronic use of glucocorticoids** beyond this duration produces **adrenal suppression** and can cause iatrogenic Cushing syndrome. The metabolic sequelae of **Cushing syndrome**⑭ include **fat redistribution (buffalo hump and moon facies)**, **hyperglycemia**⑮, and **elevations in insulin secretion leading to frank diabetes**. Continued protein degradation can cause **myopathy**⑯ and **muscle wasting**⑰, and **thinning of the skin**⑱ that becomes prone to **bruising and striae**. **Immunosuppression**⑲ leads to susceptibility to infection and poor wound healing. **Peptic ulcers and osteoporosis**⑳ are other potential consequences of glucocorticoid use. **Adrenal suppression** occurs with chronic glucocorticoid use as a result of continuous suppression of ACTH production by the pituitary. The absence of the trophic hormone leads to adrenal atrophy and an inability to respond to stress, which can be life-threatening. Neurological adverse effects include **hypomania, acute psychosis, and depression**㉑. At sufficient doses all glucocorticoids have some mineralocorticoid activity that can lead to **electrolyte imbalances and water retention**㉒.

Mineralocorticoids

Aldosterone is the naturally occurring mineralocorticoid. It is secreted by the **zona glomerulosa of the adrenal cortex. Secretion of aldosterone is increased by angiotensin II and K^+, especially when serum Na^+ is low**. The physiologic action of aldosterone is to **increase Na^+ reabsorption**㉓ in the distal convoluted tubule and cortical collecting tubule via the amiloride-sensitive Na^+ channel. As Na^+ is reabsorbed, K^+ or H^+ is secreted into the urine and water is retained. Aldosterone also causes Na^+ reabsorption in the salivary and sweat glands and the mucosa of the gastrointestinal tract. Aldosterone is not useful as an oral agent because of a nearly 100 percent first-pass effect by the liver. **Fludrocortisone**㉔ (see Table 41-1) has both glucocorticoid and mineralocorticoid activity. An alternative to fludrocortisone is **deoxycorticosterone**㉕ (**DOC**) which is a potent mineralocorticoid.

Structure

Synthetic glucocorticoids are all analogs of the natural occurring cortisol. Various modifications of the steroid nucleus have important pharmacokinetic effects to increase glucocorticoid potency relative to mineralocorticoid potency, to decrease first-pass effect and increase half life, and to decrease binding to CBG. Aldosterone has a unique epoxide structure in the "D" ring that prevents its inactivation.

Mechanism of Action

Both the **glucocorticoids and the mineralocorticoids** bind to **specific nuclear receptors within target cells**. The **glucocorticoid receptor** is in an inactive state in the cytoplasm of target cells bound to a variety of heat shock proteins, especially HSP 90. On binding a glucocorticoid, the heat shock proteins dissociate, the GR forms a homodimer and **translocates to the nucleus**㉖ and binds to the **promoter region of specific target genes**㉗. Via the process of coactivator or corepressor recruitment, transcription of these specific target genes is either increased or decreased. The mineralocorticoid receptor MR is expressed in the kidney, salivary glands and gastrointestinal tract. It binds aldosterone with high affinity but also binds cortisol with nearly the same affinity. Cortisol is prevented from binding to MR by rapid inactivation to cortisone by the enzyme hydroxysteroid dehydrogenase Type II which is expressed in mineralocorticoid target tissues.

Administration

Glucocorticoids can be administered orally, by injection, by inhalation (especially for use in asthma), rectally, and topically. Patients taking glucocorticoids for longer than 2 weeks must be slowly tapered off the drug so that adrenal function can be restored.

Pharmacokinetics

The half-life and duration of action of glucocorticoids depends on the route of administration and the particular agent. In general, glucocorticoid effects are seen within 4-6 hours. Most corticosteroids are metabolized in the liver to sterol ketones or hydroxides and eliminated by the kidney.

Glucocorticoid and Mineralocorticoid Antagonists

There are some clinical circumstances such as inoperable adrenal tumors, prior to surgery, and for diagnostic use where **inhibition of glucocorticoid action** is desirable. **Metyrapone**[28] is a **specific inhibitor of 11-hydroxylation**[29], and can thereby inhibit **the synthesis of corticosterone and cortisol**[30]. In the presence of normal pituitary function there is a **compensatory increase in 11-deoxycortisol production**. **Metyrapone is also useful in the assessment of adrenal function**. Following metyrapone administration, urinary 17-hydroxysteroids, metabolites of adrenal glucocorticoid synthesis, typically double if the adrenals are functioning normally. **Chronic metyrapone can cause hirsutism, nausea, sedation, and rash**[31].

Aminoglutheamide[32] **blocks the conversion of cholesterol to pregnenolone**. This **inhibits the synthesis of all hormonally active steroids**. It has been used to reduce glucocorticoid levels in patients with Cushing syndrome because of adrenal tumors or excessive ectopic production of ACTH. It has also been used to treat estrogen-dependent breast cancer and prostate cancer. Adverse effects are common and include gastrointestinal upset and neurological disturbances.

Ketoconazole[33] is an **antifungal agent**; at high doses **it nonspecifically blocks several enzymes, especially P_{450} enzymes**, that are involved in adrenal and gonadal steroidogenesis. It is the most effective inhibitor of steroid hormone biosynthesis available in patients with Cushing disease. **Adverse effects include hepatic dysfunction with increased transaminases and liver failure.**

Mifepristone[34] is a 19-nor steroid that is a potent antagonist of both the glucocorticoid and progesterone receptors. It has been used to reduce the activity of glucocorticoids in patients with ectopic ACTH production or adrenal carcinoma. The main use of mifepristone is as an antiprogestin (Case 40) as an abortifacient when combined with prostaglandin E_1.

Two mineralocorticoid antagonists are available, spironolactone and eplerenone[35]. **Spironolactone antagonizes the mineralocorticoid and the androgen receptor. It is used to treat hypertension**(see Case 12)usually in combination with a thiazide or a loop diuretic. It can be used diagnostically to restore potassium levels to normal in patients with hypokalemia secondary to hyperaldosteronism. Based on its **antiandrogen activity**, it has been **used to treat hirsutism in women.** Adverse effects include **hyperkalemia, sedation, cardiac arrhythmias, gynecomastia, sedation, headache, and gastrointestinal upset**[36].

Eplerenone is a **new generation, aldosterone receptor specific antagonist.** It is approved for use in **congestive heart failure, post myocardial infarction, and hypertension**[37]. It **avoids the antiandrogen activity of spironolactone. Adverse effects** include mild **hyperkalemia**, but clinical experience is limited.

Comprehension Questions

[41.1] Which of the following best describes appropriate protocols for withdrawal of glucocorticoids from a patient who has been taking large doses for 6 months?

A. Maintain dose of glucocorticoids and add metyrapone.

B. Maintain dose of glucocorticoids and add spironolactone.

C. An alternate-day dosage regimen of glucocorticoids should be begun.

D. Slow reduction of the glucocorticoid dose over 1-2 weeks.

[41.2] A patient with severe shoulder pain resulting from inflammation is not responding to treatment with naproxen. You elect to begin a course of treatment with oral dexamethasone. What is the basis that the glucocorticoid will be a more effective as an antiinflammatory agent?

A. Glucocorticoids inhibit both prostaglandin production and inflammatory cells.

B. Glucocorticoids are more potent inhibitors of cyclooxygenase than naproxen.

C. Glucocorticoids inhibit biosynthesis of both COX-1 and COX-2.

D. Glucocorticoids will reduce the edema in the inflamed area.

[41.3] A 32-year-old woman is prescribed a pill for her excessive hair on her face and arms. She notes that she has been going to the bathroom at night more often. What is the most likely explanation for the nocturia?

A. Diabetes insipidus effect of the medication

B. Osmotic load to the kidney from the medication delivery system

C. Distal renal tubule effect of the medication

D. Hyperglycemic effect from the medication

Answers

[41.1] **D.** Long-term use of glucocorticoids results in adrenal suppression and atrophy. A slow "weaning" from the drug is necessary so that the adrenals can recover.

[41.2] **A.** Glucocorticoids reduce prostaglandin production like NSAIDs and they also inhibit most of the cells that are involved in the inflammatory process.

[41.3] **C.** The medication is probably spironolactone, which has is a competitive inhibitor of androgens at the receptor level, and also an antimineralcorticoid effect at the distal tubule, inhibiting free water resorption. As such, it is a potassium sparing diuretic agent.

PHARMACOLOGY PEARLS

❖ Adverse effects, especially adrenal suppression, seriously limit the use of glucocorticoids to 2 weeks or less.

❖ Spironolactone antagonizes the mineralocorticoid and the androgen receptor. Adverse effects include hyperkalemia, sedation, cardiac arrhythmias, gynecomastia, sedation, headache, and gastrointestinal upset.

❖ Eplerenone is a new generation, aldosterone receptor specific antagonist without the antiandrogen component.

❖ Metyrapone is a specific inhibitor of 11-hydroxylation that inhibits the synthesis of corticosterone and cortisol.

REFERENCES

Boers M. Glucocorticoids in rheumatoid arthritis: a senescent research agenda on the brink of rejuvenation? Best Pract Res Clin Rheumatol 2004; 18: 21-9.

Trence DL. Management of patients on chronic glucocorticoid therapy: an endocrine perspective. Prim Care 2003; 30: 593-605.

词汇

1. glucocorticoids[糖皮质激素]
2. mineralocorticoids[盐皮质激素]

3. aldosterone[醛固酮]
4. CRH(corticotrophin-releasing hormone)[促肾上腺皮质激素释放激素]
5. circadian rhythm[生理节律]
6. adrenal cortex[肾上腺皮质]
7. zona fasciculate and reticularis[束状带和网状带(肾上腺皮质)]
8. androstenedione[雄烯二酮]
9. zona glomerulosa[球状带]
10. metabolism, catabolism, and immunity[新陈代谢,异化作用和免疫作用]
11. antiinflammatory agents[抗炎药物]
12. prostaglandin[前列腺素]
13. leukocytes and macrophages[白细胞和巨噬细胞]
14. cushing syndrome[库欣综合征]
15. fat redistribution (buffalo hump and moon facies), hyperglycemia[脂肪的重新分布(满月脸和水牛背),高血糖]
16. myopathy[肌病]
17. muscle wasting[肌肉萎缩]
18. thinning of the skin[皮肤变薄]
19. immunosuppression[免疫抑制]
20. peptic ulcers and osteoporosis[消化系统溃疡和骨质疏松症]
21. hypomania, acute psychosis, and depression[躁狂,急性精神病,抑郁]
22. electrolyte imbalances and water retention[电解质紊乱和水潴留]
23. increase Na^+ reabsorption[增加 Na^+ 重吸收]
24. fludrocortisone[氟氢可的松]
25. deoxycorticosterone[去氧皮质酮]
26. translocates to the nucleus[易位进入细胞核]
27. promoter region of specific target genes[特殊靶基因的启动子序列]
28. metyrapone[美替拉酮]
29. 11-hydroxylation[11-羟化反应]
30. corticosterone and cortisol[皮质酮和皮质醇]
31. hirsutism, nausea, sedation, and rash[多毛症,眩晕,镇静和皮疹]
32. aminoglutethimide[氨鲁米特]
33. ketoconazole[酮康唑]
34. mifepristone[米非司酮]
35. spironolactone and eplerenone[安体舒通和依普利酮]
36. hyperkalemia, sedation, cardiac arrhythmias, gynecomastia, headache, and gastrointestinal upset[高血钾,镇静,心律不齐,男性乳腺发育,头痛以及消化道反应]
37. congestive heart failure, post myocardial infarction, and hypertension[充血性心力衰竭,心肌梗死以及高血压]

注 1

皮质醇增多症，又称 Cushing 综合征，是由于肾上腺皮质分泌过量糖皮质激素(主要是皮质醇)，导致人体代谢明显紊乱，从而出现一系列相应的临床表现。

病因可分为：①下丘脑-垂体性皮质醇症，由于下丘脑-垂体释放促肾上腺皮质激素过多而引起肾上腺皮质增生所致，多数患者伴有垂体 ACTH(促肾上腺皮质激素)微腺瘤，占本病的70%左右。②肾上腺腺瘤，包括肾上腺皮质腺瘤和癌。③异源促肾上腺皮质激素综合征，因垂体、肾上腺以外的肿瘤(如肺癌、胰腺癌等)产生具有促肾上腺皮质激素活性的物质，刺激肾上腺皮质增生所致。至于医源性皮质醇症则是临床上应用此组激素过量的后果。

注 2

库欣综合征的诊断中，需要检查病人垂体肾上腺轴的反应性，临床应用较多，最经典的是地塞米松抑制试验。地塞米松是人工合成的糖皮质激素中生物作用最强的激素之一，仅需要很小的量即能达到与天然皮质醇相似的作用，因为含量小，且分布在血中浓度很低，故难以用常规的放射免疫定量测定法测出其值，故对测定自身皮质醇分泌量无影响。地塞米松抑制实验利用地塞米松这一特性，通过其对垂体、下丘脑分泌的促肾上腺皮质激素和促肾上腺皮质激素释放激素的抑制作用，及由此引起肾上腺皮质激素分泌减少的程度，来了解下丘脑-垂体-肾上腺轴功能是否高于正常，其可能的病变在那个器官。

地塞米松抑制实验分为大剂量和小剂量地塞米松抑制实验。小剂量地塞米松抑制实验主要用于与单纯性肥胖鉴别，而大剂量地塞米松抑制实验主要用于与肾上腺瘤和肾上腺癌区别。

点评

本病例有典型的体重增加，满月脸，水牛背，上呼吸道感染，及面部痤疮。另外患者还有血压升高，血糖升高等，且患者水，电解质，肾及甲状腺功能检查等均正常。这些都是库欣综合征糖皮质激素增多后的一些典型表现。引起库欣综合征的病因有很多，不同的病因需有不同的治疗，因此需进行地塞米松抑制实验与其他疾病相鉴别，才可以确诊。

常用的地塞米松抑制实验方法有：1. 小剂量地塞米松抑制试验：(1)1mg 地塞米松抑制试验：午夜一次口服地塞米松 1mg，次晨 8 时测血皮质醇，正常人血游离皮质醇(F)抑制率超过 50%，当 1mg 地塞米松不能抑制到对照值 50% 以上时提示有库欣综合征的可能。(2)2mg 地塞米松抑制试验：口服地塞米松每次 0.5mg，每日 4 次，或每次 0.75mg，每日 3 次，连服两天，分别测定服药后的血 F 和 24 小时尿 F，正常人抑制率可超过 50%，不能抑制到 50% 提示库欣综合征可能。2. 大剂量地塞米松(8mg)抑制试验：服用地塞米松每次 2mg，每日 4 次，连续两天，测定服药后血 F 及 24 小时尿 F，多数增生患者在服药后可抑制到对照值 50% 以上，肾上腺肿瘤或异位 ACTH 分泌综合征则多不能达到满意的抑制。3. 极大剂量地塞米松抑制试验：第一天上午 8 时采血测 ACTH 和皮质醇，午夜口服地塞米松 8mg，次日上午 8 时、下午 4 时、午夜 12 时各服 8mg，第二、第三日上午 8 时采血测 ACTH 和皮质醇，第二日上午 7 时至第三日上午 7 时留尿测游离皮质醇。阳性率明显高于 8mg 地塞米松抑制试验。

王毅群　姚明辉

❖ CASE 42

A 44-year-old woman presents to the office because of fatigue①. She has felt sluggish② for months and thinks she may be anemic③. She has started taking iron pills but isn't feeling any better. She has been sleeping well and doesn't feel depressed. She has noticed some thinning of her hair and feels as if her skin is dry. She takes a multivitamin and iron supplement, otherwise no medications. She has smoked a pack of cigarettes a day for about 20 years, occasionally drinks alcohol, and doesn't exercise. Her mother takes some kind of thyroid pill and has diabetes. On examination, her blood pressure and pulse are normal. Her hair is thinned but there are no focal patches of alopecia④ or scarring⑤ of the scalp. Her skin is diffusely dry. Her thyroid gland⑥ feels diffusely enlarged, is nontender⑦, and has no nodules⑧. The remainder of her exam is unremarkable. Lab tests show a normal complete blood count (CBC), glucose, and electrolytes. Her thyroid-stimulating hormone (TSH)⑨ level is elevated, and T_4 level is reduced. You diagnose her with hypothyroidism⑩ and start her on oral levothyroxine⑪ sodium.

◆ **What is levothyroxine sodium?**

◆ **How is triiodothyronine (T_3) produced in the body?**

◆ **What is the mechanism of action of thyroid hormones?**

ANSWERS TO CASE 42: Thyroid Hormones

Summary: A 44-year-old woman is diagnosed with hypothyroidism and prescribed levothyroxine.

- **Levothyroxine sodium is**: Synthetic sodium salt of thyroxine (T_4).

- **Derivation of T_3 in the body**: Approximately 75 percent from the deiodination[12] of T_4; also produced by the coupling of monoiodotyrosine (MIT)[13] and diiodotyrosine (DIT)[14].

- **Mechanism of action of thyroid hormones**: Bind with receptors in nuclei of target cells and alter synthesis rates of specific messenger ribonucleoprotein acids (mRNAs), increasing production of certain proteins including Na^+, K^+-ATPase.

CLINICAL CORRELATION

Thyroid hormones have wide-ranging effects of tissues throughout the body. They are involved primarily in the regulation of metabolism. The hypothalamicpituitary-thyroid axis[15] regulates release of active hormone from the thyroid via a feedback loop. Thyrotropin-releasing hormone (TRH)[16] is produced in the hypothalamus[17] and stimulates the release of thyroid-stimulating hormone (TSH) from the anterior pituitary[18]. TSH binds to membrane receptors in the thyroid and stimulates the production and release of T_4 and T_3 via a cyclic adenosine monophosphate (cAMP)-mediated system. Synthesis of T_4 exceeds T_3 by about fourfold; most circulating T_3 comes from the deiodination of T_4. T_4 is almost entirely protein bound, whereas over 90 percent of circulating T_3 is not. Unbound thyroid hormone binds to receptors located in the nuclei of target cells. This alters the rate of synthesis of specific mRNAs which lead to the increased production of proteins, including Na^+, K^+-ATPase. This results in a net increase in ATP and oxygen consumption, raising the metabolic rate. Hypothyroidism occurs when there is inadequate thyroid hormone production and release to meet the body's metabolic demands. In primary hypothyroidism the thyroid gland is unable to synthesize adequate amounts of thyroid hormone. The pituitary releases increasing amounts of TSH to try to stimulate production, leading to the characteristic laboratory findings of low circulating levels of thyroid hormones with an elevated TSH. Conversely, primary hyperthyroidism is diagnosed by the presence of elevated thyroid hormone levels and a suppressed level of TSH. Hypothyroidism is most often treated by the oral administration of synthetic T_4 in the form of levothyroxine sodium. This replaces both T_4 and, by deiodination, T_3.

Pharmacology of Thyroid Drugs

Objectives

1. List the hormones involved in the hypothalamic-pituitary-thyroid axis and the synthesis of thyroid hormones.
2. Know the actions of thyroid hormones.
3. List the thyroid hormone preparations, their therapeutic uses, actions, and adverse effects.
4. Describe the antithyroid agents, their mechanisms of action, therapeutic uses, and adverse effects.

Definitions

Myxedema[19]: Serious hypothyroidism.

Thyrotoxicosis[20]: Hyperthyroidism.

Discussion of Class

Thyroid Agonists

Thyroid hormones are required for optimum development, growth, and maintenance of function of virtually every tissue of the body. Either hypoor hyperthyroidism leads to untoward symptoms that need to be treated. The **thyroid gland produces both thyroxine (T_4) and triiodothyronine (T_3).** Adequate dietary intake of sufficient **iodide**[21] **(I^-) is essential** to maintain normal biosynthesis of thyroid hormones. **Iodide is transported into the thyroid cell by a sodium-iodide symporter**[22] **(NIS)** and then transported through the **apical plasma membrane into the colloid of the thyroid** gland. Within the colloid[23], **iodide is oxidized to iodine**[24] **by thyroidal peroxidase**[25]. The process called organification involves the iodination of tyrosine residues of the colloidal protein thyroglobulin[26] to form **monoiodotyrosine (MIT) and diiodotyrosine (DIT)**. The coupling of two molecules of DIT forms T_4 and the coupling of one molecule of MIT, and one molecule of DIT forms T_3. Under normal circumstances and sufficient iodide, the ratio of T_4 to T_3 is 4:1. T_3 can also be formed by the removal of an iodide molecule from T_4 by the action of 5′-deiodinase, which is present within the thyroid gland and in peripheral tissues.

Iodinated thyroglobulin undergoes endocytosis at the apical border and then extensively degraded within the thyroid cells by proteolysis[27] prior to secretion of T_4 and T_3. Although T_3 is produced with the thyroid, **about 80 percent of circulating levels of T_3 are produced by the action of 5′-deiodinase in the periphery**, especially the **liver**. Alternatively T_4 can be *degraded* by the action of deiodinase to reverse T_3, which is an inactive metabolite. Normally about 40 percent of T_4 is converted to T_3, 38 percent is converted to rT_3, and the remainder is degraded by other, typically hepatic pathways. Greater than 99 percent of both T_4 and T_3 are bound in the plasma to TBG; T_4 binds to TBG much more avidly. **Only the unbound "free" hormone exerts physiological effects.**

Secretion of thyroid hormones is regulated by a **classical hypothalamuspituitary-thyroid negative feedback loop. TRH is produced within hypothalamus.** It acts on **thyrotrophs[28] in the pituitary to cause the release of thyrotropin (TSH)**, which in turn stimulates all steps in the **biosynthesis and secretion of thyroid hormones.** Circulating levels of thyroid hormone decrease the amount of TRH that is released from the hypothalamus, completing the feedback loop.

Thyroid hormone is critical for normal brain development. The **absence of normal thyroid hormone function in the first months of the infant leads to irreversible cretinism[29].** [注1] Thyroid hormone induces myelin basic protein[30], and hypothyroidism leads to decreased production of this protein and defective neuronal myelination[31]. Thyroid hormones have an important effect on oxygen consumption in many tissues including heart, skeletal muscle, kidney and liver; brain gonads[32], and spleen are not affected. This calorigenic effect[33] is important to normal thermogenesis. Thyroid hormones also increase lipolysis[34].

Thyroid hormone has direct actions on the heart and vascular system. Hyperthyroidism leads to tachycardia, increased stroke volume, increased pulse pressure, and decreased vascular resistance. Hypothyroidism leads to bradycardia[35], and reversal of the above effects. Thyroid hormones increase the conversion of cholesterol to bile and increase LDL uptake by the liver and thereby reduce plasma cholesterol concentrations. [注2]

Hypothyroidism is can be treated effectively by hormone replacement. Common causes of hypothyroidism include **autoimmune destruction[36]** of the thyroid gland (**Hashimoto disease**), **congenital[37] hypothyroidism, or impaired pituitary or hypothalamic function.** Thyroid hormones are indicated for the treatment and prophylaxis of goiter[38] by suppressing abnormal growth of the thyroid gland. Thyroid hormones are also useful in the treatment of TSH-dependent thyroid cancers. Adverse effects of thyroid hormones is a hyperthyroid state with increased calorigenesis and oxygen demand, tachycardia, and increased cardiac workload.

Structure

Synthetic preparations of T_4 (levothyroxine), T_3 (liothyronine) and a 4∶1 mixture of

T_4/T_3 (liotrix) are preferable to desiccated preparations of thyroid prepared from animals that are more variable in biological activity.

Mechanism of Action

The actions of the thyroid hormones are mediated by nuclear thyroid receptors that act by increasing or decreasing transcription of target genes. There are three major thyroid receptors:

$TR\beta_1$, $TR\beta_2$, and $TR\alpha_1$. Whereas $TR\beta_1$ and $TR\alpha_1$ are expressed in virtually every tissue, $TR\beta_2$ is expressed exclusively in the anterior pituitary. These receptors bind T_3 in the nucleus. T_4 can bind to the receptors but at much lower affinity and with much less, if any, effect on transcription. Thyroid receptors are bound in the absence of ligand to the promoters of target genes, and in some cases the nonliganded receptor exerts a potent inhibition of basal transcription. T_3 binding to TR results in recruitment of coactivators and subsequent disinhibition and increased rates of transcription.

Mechanism of Action

All the above preparation of thyroid hormone can be administered orally. Levothyroxine and liothyronine are also available for parenteral administration. Doses are individualized and monitored by measuring the level of circulating TSH.

Pharmacokinetics

T_4 has a very long half-life (7 days), in large part because of its extensive binding to TBG. The half-life of T_4 is lengthened to 9-10 days in hypothyroidism and decreased to 3-4 days in hyperthyroidism. Thyroid hormones are degraded mostly by the liver and excreted in the bile.

Thyroid Antagonists

Hyperthyroidism can be treated with agents that **decrease the biosynthesis of thyroid hormones** that **decrease cellular response to thyroid hormones**, or **destruction** of the **thyroid gland with radioactive isotopes** of thyroid hormones or surgery. The **thioamides**[39], **methimazole**[40] **and propylthiouracil**[41], are the major drugs for treating hyperthyroidism. These drugs act by **inhibiting peroxidation of iodide and organification of thyroglobulin**. **Propylthiouracil** also acts to **inhibit the coupling reaction that forms MIT and DIT**. Adverse effects of **thioamides** include a **maculopapular rash**, **and less commonly arthralgia**, **skin rashes**, **hepatoxicity**, **cholestatic jaundice**, **and a lupus-like syndrome**. Potentially life-threatening **agranulocytosis** has occurred with their use.

Historically, iodides were the major antithyroid agents. Large oral doses of iodide inhibit organification and the secretion of thyroid hormones. **Iodide is useful in treating acute thyrotoxicosis (thyroid storm)**, and reduce the size, vascularity, and fragility of a hyperplastic thyroid preoperatively. Most patients will escape the blocking effects of iodide in 2-8 weeks.

Monovalent anions such as perchlorate (ClO_4^-), thiocyanate (SCN^-), and pertechnetate (TcO_4^-) are competitive inhibitors of the iodide transport mechanism.

Radioactive 131 iodine is rapidly trapped and concentrated in the colloid of the thyroid gland exactly as occurs with the stable ^{127}I. Radiation is nearly exclusively delivered to the parenchymal cells of the thyroid and leads to a dose-dependent destruction of part or all of the gland. In many circumstances it is considered the treatment of choice for chronic hyperthyroidism. It should not be used in patients who are pregnant because of its action on the thyroid of the fetus.

Comprehension Questions

[42.1] A woman enters your clinic with an enlarged thyroid and you suspect simple adenomatous goiter. The best treatment for this condition would be

A. Intravenous infusion of TSH

B. Levothyroxine

C. Propylthiouracil

D. Thyroid ablation with ^{131}I

[42.2] The mechanism by which thiocyanate reduces synthesis of thyroid hormones is by inhibition of

A. Iodine oxidation

B. Iodide transport

C. TSH biosynthesis

D. TRβ

[42.3] A 33-year-old man is noted to have tachycardia, heat intolerance, weight loss, and an enlarged thyroid gland. Which of the following is the probable ultimate treatment for this patient?

A. Long-term corticosteroid therapy

B. Propranolol therapy

C. Radioactive iodine

D. Surgical resection

Answers

[42.1] **B.** Goiter is an indication for thyroid hormone replacement.

[42.2] **B.** Anions such as perchlorate and thiocyanate inhibit the transport of iodide into thyroid cells.

[42.3] **C.** This patient likely has Graves disease, the most common cause of hyperthyroidism in the United States, typically presenting with a painless goiter and symptoms of hyperthyroidism. The treatment of choice is radioactive iodine.

PHARMACOLOGY PEARLS

- Levothyroxine is the drug of choice for treatment of hypothyroidism.
- The free, unbound thyroid hormone is the active component.
- The thioamides methimazole and propylthiouracil are the major drugs for treating hyperthyroidism, and act by inhibiting peroxidation of iodide and organification of thyroglobulin. Propylthiouracil also acts to inhibit the coupling reaction that forms MIT and DIT.

REFERENCES

Klein I, Danzi S. Evaluation of the therapeutic efficacy of different levothyroxine preparations in the treatment of human thyroid disease. Thyroid 2003; 13: 1127-32.

Wiersinga WM. Thyroid hormone replacement therapy. Horm Res 2001; 56 (suppl 1): 74-81.

词汇

1. fatigue[疲劳]
2. sluggish[缓慢的,迟钝的]
3. anemic[贫血的]
4. alopecia[秃头,脱发]
5. scarring[瘢痕化]
6. thyroid gland[甲状腺]
7. nontender[无触痛的]
8. nodule[小结节]
9. thyroid-stimulating hormone (TSH)[促甲状腺激素]
10. hypothyroidism[甲状腺功能减退]
11. levothyroxine[左旋甲状腺素]
12. deiodination[脱碘(作用)]
13. monoiodotyrosine (MIT)[一碘酪氨酸]
14. diiodotyrosine (DIT)[二碘酪氨酸]
15. hypothalamic-pituitary-thyroid axis[下丘脑-垂体-甲状腺轴]
16. thyrotropin-releasing hormone (TRH)[促甲状腺激素释放激素]
17. hypothalamus[下丘脑]
18. anterior pituitary[垂体前部]
19. myxedema[粘液(性)水肿]
20. thyrotoxicosis[甲状腺毒症]
21. iodide[碘化物]
22. symporter[共输送体]
23. colloid[胶体,胶质]
24. iodine[碘]
25. thyroidal peroxidase[甲状腺过氧化物酶]
26. thyroglobulin[甲状腺球蛋白]
27. proteolysis[蛋白水解作用]
28. thyrotroph[促甲状腺细胞]
29. cretinism[呆小病]
30. myelin basic protein[髓磷脂碱性蛋白]
31. myelination[髓鞘形成]

32. gonad[生殖腺]
33. calorigenic effect[产热作用]
34. lipolysis[脂解作用]
35. bradycardia[心动过缓]
36. autoimmune destruction[自身免疫破坏]
37. congenital[先天性的]
38. goiter[甲状腺肿]
39. thioamide[硫金黄菌素]
40. methimazole[甲巯咪唑]
41. propylthiouracil[丙基硫氧嘧啶]

注 1

发病开始于胎儿或新生儿期的甲减应尽早治疗，常用甲状腺片。从小剂量开始逐渐增加剂量，临床症状缓解后改用维持量。呆小病的疗效与开始治疗的时间有关。

注 2

甲状腺激素可促进脂肪组织对肾上腺素和高血糖素的敏感性，使脂肪酶活性增加，血浆非酯化脂肪酸水平升高；同时可加速胆固醇转变为脂肪酸，使血浆胆固醇水平降低，故甲状腺功能减退的病人可能出现高胆固醇血症。

点评

病例为 44 岁中年妇女，出现疲劳、行动迟缓、皮肤干燥、毛发稀疏，但无斑秃等征兆，患者血糖和电解质结果正常，完全血细胞计数正常，可基本排除贫血引起。体检发现病人甲状腺弥散性肿大，无触痛、无结节，实验室检查发现其 T_4 水平降低而 TSH 水平增高，诊断为甲状腺功能减退症。其母亲曾服用甲状腺素片，说明可能有家族史。给予左甲状腺素钠口服替代治疗，甲状腺素钠是人工合成品，左旋比右旋型作用强 8 ~ 10 倍，左旋型是最常用于治疗甲状腺功能减退的药品。优点是作用强度稳定，无抗原性。口服吸收 60 % 左右。T_4 吸收入血后绝大部分与血浆蛋白结合，仅 0.03%~ 0.05% 以游离形式存在，口服 1 ~ 2 周疗效达高峰，静脉注射因游离浓度低而作用并不比口服快。停药后作用可维持 1 ~ 3 周，$t_{1/2}$ 较长，故作用缓慢持久，反复用药易蓄积中毒。不易透过胎盘，故甲状腺机能减退合并妊娠时无须停药。可用于用于各种原因所致甲状腺功能减退症。也用于甲亢治疗时的辅助治疗，以防止发生甲状腺机能减退和甲状腺肿大。

张 伟

❖ CASE 43

A 12-year-old boy is brought to the office by his parents because of abdominal pain① for the past day. Prior to this, the parents noted that he was drinking a lot of water and going to the bathroom frequently. He said that his mouth was very dry and he was very thirsty. Until the past day or two he was eating more than usual but was losing weight. He has no significant medical history, and the family history is unremarkable. On exam, he appears moderately ill, and his blood pressure is normal, but he is tachycardic. His mucous membranes② are dry. His abdomen is diffusely tender but without rebound or guarding. A urine dipstick test③ in the office reveals the presence of large ketones and glucose. A glucose measurement from a drop of blood obtained by fingerstick is markedly elevated at 550 mg/dL. You immediately admit the patient to the hospital for newly diagnosed type I diabetes[注1] mellitus in ketoacidosis④ and start an infusion of IV fluids and regular insulin.

◆ **What is the structure of natural human insulin?**

◆ **What effect does insulin have on potassium?**

◆ **What is the effect of α-adrenergic stimulation on insulin secretion?**

◆ **What is the effect of β-adrenergic stimulation on insulin secretion?**

ANSWERS TO CASE 43: The Pancreas and Glucose Homeostasis

Summary: A 12-year-old with newly diagnosed type I diabetes mellitus has ketoacidosis.

- **Structure of human insulin**: A 51-amino acid polypeptide that consists of two chains linked by two disulfide bridges.
- **Effect of insulin on potassium**: Promotes cellular K^+ uptake.
- **Effect of α-adrenergic stimulation**: Inhibition of insulin secretion.
- **Effect of β-adrenergic stimulation**: Increased insulin secretion.

CLINICAL CORRELATION

Insulin is a 51-amino acid polypeptide that is produced in pancreatic β-cells and stored as a complex with Zn^{2+}. The primary stimulus for insulin release is glucose, but amino acids, fatty acids, and ketone bodies may stimulate its release. Glucagon and somatostatin⑤ also may modulate its secretion. α-adrenergic stimulation is a predominant inhibitory mechanism, whereas β-adrenergic stimulation increases its release. Insulin acts by binding to specific membrane receptors with tyrosine kinase⑥ activity. Tyrosine in the receptor becomes phosphorylated⑦ and allows for glucose transport into the cell. In muscle and adipose tissue, glucose transport is mediated by the recruitment of hexose⑧ transport molecules into the plasma membrane. Among its many actions, insulin increases glucose transport, glycogen synthesis and deposition, lipogenesis, and protein synthesis. It decreases intracellular lipolysis and hepatic gluconeogenesis. Insulin also stimulates cellular potassium uptake. Type I diabetes mellitus is a disease in which pancreatic β-cells fail to produce adequate amounts of insulin. Insulin must then be supplemented. Most currently used insulin preparations are human insulin produced by recombinant deoxyribonucleic acid (DNA) techniques. There are short-, intermediate-, and long-acting insulin preparations available. All currently available products must be given by injection, usually requiring one to four subcutaneous injections⑨ a day or continuous subcutaneous infusion with an insulin pump. Regular insulin can also be given intravenously in the setting of diabetic ketoacidosis. Insulin injections are also used in type II diabetics who cannot achieve adequate control with oral agents. The most significant risk of insulin therapy is the induction of hypoglycemia. Hypoglycemia may produce tachycardia, sweating, and confusion. In severe cases, hypoglycemia may progress to coma⑩, seizures⑪, or even death.

Pharmacology of Insulin and Oral Hypoglycemic Agents

Definitions

Type I diabetes: Historically called juvenile onset diabetes or insulindependent diabetes mellitus (IDDM) is a hyperglycemic condition caused by inadequate production of insulin by B cells of the pancreas.

Type II diabetes: A condition of hyperglycemia caused by resistance to circulating levels of insulin. Also called non-insulin-dependent diabetes mellitus (NIDDM). The incidence of this condition is increasing markedly in the United States and is especially prevalent in the Hispanic population.

Objectives

1. List the structure and function of endogenous insulin.
2. Know the characteristics, therapeutic uses, and adverse effects of insulin preparations.
3. Understand the mechanisms of action, uses, and adverse effects of oral hypoglycemic agents.
4. Understand the mechanisms of action, uses, and adverse effects of agents used to raise blood sugar levels.

Pharmacology of Class

Insulin is secreted by the B cells of the pancreas. The islet of Langerhans within the pancreas is made of four cell types, each secretes a distinct polypeptide. The **B (or β) cells secrete insulin**, the **A (or α) cells secrete glucagon**, the **D (or δ) cells secrete somatostatin**, and the PP or F cells secrete pancreatic polypeptide. **Human insulin comprises two chains, the A and B chains**, that are produced by the formation of **one intrapeptide and two interpeptide disulfide bonds** from a 110-amino acid precursor[12] called **preproinsulin**. This precursor is cleaved within the endoplasmic reticulum and Golgi complex to form mature insulin and C-peptide. Insulin secretion is a tightly regulated process that normally maintains a stable concentration of plasma glucose through both postprandial periods and periods of fasting. **Glucose is the most important stimulus to insulin secretion in humans**. Insulin secretion is also stimulated by gastrointestinal inhibitory polypeptide 1, glucagon-like peptide 1, gastrin[13], secretin[14], cholecystokinin[15], vasoactive intestinal polypeptide gastrinreleasing peptide and enteroglucagon. Neural input via catecholamines also regulate insulin secretion as stated above. **Glucose enters the pancreas via a specific transporter, GLUT-2**, and is **rapidly phosphorylated by glucokinase**. Glucokinase is considered to be the glucose sensor within the B cell and its activity ultimately leads to increased intracellular Ca^{2+} within the B cell and this causes insulin secretion. Insulin promotes the uptake of carbohydrates, proteins, and fats in most tissues. It influences metabolism by stimulating protein and free fatty acid biosynthesis and inhibits the release of fatty acids from adipose cells. Insulin stimulates the production of glycogen and triglycerides.

Insulin is the mainstay for the treatment of virtually all type I diabetics and many type II diabetics. There are four principal types available that differ in their onset and duration of action (Table 43-1).

Table 43-1

INSULIN PREPARATIONS

AGENT	TIME TO ONSET	DURATION OF ACTION
Rapid acting(lispro)	5-15min	3-5h
Short acting(regular insulin)	30min	5-8h
Immediate acting(lente)	1-2h	18-24h
NPH insulin	1-2	18-24
Long-acting(ultralente)	4-6h	20-36

The **goal of insulin therapy is to control plasma glucose levels as tightly as possible**. Most of the sequelae[16] of diabetes such as **retinopathy, renal damage, and neuropathy** are caused by the **hyperglycemic condition** rather than the absence of insulin. Current regimens generally use an intermediate or long acting preparation supplemented with injections of short or rapid acting preparations to meet postprandial needs. Premixed mixtures of different types of insulins are also available. The most common adverse effect of insulin administration is **hypoglycemia**.

Structure

Human insulin derived by recombinant technology in bacteria or yeast has supplanted the use of bovine or pork insulins.

Mechanism of Action

All of insulin's activities are mediated by the insulin receptor which is expressed in most tissue types. The insulin receptor consists of an extracellular α-subunit that forms the insulin binding site and a transmembrane β-subunit that possesses tyrosine kinase activity. The mature insulin receptor is a dimer composed of 2 α-and 2 β-subunits. Insulin binds its receptor in the picomolar range within a binding pocket formed by the two α-subunits. Binding produces conformational changes in the receptor that activate intrinsic tyrosine kinase activity that results in autophosphorylation of one β-subunit by the other. This autophosphorylation increases the tyrosine kinase activity of the receptor towards other substrates, especially the docking proteins insulin-receptor substrate 1 (IRS-1) and IRS-2. Phosphorylation of IRS-1 and IRS-2 results in further downstream phosphorylation and activation of MAP kinase and phosphatidylinositol-3-kinase. This network of phosphorylation ultimately leads to translocation of glucose transporters, especially GLUT-4 to the plasma membrane. This results in an increase in glucose transport into muscle and adipose tissue. Phosphorylation of various substrates in this insulin pathway also increases glycogen synthesis, lipogenesis, protein synthesis, and activation of transcription factors that mediate effects on cell growth and division.

Administration

All currently available preparations are injected subcutaneously or delivered by continuous infusion. Short-acting soluble insulin is the only form that should be administered intravenously.

Oral Hypoglycemic Agents

Oral hypoglycemic agents increase the secretion of insulin by the pancreas or alter tissue sensitivity to insulin. These agents are typically used to control hyperglycemia in patients with type II diabetes (Table 43-2).

Sulfonylureas

Sulfonylureas act to **increase the release of insulin from the pancreas**. **First-generation sulfonylureas** include tolbutamide, chlorpropamide, tolazamide, and acetohexamide. **Second-generation agents** include glyburide, glipizide, gliclazide, and glimepiride, which are considerably **more potent** than the earlier agents. All are **substituted arylsulfonylureas** with different substitutions on the benzene ring[17] and at one nitrogen residue of the urea moiety[18]. Sulfonylureas are used to control glucose levels in type II diabetics who cannot achieve adequate control with diet alone. A limitation in the use of the sulfonylureas is secondary failure,[注2] that is, failure to maintain glucose levels with chronic use. **Adverse effects of sulfonylureas include hypoglycemia, nausea and vomiting, anemia, and dermatological reactions.**

Mechanism of Action

Sulfonylureas bind to a high-affinity sulfonylurea receptor on B cells that inhibits a K^+-efflux channel. This leads to **depolarization of the cell with an increase in Ca^{2+} entry** through voltage-gated Ca^{2+} channels. The increased intracellular Ca^{2+} causes an increase in insulin secretion. Sulfonylureas **also stimulate the release of pancreatic somatostatin**, which can reduce the secretion of glucagon.

Administration

All of the sulfonylureas are administered orally.

Table 43-2

COMMON AGENTS FOR DIABETES

MEDICATION	MECHANISM OF ACTION/INDICATIONS	SPECIAL CONSIDERATIONS	COST
Insulin	Supplement patient's own insulin production.	Must check blood glucose frequently to monitor therapy and prevent complications.	$
Sulfonylurea	Augments patient's own insulin production, works at the pancreatic B-cells.	Can cause hypoglycemia, can accumulate in renal insufficiency and cause prolonged hypoglycemia. Best for young patients with FPG <300mg/dl.	$
Metformin	Deceases gluconeogensis in the liver, decreases insulin resistance.	In patients with renal insufficiency, or liver dysfunction, may cause lactic acidosis.	$$ – $$$
α-Glucosidase	Inhibits breakdown of complex carbohydrates in the GI tract.	Can cause GI distress, and must be taken TID with meals. Dose-dependent hepatotoxicity.	$$
Pioglitazone Rosiglitazone	Promote skeletal muscle glucose uptake, decrease insulin resistance.	Hepatoxicity. Edema.	$$$ – $$$$
Repaglinide	Nonsulfonylurea—but works in a similar manner—rapid onset of action. Monotherapy or in combination with metformin.	Caution in elderly, renal, or hepatic insufficiency. Must dose TID with meals.	$$

With permission, from Case Files: Internal Medicine, 2004.

Pharmacokinetics

First-generation sulfonylureas have relatively long half-lives: Chlorpropamide is 32 hours, tolazamide is 7 hours, tolbutamide is 5 hours. The second-generation agents tend to have shorter half-lives (about 4 hours) which makes them less prone to causing hypoglycemia.

Other Insulin Secretagogues

Two relatively new insulin secretagogues, repaglinide and nateglinide, are approved for use in **type II diabetics**. Both of these agents act by **decreasing the activity of K^+ channels as described for the sulfonylureas**. This increases insulin release. Chemically, **repaglinide** is a **meglitinide**, **nateglinide** is a **Dphenylalanine**[19] **derivative**. Repaglinide has a half-life of about 1 hour and a very rapid onset of action that make it well suited to control postprandial increases in plasma glucose. It should be taken about 10 minutes before a meal. It is metabolized in the kidney and should be used cautiously in patients with renal impairment. Nateglinide is also used to control plasma glucose after meals. It should be taken 1-10 minutes prior to eating. Both these drugs can cause hypoglycemia but nateglinide has the lowest incidence of this adverse effect.

Insulin Sensitizers

Thiazolidinediones

A **hallmark of type II diabetes is insulin resistance**. The hormone is present at significant plasma concentrations but is ineffective in reducing plasma glucose. **Thiazolidinediones (TZDs) act to increase tissue sensitivity to insulin**. TZDs appear to **increase glucose uptake in adipose and muscle tissues**. Two TZDs are approved for use: **pioglitazone and rosiglitazone**. The effect of the TZDs are mediated by agonist activity at the peroxisomal proliferator-activated receptor γ (PPAR-γ). PPARs are members of the nuclear receptor family that are present in the nucleus of cells tethered to the promoters of target genes. PPARs bind a rather diverse group of ligands including fibrates and TZDs. There are three members of PPAR receptors, PPARα, PPARβ, and PPARγ; the latter mediates the effects of the TZDs. TZDs are effective in about 70 percent of type II diabetics. TZDs alter plasma lipid levels by reducing triglycerides, high-density lipoprotein (HDL) and low-density lipoprotein (LDL) cholesterol.

Biguanides

Metformin lowers plasma glucose levels in the absence of functioning B cells, it does not increase insulin secretion but **decreases insulin resistance** by an unknown mechanism. It is useful in patients with type II diabetes and **does not cause weight gain** or provoke hypoglycemia as do the sulfonylureas. Biguanides are frequently used in combination with TZDs or insulin secretagogues when monotherapy has not provided adequate glycemic control. **Common adverse effects include nausea, vomiting, diarrhea, and abdominal pain**. Biguanides are **cleared by the kidney** and are **contraindicated in patients with renal disease**.

Enzyme Inhibitors

Monosaccharides[20] such as **glucose and fructose**[21] can be absorbed across the intestine and into the portal circulation. Complex disaccharides[22], starches and disaccharides that comprise a significant percentage of the carbohydrates ingested, must be broken into monosaccharides before they can be absorbed. Pancreatic α-amylase[23] and α-glucosidases[24] are primarily responsible for this hydrolysis of more complex carbohydrates. **Inhibitors of α-glucosidase such as acarbose and miglitol inhibit the intestinal breakdown of complex carbohydrates. Acarbose** inhibits the α-glucosidases, sucrase[25], maltase[26], glucoamylase, dextranase. It weakly inhibits α-amylase. **Miglitol**[27] is 5 to 6 times more potent than acarbose and inhibits the same α-glucosidase, as well as isomaltase and β-glucosidases (responsible for hydrolysis of lactose) as well. Inhibition of these digestive enzymes reduces postprandial absorption of complex carbohydrates and thereby reduces plasma glucose levels. They are approved for treatment of type II diabetes as monotherapy or combined with a sulfonylurea if additional hypoglycemic effect is needed. [注3] **Adverse effects include flatulence, diarrhea, and abdominal pain**, most likely caused by the increase in carbohydrates in the distal small intestine and colon. α-glucosidase inhibitors prevented the progression from a prediabetic state into new cases of type II diabetes and this may become a new indication for these drugs.

Agents That Increase Plasma Glucose

Glucagon is useful for the **emergency treatment of severe hypoglycemia** when **unconsciousness prevents oral administration of nutrients and IV glucose is unavailable**. Glucagon binds to specific receptors in the **liver** that **increase cAMP** and promote the catabolism of glycogen into glucose. Glucagon must be administered parenterally.

Comprehension Questions

[43.1] The goal of insulin therapy is to

A. Control serum glucose as tightly as possible

B. Control triglyceride biosynthesis

C. Maintain adequate hepatic glycogen stores

D. Maintain serum K^+ homeostasis

[43.2] The thiazolidinediones are useful in treating type II diabetes because they

A. Decrease the degradation of insulin

B. Increase insulin release

C. Increase glucose utilization

D. Increase glucose uptake in muscle cells

[43.3] A 42-year-old man is diagnosed with diabetes mellitus. He has tried diet and exercise without success. A second-generation sulfonylurea agent is prescribed. Which of the following is the most likely side effect he will experience?

A. Agranulocytosis
B. Hypoglycemia
C. Lactic acidosis
D. Myositis

Answers

[43.1] **A.** The goal in treating diabetes is tight control of serum glucose to avoid the complications of hyperglycemia.

[43.2] **D.** The TZDs are insulin sensitizers; they do not alter insulin secretion or degradation but act to increase glucose uptake in adipose and muscle.

[43.3] **B.** In general, the most common adverse effect of the agents for diabetes is hypoglycemia.

PHARMACOLOGY PEARLS

- The goal in treating diabetes is tight glucose control to prevent the micro and macrovascular complications.
- Human recombinant insulin is preferable to either bovine or porcine insulin.
- Biguanides such as metformin are cleared by the kidney and are contraindicated in patients with renal disease.
- Glucagon is useful for the emergency treatment of severe hypoglycemia when unconsciousness prevents oral administration of nutrients and IV glucose in unavailable.

REFERENCES

Inzucchi SE. Oral antihyperglycemic therapy for type 2 diabetes: scientific review. JAMA 2002; 287: 360-72.

Quinn L. Type 2 diabetes: epidemiology, pathophysiology, and diagnosis. Nurs Clin North Am 2001; 36: 175-92.

词汇

1. abdominal pain[腹痛]
2. mucous membrane[黏膜]
3. dipstick test[浸渍检查法]
4. ketoacidosis[酮症酸中毒]
5. somatostatin[生长抑素]
6. tyrosine kinase[酪氨酸激酶]
7. phosphorylate[磷酸化(作用)]
8. hexose[己糖]
9. subcutaneous injection[皮下注射(剂)]
10. coma[昏迷]
11. seizure[癫痫发作]
12. precursor[前体,先质]

13. gastrin[胃泌素]
14. secretin[促胰液素]
15. cholecystokinin[胆囊收缩素]
16. sequelae[后遗症]
17. benzene ring[苯环]
18. moiety[等份,部分]
19. Dphenylalanine[苯丙氨酸]
20. monosaccharide[单糖]
21. fructose[果糖]
22. disaccharide[双糖,二糖]
23. α-amylase[α-淀粉酶]
24. α-glucosidase[α-糖苷酶]
25. sucrase[蔗糖酶]
26. maltase[麦芽糖酶]
27. miglitol[米格列醇(降血糖药)]

注 1

1 型为胰岛素依赖性糖尿病(insulin-dependent diabetes mellitus,IDDM)，是源于多种因素引起的自身免疫机制紊乱所导致的胰岛 β 细胞破坏、胰岛素分泌缺乏，为儿童及青少年最常见的内分泌疾病。胰岛素是治疗 1 型为胰岛素依赖性糖尿病的唯一手段。低血糖反应是胰岛素治疗中最易发生的并发症，应教会病人熟知反应症状，以便及早发现和及时引用糖水；患者应随时备有甜食；严重者应立即静脉注射 50% 葡萄糖。

注 2

磺脲类药物继发失效是指 2 型糖尿病患者曾有效地使用某种磺脲类降糖药 1 个月或更长时间，但后来虽剂量充足，疗程 1 个月以上，仍无效或效果很差。磺脲类降糖药继发失效的判定标准是：每日应用最大剂量的磺脲类降糖药(如优降糖 15mg/日,疗程 3 个月)，空腹血糖仍 >10mmol/L，糖化血红蛋白 >9.5%。研究认为，高浓度的磺脲类药物持续刺激 B 细胞可能减弱 B 细胞对磺脲类药物的反应。这时应考虑加用胰岛素或改用胰岛素治疗。

注 3

胰岛素促分泌剂(如磺脲类、瑞格列奈和那格列奈等)其降血糖作用有赖于有功能的胰岛 B 细胞(>30%)，因此仅限于胰岛功能尚存的 2 型糖尿病患者。

点评

病例具有典型的 1 型糖尿病特征，发病早(为 12 岁儿童)，表现为“三多一少”即多尿、多饮、多食、消瘦。除上述临床表现外，伴有急腹症(表现为全腹压痛,无反跳痛和肌紧张)，血糖≥300mg/dl(患儿血糖为 550mg/dL)，同时尿酮体及尿糖阳性，诊断为 1 型糖尿病伴酮症酸中毒；当腹痛剧烈时，极易与小儿急腹症，如急性阑尾炎相混淆，应注意酮症酸中毒病人的腹疼部位不固定，多表现为全腹压痛，一般不具备疼痛持续的特点。

确诊后应及时给予常规胰岛素治疗，原则是提供充足的胰岛素，覆盖 24 小时的基础需要，给予较大剂量胰岛素以尽量与进餐后引起的血糖变化相匹配，尽量模仿正常生理状况。

胰岛素的药理作用主要体现在以下几点：(1)糖代谢：促进糖原的合成和贮存，加速葡萄糖的氧化、酵解，并抑制糖原分解和异生而降低血糖。此外，胰岛素可使葡萄糖转运体从胞内重新分布到胞膜(如 GLUT4)，增加转运体的合成并提高其活性，从而加速葡萄糖的转运；(2)脂肪代谢：促进脂肪合成，抑制脂肪分解，减少游离脂肪酸和酮体的生成，增加脂肪酸和葡萄糖的转运，使其利用增加；(3)蛋白质代谢：增加氨基酸的转运，促进核酸、蛋白质的合成，抑制蛋白质的分解。

低血糖症是胰岛素应用时最常见的不良反应，多发生于胰岛素剂量过大、未按时进餐、肝肾功能不全、升血糖反应有缺陷者。当血糖降至一定程度时，患者可出现饥饿感、心跳加快、出汗、焦虑、震颤等症状。严重者可出现昏迷、惊厥及低血糖休克，甚至脑损伤及死亡。为防止低血糖症的严重后果，应告知病人反应症状，以便及早发现和进餐。发生低血糖后，轻者可口服糖水，严重者应立即静脉注射50%葡萄糖。

张 伟

❖ CASE 44

A 66-year-old woman presents for an annual health maintenance visit. She is generally feeling well and has no specific complaints. She takes hydrochlorothiazide① for hypertension, levothyroxine sodium for hypothyroidism, and a multivitamin. She went through menopause at age 48 and never took hormone replacement therapy. She is a former cigarette smoker, having a 30 pack-year history and having quit 20 years ago. She occasionally has a glass of wine with dinner and walks three or four times a week for exercise. On examination you note that her height is 1 inch less than it was 3 years ago. Her vital signs are normal. She has a prominent kyphoscoliosis② of the spine. Her examination is otherwise unremarkable. Blood work reveals a normal electrolytes, renal function, blood count, calcium, and thyroid-stimulating hormone (TSH) levels. You order a bone density test, which shows a significant reduction of density in the spine and hips. You diagnose her with osteoporosis③ and start her on alendronate sodium④.[注1]

◆ **What is the mechanism of action of parathyroid hormone on the bone? In the kidney?**

◆ **What is the mechanism of action of alendronate sodium?**

ANSWERS TO CASE 44: Agents Affecting Calcium Homeostasis

Summary: A 66-year-old woman with osteoporosis is prescribed alendronate.

- **Mechanism of action of parathyroid hormone[5] on the bone**: Increase in number and activity of osteoclasts[6], resulting in bone resorption[7].
- **Mechanism of action of parathyroid hormone in the kidney**: Increases reabsorption of Ca^{2+} and Mg^{2+} and increases production of calcitriol and dihydrotachysterol; decreases reabsorption of phosphate, bicarbonate, amino acids, sulfate, sodium, and chloride.
- **Mechanism of action of alendronate**: Inhibition of osteoclastic activity in bone, which reduces bone reabsorption.

CLINICAL CORRELATION

Parathyroid hormone (PTH) has multiple actions on bone. Chronic elevations in PTH, for example, from a tumor, stimulate the resorption of bone via its stimulation of the number and activity of osteoclasts. This is mediated by specific PTH receptors in the bone, coupled to an increase in cyclic adenosine monophosphate (cAMP). Intermittent administration of PTH stimulates bone growth. Estrogen is an indirect inhibitor of PTH activity in the bone. This effect allows premenopausal women to maintain higher levels of bone density. Following menopause, and the resultant decrease in circulating estrogen levels, there is a relative increase in osteoclastic activity and resorption of bone, with a net loss of bone mineral density. Alendronate sodium is an analog of pyrophosphate[8] that directly binds to bone. It inhibits osteoclastic activity, reducing the resorption of bone. This retards the progression of bone density loss and may allow for increases in density, because osteoblastic[9] activity is not affected. It is administered orally, and its most common adverse effects are gastrointestinal (GI). It may produce esophagitis[10], and even esophageal perforation[11], if the pill were to get caught in the esophagus while swallowing. For that reason, patients taking alendronate are instructed to take it on an empty stomach with a full glass of water and to remain upright for at least 30 minutes after ingesting the medication.

Pharmacology of Agents Regulating Calcium Homeostatis

Objectives

1. Know the structure, actions, and uses of parathyroid hormone (PTH).
2. Describe the structure, actions, and uses of calcitonin[12].
3. Describe the structure, synthesis, actions, and uses of vitamin D and its metabo-

lites.

4. Know the secondary agents that affect calcium homeostasis and their characteristics.

Definitions

Osteocyte: A bone-maintaining cell, an embedded osteoblast.

Osteoblast: Bone forming cells derived from the stroma of bone.

Osteoclast: Bone-resorptive cell derived from myeloid⑬ lineages.

OPG (osteoprotegerin): A member of the OPG, OPGL (osteoprotegerin⑭ ligand), RANK (receptor activator of nuclear factor-κB) signal transduction cascade that is central to bone metabolism.

Pharmacology of Class

Calcium is the major extracellular divalent ion. It has diverse roles— including enzyme activation, secretion, excitation-contraction coupling in all muscle types, and neuronal function—and is a critical structural element in bone and teeth.

About **40-50 percent of serum calcium exists as free, ionized Ca^{2+}**. This is **the biologically active fraction**, and it is maintained at about 2.5 mM in the serum. An additional **40 percent is bound to serum proteins** and the remainder is complexed to ions such as phosphate, citrate, and bicarbonate. The serum concentration of Ca^{2+} is tightly regulated by several endocrine systems and three major tissues: the **gut, kidney, and bone**.

Bone is the **storage depot** for over **99 percent of calcium in the body**, and most of the calcium is in the form of **hydroxyapatite**: $[Ca_{10}(PO_4)_6(OH)_2]$. Bone is a remarkably dynamic tissue and bone remodeling is a continuous process. Normal bone is continuously **reabsorbed by the action of osteoclasts**, and **new bone is formed by the action of osteoblasts**; if these two processes are not equal in magnitude, excess bone can be lost, as in osteoporosis, or too much bone can be formed. **Coupling of the actions of osteoblasts and osteoclasts is largely under the control of the OPG/OPGL signaling system** (Figs. 44-1A and 44-1B).

Osteoblasts produce **OPGL**, a polypeptide that binds to receptors on osteoclasts termed **RANK**. **Stimulation of RANK-R** leads to increased **proliferation, maturation, and activation** of **osteoclasts**. **Osteoblasts** also elaborate **osteoprotegerin**, which is a **molecular antagonist of OPGL**. OPG can bind OPGL before it can activate the RANK receptor on osteoclasts. Osteoclast activation is thus controlled by the ratio of OPG/OPGL that is secreted by osteoblasts. Most drugs that act to alter calcium homeostasis in bone do so by altering OPG/OPGL.

Parathyroid hormone (PTH) is an 84-amino acid peptide synthesized in the **par-**

athyroid glands and is **secreted in response to low serum ionized Ca^{2+}**. PTH 1-34 has full biological activity. In the **kidney it acts to increase Ca^{2+} reabsorption** and **promotes phosphate (PO_4^{2-}) excretion**. It has indirect effects on the **gastrointestinal**

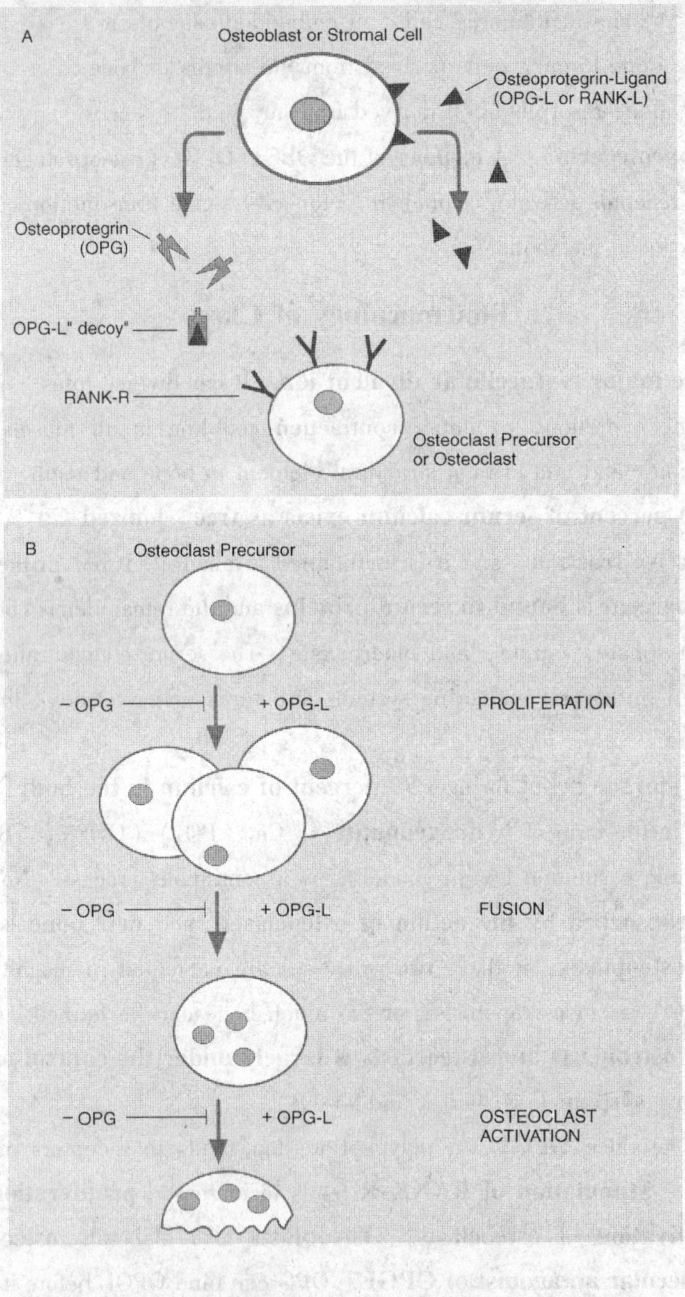

Figure 44-1. Osteoblast (A) and osteoclast (B). The OPG/OPGL signaling system controls the number and activity of osteoclasts. Osteoblasts secrete both OPG and OPGL. PGL stimulates proliferation and activation of osteoclasts. OPG is a "decoy" that binds OPG-L in the interstitial space and prevents its association with its receptor (RANK-R).

system to **increase Ca^{2+} absorption.** The effects of PTH on bone are complex and dependent on the temporal nature of its release or administration. **Continuously elevated PTH, as in hyperparathyroidism, increases osteoclast activity via increased OPGL and results in increased bone resorption. Pulsatile release of PTH** activates **osteoblasts** and increases bone formation.

Calcitonin (CT) is a 32-amino acid polypeptide produced in the **parafollicular cells** of the **thyroid**. It is secreted in response to elevated serum Ca^{2+} levels. **CT increases OPG and decreases OPG-L release** from **osteoblasts**, and its action on bone is to **reduce bone turnover**. In response to CT, osteoclasts withdraw reabsorptive processes, shrink in size, and retract the ruffled border from the surface of bone; CT effectively prevents all stages of osteoclastic-dependent bone resorption. It **increases renal excretion of Ca^{2+}, PO_4^{2-}, Mg^{2+}, Cl^-, and K^+ by decreasing reabsorption of these ions.**

The **third endocrine system** that has effects on **bone** is **vitamin D_3** and its **metabolites**. Vitamin D_3 (not a true vitamin in a nutritional sense) is a **prehormone**[15] that undergoes a series of metabolic alterations to the final agonist in the pathway, 1,25-$(OH)_2$ vitamin D_3. **Vitamin D_3 is synthesized from cholesterol** in the skin in a **two-step photo-dependent reaction.** Vitamin D_3 is converted by the **liver enzyme 25-hydroxylase to 25-(OH)D_3**; in the **kidney** the enzyme **1-hydroxylase metabolizes 25-(OH)D_3 to 1,25-$(OH)_2$ D_3. 1,25-$(OH)_2$ D_3** acts on the intestine to **increase intestinal absorption of Ca^{2+}**. In the **kidney**, 1,25-$(OH)_2$ D_3 acts to **increase the absorption** of both **Ca^{2+}** and **PO_4^{2-}**. 1,25-$(OH)_2$ D_3 stimulates Ca^{2+} mobilization from bone and enhances the resorptive action of PTH on bone. However, **1,25-$(OH)_2$ D_3** also induces **osteocalcin** and **osteopontin**, **two matrix proteins** important in bone formation.

Treatment of Hypocalcemia

Calcium Salts

A wide variety of preparations are available for both intravenous and oral administration for treating **acute hypocalcemic tetany**[16]. These include **calcium gluconate**[17], **calcium lactate**[18], **calcium carbonate**[19], **and calcium citrate**[20]. They vary in the percentage of calcium by weight from a low of 9 percent for calcium gluconate to a high of 40 percent for calcium carbonate.

Vitamin D

Several vitamin D or vitamin D-related agents are available for use for hypocalcemia and osteoporosis (Table 44-1). Selection of which agent to use depends on the desired onset of action, duration of effect and the presence of underlying liver or kidney disease. Thiazide diuretics act on the kidney to increase Ca^{2+} reabsorption in the distal convoluted tubule and can be used in the treatment of hypocalcemia.

Table 44-1

VITAMIN D-RELATED AGENTS

AGENT	CHEMICAL NATURE	TIME TO MAXIMUM EFFECT	DURATION OF ACTION	REQUIREMENT FOR METABOLISM
Cholecalciferol	Vit D_3	4wks	8wks	liver, kidney
Ergocalciferol	Vit D_2	4wks	8wks	liver, kidney
Dihydrotachysterol	1-(OH)D_3	1-2wks	1-2wks	liver
Doxercalciferol	1-(OH)D_2	1-2wks	1-2wks	liver
Calcifidiol	25-(OH)D_3	2-3wks	2-3wks	kidney
Paricalcitol	25-(OH)D_2	2-3wks	2-3wks	kidney
Calcitriol	1,25-$(OH)_2D_3$	24h	3-5d	none

Treatment of Hypercalcemia

Hypercalcemia㉑ has a number of pathophysiological causes including **hyperparathyroidism, Paget disease**[注2]**, and hypercalcemia of malignancy**㉒. **Calcitonin** is useful for **short-term treatment of hypercalcemia**. Salmon calcitonin is more potent and has a longer half-life than human calcitonin and is the form used therapeutically. Calcitonin has few side effects but **refractoriness**㉓ frequently develops. Calcitonin is available for parenteral and nasal administration. Peak plasma concentration after an inhaled dose is about 30 minutes after administration, but normalization of the rate of bone turnover as in Paget disease may take several months.

Bisphosphonates are **analogs of pyrophosphate in which the phosphodiester bond (P-O-P) is replaced by a nonhydrolyzable bisphosphonate (P-C-P) bond**. First-generation bisphosphonates included sodium **etidronate**. Second-generation bisphosphonates have been made that **include an amino group**; these include **risedronate**㉔, **alendronate, pamidronate, tiludronate, clodronate, and zoledronate**. The two classes of bisphosphonates have different mechanisms of action and different potencies. For example, **risedronate** is 1000 times more potent as an inhibitor of bone resorption than etidronate㉕. All bisphosphonates bind to and accumulate in bone, and this provides a measure of tissue specificity. The first-generation nonnitrogenous bisphosphonates are converted into an adenosine triphosphate (ATP) analog that cannot be internalized. This metabolite impairs osteoclast function and triggers osteoclast apoptosis. The amino-bisphosphonates[26] are not converted into an ATP analog; rather they interfere with mevalonate and ubiquitin metabolism (similar to statins). This leads to impaired posttranslational modification of a number of proteins that are critical to osteoclast function. Ultimately, the aminobisphosphonates lead to osteoclast hypofunction. **Etidronate** is available for oral use, the amino-bisphosphonates may be administered orally or by infusion. Administered orally, all the bisphosphonates have **very poor (approximately 5%) bioavailability**, but sufficient drug is absorbed to achieve therapeutic concentrations in bone. All bisphosphonates are approved for treatment of **Paget disease**; **alendronate** and risendronate are also approved for **prevention and treatment of osteoporosis**. The remaining aminobisphosphonates are used to treat hypercalcemia of malignancy. Adverse effects of bisphosphonates include **gastrointestinal upset, diarrhea, and nausea**. Bisphosphonates are associated with **lower esophageal erosion**, and the recommendation with alendronate and risedronate is to **avoid lying down for 30 minutes after oral administration to avoid reflux.**

Loop diuretics increase the amount of Ca^{2+} excreted and can be used in the acute management of hypercalcemia.

Treatment of Osteoporosis

Osteoporosis, loss of bone mass, affects nearly 30 percent of women age 65 years and older and a smaller percentage of men. Historically, osteoporosis has been divided into **postmenopausal osteoporosis**, which occurs in women and is related to the loss of ovarian hormones after menopause, and **senile**[27] **osteoporosis**, which is age related and affects both sexes. Histologically and biochemically, they seem indistinguishable disorders of bone metabolism caused by excessive bone reabsorption. Adequate dietary Ca^{2+} and vitamin D (to facilitate Ca^{2+} absorption) is critical in patients at risk for osteoporosis. The recommended daily allowance (RDA) for Ca^{2+} in patients at risk is **1200mg/day**.

Teriparatide[28] (PTH 1-34) has recently been approved for the treatment of osteoporosis. Administered intermittently, once a day by injection, teriparatide **increases bone formation in excess of resorption**. This treatment has been shown to increase bone mass and decrease the incidence of fractures. Studies in **rats** receiving very high doses of teriparatide for 2 years demonstrated an **increased frequency of osteosarcoma**. It is **contraindicated in patients with bone malignancy or in pediatric**[29] **patients**. Major adverse effects are **hypotension, hypocalcemia, dizziness, and nausea**.

Estrogens (see Case 40) have been shown to reduce the rate of bone loss in the postmenopausal period when the rate of loss can be as high as 10 percent per year. Estrogens increase bone mineral density and decrease the incidence of vertebral and nonvertebral fractures. However, estrogens do not increase net bone formation.

Selective estrogen receptor modifiers (SERMs) are compounds whose estrogenic activities are tissue-selective. Three SERMS are currently approved for use: **tamoxifen, raloxifene, and toremifene**. **Raloxifene** is approved for the prevention and treatment of osteoporosis; tamoxifen and toremifene are used to treat breast cancer. Raloxifene is a polyhydroxylated nonsteroidal compound that binds to the estrogen receptor, but it has estrogen-agonist activity only in bone and the liver; it has no effect on the uterus[30], and it is an estrogen antagonist in breast tissue and in the brain. It has antiresorptive activity in bone. It increases bone mineral density and has been shown to decrease the incidence of vertebral and nonvertebral fractures. Adverse effects include hot flashes and leg cramps[31]. More serious adverse effects include about a threefold increase in deep vein thrombosis and pulmonary embolism[32].

Sodium fluoride[33] has been examined in a number of clinical trials for the treatment of osteoporosis. Early studies using relatively high doses reported an increase in bone mineral density but no decrease in the incidence of fractures, probably because of the formation of abnormal hydroxylapatite crystals[34] in bone. More recent studies using slow-release monofluoride have suggested a decrease in fracture rates but fluoride is not yet approved for the treatment of osteoporosis.

Comprehension Questions

[44.1] Which of the following vitamin D preparations would be the most appropriate in a patient with poor renal function?

A. Calcifediol
B. Calcitriol
C. Cholecalciferol
D. Ergocalciferol

[44.2] Intermittent administration of PTH produces which of the following?

A. Impaired Ca^{2+} absorption in the gut
B. Inhibition of 1-hydroxylase
C. Net increase in bone formation
D. Net increase in bone resorption

[44.3] A 53-year-old woman who is being treated for metastatic breast cancer is noted to have some lethargy, fatigue, and an elevated serum calcium level. She is brought into the emergency department for near comatose state, thought to be caused by the hypercalcemia. After addressing the ABCs (airway, breathing, circulation), what is the best therapy for this patient?

A. Bisphosphonates
B. Calcitonin

C. Intravenous estrogen therapy D. Saline infusion and furosemide

Answers

[44.1] **B.** 1-hydroxylase activity must be adequate to produce $1,25(OH)_2D_3$. Calcitriol is the only choice that is already 1-hydroxylated.

[44.2] **C.** Intermittent administration of PTH on its analogs will result in bone formation. Continuous dosing or a PTH secreting tumor will cause bone resorption.

[44.3] **D.** Loop diuretics are the best choice in a patient with acute onset hypercalcemia.

PHARMACOLOGY PEARLS

- ❖ Teriparatide (PTH 1-34) is the only agent on the market that promotes new bone formation.
- ❖ Estrogens slow the rate of resorption but do not increase bone formation.
- ❖ Thiazide diuretics promote renal reabsorption of Ca^{2+}; loop diuretics have the opposite effect.
- ❖ Bisphosphonates can lead to severe esophageal erosions; patients are advised to not lie down for 30 minutes after taking them.

REFERENCES

Ariyan CE, Sosa JA. Assessment and management of patients with abnormal calcium. Crit Care Med 2004; 32(4 suppl): S146-54.

Stepan JJ, Alenfeld F, Boivin G, Feyen JH, Lakatos P. Mechanisms of action of antiresorptive therapies of postmenopausal osteoporosis. Endocr Regul 2003; 37: 225-38.

词汇

1. hydrochlorothiazide[氢氯噻嗪,双氢克尿塞]
2. kyphoscoliosis[脊柱后侧凸]
3. osteoporosis[骨质疏松症]
4. alendronate sodium[阿仑膦酸钠 <骨吸收抑制药>]
5. parathyroid hormone[甲状旁腺素]
6. osteoclast[破骨细胞]
7. resorption[再吸收]
8. pyrophosphate[焦磷酸盐]
9. osteoblastic[成骨细胞的]
10. esophagitis[食管炎]
11. esophageal perforation[食管穿孔]
12. calcitonin[降钙素]
13. myeloid[来自骨髓的]
14. osteoprotegerin[骨保护素]
15. prehormone[前激素]
16. tetany[手足搐搦]
17. calcium gluconate[葡糖酸钙]
18. calcium lactate[乳酸钙]
19. calcium carbonate[碳酸钙]

20. calcium citrate[柠檬酸钙]
21. hypocalcemia[低钙血症]
22. malignancy[恶性肿瘤]
23. refractoriness[脱敏感]
24. risedronate[利塞膦酸盐]
25. etidronate[1-羟基-亚乙基-1,1-二膦酸]
26. amino-bisphosphonate[氨基酰二碳磷酸盐化合物]
27. senile[老年的]
28. teriparatide[特立帕肽]
29. pediatric[儿科的]
30. uterus[子宫]
31. cramp[痉挛]
32. pulmonary embolism[肺栓塞]
33. fluoride[氟化物]
34. hydroxylapatite crystal[羟(基)磷灰石结晶]

注 1

阿仑膦酸钠盐口服难以吸收，对上消化道刺激症状较重，尤其对食管粘膜的损伤更为明显，可致食管炎、食管糜烂、食管溃疡、罕见食管狭窄等。有研究表明，服用该药的病人中约有 1.5% 发生食管炎或溃疡，并认为其机制是该药可能引起食管局部粘膜酸烧伤或由于该药的相关复合因素所致。因此应使该药尽可能短时间接触食管，尽快地通过胃，减少该药随胃食管反流而进入食管，防止食管不良反应。

注 2

Paget 骨病又称变形性骨炎，是一种成人的慢性骨骼病，其特征为骨局部代谢过强，骨组织被软化和增大的骨性结构取代。病因未明，电镜下 Paget 破骨细胞核的“指纹”型提示为病毒感染。本病常有家族性，但其特异性基因仍不清楚，年龄大于 40 岁者约 3% 患本病，男女比率为 3:2，东欧、西欧、英格兰、澳大利亚和新西兰多见。

点评

本病例为老年妇女(66 岁)，自 48 岁绝经后未曾服用雌激素替代治疗(提示雌激素的减退可能是骨质疏松的重要原因之一)，体检发现脊柱后侧凸，骨密度检查发现脊椎骨和髋骨密度显著降低，其余血液学检查如血细胞计数、电解质、肾功能、TSH 均正常，诊断为骨质疏松症并给予阿仑膦酸钠盐口服治疗，该类药物与焦磷酸相似，可选择性地抑制骨吸收，对骨骼中的羟磷灰石结晶有高度的亲和力，可牢固地吸附在骨小梁的表面并逐渐被破骨细胞吸收入细胞内，导致破骨细胞产生形态学改变，使破骨细胞功能下降甚至失活，从而抑制骨的再吸收过程。亦可与骨基质中的羟基磷灰石晶体结合，形成一层保护膜，阻止破骨前体细胞吸附于骨及随后被转化为成熟的破骨细胞，从而抑制破骨细胞性骨溶解。由于雌激素替代疗法在部分病人中可增高罹患子宫内膜癌或乳腺癌的风险，且并不适用于男性病人，阿仑膦酸钠盐类药物的应用成为绝经后及老年性骨质疏松症的有效治疗手段。

张 伟

❖ CASE 45

A 48-year-old man comes to your office with a 6-day history of worsening cough productive of green sputum. He has had fever and chills. He complains of pain in the right midback with deep breathing or coughing. Further history reveals that he has smoked one pack of cigarettes a day for 30 years. He has no other significant medical history. On examination, his temperature is 38.1℃ (100.5℉), his respiratory rate is 24 breaths per minute; pulse, 98 beats per minute; blood pressure, 120/75 mmHg; and saturation of oxygen, 96 percent on room air by pulse oximetry. Auscultation of his lungs reveals rales in the right lower-posterior lung field. The remainder of his examination is within normal limits. A posterior-to-anterior (PA) and lateral chest x-ray show a right lower-lobe infiltrate. A sputum Gram-stain reveals Gram-positive cocci, and subsequent sputum and blood culture results confirm the diagnosis of pneumonia[注1] caused by *streptococcus pneumoniae* (pneumococcus). You treat him with a combination of amoxicillin and clavulanic acid.[注2]

◆ **What is the mechanism of action of amoxicillin?**

◆ **What is the mechanism of action of clavulanic acid?**

ANSWERS TO CASE 45: Antibacterial Agents

Summary: A 48-year-old man with pneumococcal pneumonia is being treated with amoxicillin and clavulanic acid.

- **Mechanism of action of amoxicillin**: Inactivation of bacterial transpeptidases and prevention of cross-linking of peptidoglycan polymers necessary for cell-wall integrity, resulting in loss of cell-wall rigidity and cell rupture; also inhibition of cell-wall synthesis.
- **Mechanism of action of clavulanic acid**: Irreversible inhibition of β-lactamase.

CLINICAL CORRELATION

Penicillin is the prototype antibiotic in the β-lactam class. **β-lactam antibiotics inactivate bacterial transpeptidases**① and **prevent the cross-linking of peptidoglycan**② polymers essential for **cell-wall integrity**③. They also inactivate penicillin binding proteins that are involved in cell-wall synthesis. β-lactam antibiotics are **bactericidal**④ in growing cells, with Gram-positive bacteria being particularly susceptible. Penicillin has activity against many Gram-positive aerobic organisms, some Gram-negative aerobes and anaerobic organisms. It does not have significant activity against Gram-negative rods. Amoxicillin is an extended-spectrum penicillin with better activity against Gram-negative rods and similar activity against other organisms. **Both penicillin and amoxicillin are susceptible to β-lactamases**⑤, which cleave the β-lactam ring required for antibacterial action. Clavulanic acid is structurally similar to penicillin. It has no antimicrobial activity of its own but it irreversibly inhibits β-lactamases. It frequently is given in combination with amoxicillin, thus allowing it to be used to treat β-lactamase producing organisms. Penicillins can cause hypersensitivity reactions in susceptible persons. Approximately 5-10 percent of penicillin allergic persons will have a cross-sensitivity to cephalosporin drugs as well. Penicillins also have gastrointestinal side effects, and the addition of clavulanic acid significantly increases the incidence of diarrhea.

Pharmacology of Antibacterial Agents

Objectives

1. Describe the factors in choosing appropriate antibiotic agents.
2. List the classes of antibiotics, and describe their mechanisms of action, therapeutic uses, and adverse effects.
3. Outline mechanism of development of bacterial drug resistance.

Definitions

Chemotherapy: Therapeutic use of chemical agents that selectively act on microbes and cancer.

Plasmids: Extrachromosomal genetic elements that may be transferred between bacteria.

Discussion of Class

The basic principles for the selection of **antibacterial therapy**⑥ include consideration of factors such as the **likelihood that the infection is bacterial**⑦ and the identification of the **likely infecting organism**⑧ to support a rational selection of an antibiotic. Consideration of host and drug factors that could influence antibiotic selection include identification of the site of infection, which will influence the selection of the antibiotic and its route of administration; recognition of concomitant diseases such as AIDS; recognition of the likelihood of drug allergies; recognition of hepatic or renal dysfunction that could alter antibiotic clearance; and recognition of drug toxicity, drug-drug interactions, drug resistance, the patient's age or pregnancy or maternal status; and drug cost.

Antibacterial agents, which target specific components of microorganisms that are unique or more essential to their function than they are to humans, are classified according to their mechanisms of action. The component targets include **enzymes necessary for bacterial cell-wall synthesis, the bacterial ribosome, and enzymes necessary for nucleotide synthesis and deoxyribonucleic acid (DNA) replication**⑨.

Resistance of pathogens to antibacterial and other chemotherapeutic agents may be the result of a natural resistance or may be acquired. In either case, it occurs through mutation, adaptation, or gene transfer. The mechanism of resistance for any antibacterial agent varies, but is a result of either changes in uptake of drug into, or its removal from, the bacterial cell, or to changes in the bacterial cell target site of the drug from a gene mutation. **Multiple drug resistance**⑩ is also a major impediment to antibacterial therapy and may be **chromosomal or plasmid mediated**⑪ where genetic elements from resistant bacteria that code for enzymes that inactivate antibacterial agents are transferred to nonresistant bacteria. The emergence of drug resistance is to a large degree the result of the widespread and often unnecessary or inappropriate use of antibiotics in humans.

The **penicillins**⑫ (see above) include natural penicillins, penicillins that are resistant to staphylococcal β-lactamase, and extended-spectrum penicillins (Table 45-1).

The **cephalosporins**⑬ are classified as first to fourth generation, according to their antibacterial spectrum (Table 45-2).

Table 45-1

PARTIAL LISTING OF PENICILLINS

Natural Penicillin G (prototype) Penicillin V	*Extended-Spectrum* Aminopenicillins Ampicillin Amoxicillin Ureidopenicillins Mezlocillin Piperacillin Carboxypenicillin Ticarcillin
β-lactamase Resistant Nafcillin Oxacillin Cloxacillin Dicloxacillin	

Table 45-2

SELECTED LISTING OF CEPHALOSPORINS

REPRESENTATIVE CEPHALOSPORINS (route)	NOTES
First generation • Cefazolin (IV) • Cephalexin (PO) • Cefadroxil (PO)	Active against Gram-positive cocci, including staphylococci, pneumococci, and streptococci. They are particularly good for soft tissue and skin infection.
Second generation • Cefuroxime (PO) oral form is cefuroxime axetil • Cefotoxin (IV) • Cefotetan (IV)	These agents have marked differences in their spectrum of activity. In general, they are active against certain aerobic Gram-negative bacteria in addition to activity against many Gram-positive organisms sensitive to first-generation cephalosporins. Certain agents are active against *Haemophilus influenza* (e.g., cefuroxime), whereas others are active against *Bacteroides fragilis* (e.g., cefotoxin).
Third generation • Cefotaxime (IV) • Ceftazidime (IV) • Ceftriaxone (IV)	Expanded aerobic Gram-negative spectrum. Cross the blood-brain barrier. Useful to treat bacterial strains resistant to other drugs.
Fourth generation • Cefepime (IV)	Generally similar activity to third-generation cephalosporins but more resistance to β-lactamases.

Aztreonam[14], which is relatively β-lactamase resistant, is the only available monobactam. It is nonallergenic and is active only against aerobic gramnegative bacilli (e. g., pseudomonas, serratia). Table 45-3 lists selected agents. The **carbapenems**[15] (imipenem, meropenem, and ertapenem), which are resistant to most β-lactamases, have a wide spectrum of activity against Grampositive and Gram-negative rods and anaerobes. To **prevent its metabolism to a nephrotoxic metabolite**[16], **imipenem**[17] is administered with an **inhibitor of renal tubule dehydropeptidase**[18], **cilastatin**[19].

Vancomycin[20], which is unaffected by β-lactamases, **inhibits bacterial cellwall synthesis**[21] by covalent binding to the terminal two D-alanine residues of nascent peptidoglycan pentapeptide to prevent their elongation and crosslinking, thus increasing the susceptibility of the cell to lysis. It is **active against Gram-positive bacteria**[22].

Table 45-3

PARTIAL LISTING OF ANTIMICROBIAL AGENTS

ANTIBACTERIAL AGENTS	MECHANISM OF ACTION	ADVERSE EFFECTS
β-lactam antibiotics Penicillins Cephalosporins Monobactams • aztreonam(p) *Carbapenems* • imipenem(p) • meropenem(p) • ertapenem(p) *Vancomycin*(o,p)	Inhibit synthesis of the bacterial cell wall.	*β-lactam antibiotics*: hypersensitivity with rare potential for anaphylactic shock. *Cephalosporins*: may cause local irritation and pain from IM injection. Those with a methylthiotetrazole group, e. g., cefotetan, may cause hypoprothrombinemia and bleeding disorders. *Aztreonam*: occasionally may cause skin rashes. *Carbapenems*: may cause GI discomfort and skin rashes and seizures in patients with renal dysfunction (particularly imipenem). *Vancomycin*: relatively nontoxic. Fever, chills, and infusion-related flushing ("red-neck" syndrome) are encountered. Ototoxicity is a rare effect.

续表

ANTIBACTERIAL AGENTS	MECHANISM OF ACTION	ADVERSE EFFECTS
Chloramphenicol *Tetracyclines* • tetracycline(o,p) • oxytetracycline(o,p) • doxycycline(o,p) • methacycline(o) • minocycline(o,p) *Macrolides* • erythromycin(o,p) • clarithromycin(o) • azithromycin(o) *Ketolides* • telithromycin(o) *Oxazolidinones* • linezolid(o,p) *Aminoglycosides* *Spectinomycin(p)* *Lincomycins* • clindamycin(o,p)	Bind to bacterial ribosomes to inhibit protein synthesis.	*Chloramphenicol*: GI disturbances, reversible suppression of bone marrow, rarely aplastic anemia. *Tetracyclines*: GI disturbances and bacterial overgrowth, teeth and bone deformation in children. *Erythromycin and clarithromycin*: severe GI disturbances, hypersensitivity, hepatic P_{450} inhibition. *Telithromycin*: hepatic P_{450} inhibition. *Linezolid*: reversible thrombocytopenia. *Aminoglycosides*: ototoxicity and nephrotoxicity. *Clindamycin*: GI disturbances, hepatic dysfunction, potentiallyfatal colitis.
Sulfonamides • sulfadiazine(o) • sulfamethizole(o) • sulfamethoxazole(o) • sulfanilamide(t) • sulfisoxazole(t,o) *Trimethoprim*	*Sulfonamides*: Structural analogs of p-aminobenzoic acid that inhibit bacterial dihydropteroate synthase to block folic acid synthesis and cell growth. *Trimethoprim*: selectively inhibits dihydrofolic acid reductase to block folic acid synthesis and cell growth. Acts synergistically with sulfamethoxazole with which it is often coadministered.	*Sulfonamides*: hypersensitivity urinary tract dysfunction, hemolytic or aplastic anemia, potentially fatal Stevens-Johnson syndrome. *Trimethoprim*: blood dyscrasias.

续表

ANTIBACTERIAL AGENTS	MECHANISM OF ACTION	ADVERSE EFFECTS
Fluoroquinolones (selected) • ciprofloxacin(t,o,p) • levofloxacin(t,o,p) • ofloxacin(t,o,p) • gatifloxacin(o,p) • moxifloxacin(o,p)	Inhibit activity of bacterial topoisomerase (DNA gyrase) that is necessary for replication.	GI disturbances, reversible arthropathy, arrhythmias.

t = topical, o = oral, p = parenteral

Comprehension Questions

[45.1] Which of the following is the most likely explanation for multiple drug resistance to antibiotics that has increased from one type of bacteria to other types?

A. Adaptation
B. Decreased bioavailability
C. Gene transfer
D. Mutation

[45.2] Penicillins

A. Bind to bacterial ribosomes to inhibit protein synthesis
B. Inhibit activity of bacterial topoisomerase
C. Inhibit bacterial dihydropteroate synthase
D. Inhibit synthesis of the bacterial cell wall

[45.3] Ototoxicity and nephrotoxicity are characteristic adverse effects of

A. Aminoglycosides
B. β-lactam antibiotics
C. Chloramphenicol
D. Fluoroquinolones

Answers

[45.1] **C.** Antibiotic drug resistance can occur through bacterial cell mutation, adaptation, or gene transfer. The best route for multiple drug resistance that spreads from one type of bacteria to another is via plasmid or chromosomal gene transfer.

[45.2] **D.** Penicillins inhibit synthesis of the bacterial cell wall. Chloramphenicol, tetracyclines, macrolides, ketolides, oxazolidinones, aminoglycosides, spectinomycin, and the lincomycin bind to bacterial ribosomes to inhibit protein synthesis. The fluoroquinolones inhibit activity of bacterial topoisomerase to inhibit protein synthesis, and the sulfonamides inhibit bacterial dihydropteroate synthase to block folic acid synthesis and cell growth.

[45.3] **A.** Ototoxicity and nephrotoxicity are characteristic adverse effects of aminoglycosides. Chloramphenicol can cause gastrointestinal (GI) disturbances, reversible suppression of bone marrow, and rarely aplastic anemia. As a group, the β-lactam antibiotics can cause hypersensitivity and have the potential to cause anaphylactic shock. The fluoroquinolones can cause GI disturbances, reversible arthropathy, and arrhythmias.

PHARMACOLOGY PEARLS

- ❖ β-lactam antibiotics inactivate bacterial transpeptidases and prevent the cross-linking of peptidoglycan polymers essential for cellwall integrity.
- ❖ Both penicillin and amoxicillin are susceptible to β-lactamases.
- ❖ To prevent its metabolism to a nephrotoxic metabolite, imipenem is administered with an inhibitor of renal tubule dehydropeptidase, cilastatin.
- ❖ Vancomycin, which is unaffected by β-lactamases, is active against Gram-positive bacteria.
- ❖ Chloramphenicol can cause GI disturbances, reversible suppression of bone marrow, and rarely aplastic anemia.
- ❖ Aminoglycosides may cause ototoxicity or nephrotoxicity and should be used with caution in those patients who have renal insufficiency or who are elderly.

REFERENCES

Gale EF, Cundliffe E, Reynolds PE, et al. The molecular basis of antibiotic action, 2nd ed. London: Wiley, 1981.

Levy SB. The challenge of antimicrobial resistance. Sci Am 1998; 278(3): 46-53. Wright AJ. The penicillins. Mayo Clin Proc 1999; 74(3): 290-307.

词汇

1. β-lactam antibiotics inactivate bacterial transpeptidase[β-内酰胺抗生素抑制细菌转肽酶]
2. peptidoglycan[多糖肽]
3. cell wall integrity[细胞壁组成成分]
4. bactericidal [杀菌剂]
5. both penicillin and amoxicillin are susecptible to β-lactamaes[青霉素和阿莫西林均对β-内酰胺酶敏感]
6. antibacterial therapy[抗菌治疗]
7. likelihood that the infection is bacterial[感染可能是由细菌引起的]
8. likely infecting organism[可能感染的器官]
9. deoxyribonucleic acid(DNA) replication. [脱

氧核糖核酸复制]

10. multiple drug resistance[多重耐药]
11. chromosomal or plasmid mediated[染色体或质粒介导的]
12. penicillins[青霉素类]
13. cephalosporins[头孢菌素类]
14. aztreconam[氨曲南]
15. carbapenems [碳青霉烯类]
16. nephrotoxic metabolite[肾毒性代谢产物]
17. imipenem[亚胺培南]
18. inhibitor of renal tubule dehydropeptidase [肾小管脱氢肽酶的抑制剂]
19. cilastatin [西司他丁]
20. vancomycin[万古霉素]
21. inhibits bacterial cell-wall synthesis[抑制细菌胞壁的合成]
22. active against gram-positive bacteria[作用于革兰阳性菌]

注 1

肺炎的常见症状有：咳嗽，发热，且体温较高，X 线检查有阴影是一支持点，血培养和痰培养可确定了病原体。白细胞计数有助于诊断。对于肺炎的治疗原则是找出致病的微生物，从根本上消除病原体，需用抗菌药物，由于是肺炎链球菌感染，需选择对肺炎链球菌敏感的药物。同时根据病人情况进行对症治疗，该病人有咳嗽，且有痰，可用化痰止咳药，同时有发热，可用降低体温的药物。

注 2

阿莫西林是广谱抗生素，它可以抑制细菌转肽酶使细菌细胞壁的多糖肽不能形成，导致细胞壁的破裂，从而杀灭细菌，对革兰阴性和革兰阳性菌均有杀菌作用。阿莫西林主要用于由肺炎链球菌、嗜血流感杆菌和化脓性链球菌引起的呼吸道感染；也用于由大肠埃希菌和肠球菌引起的尿道感染，大剂量阿莫西林对沙门菌引起的伤寒、副伤寒用有效。本类药物耐酸，可口服。阿莫西林口服后约三小时达血药高峰浓度。1/3 的药物被吸收，当机体出现炎症时，在中耳炎渗出液、脑脊液、关节腔、支气管分泌液和腹水均有较高浓度，主要经肾排出。克拉维酸本身只有微弱的抗菌活性，但具有强大的广谱 β-内酰胺酶抑制作用，两者合用，可保护阿莫西林免遭细菌 β-内酰胺酶水解而增强阿莫西林的抗菌活性。

点评

肺炎是指肺实质的炎质，按病因可分为细菌性、霉菌性、病毒性和支原体性肺炎。临床上最常见的是细菌性肺炎，其中约 90%~ 95% 是由肺炎链球菌引起。临床有突发的寒战、高热、咳嗽、血痰、胸痛等症状。肺炎属于急性感染性疾病，其治疗的根本是进行抗感染。用阿莫西林与克拉维酸药物联合治疗是针对有产生 β-内酰胺酶的肺炎链球菌感染。近年由于抗菌药物的广泛使用，肺炎链球菌有较高的产酶（β-内酰胺酶）率，因此选用的抗菌药物需选择有抑制 β-内酰胺酶作用的药物。阿莫西林和克拉维酸的复方制剂的抗菌谱与阿莫西林相同，且有所扩大，同时对肺炎链球菌感染的肺炎有效。还可进一步作细菌的药敏试验，但细菌药敏试验要约一周才有结果，所以首先选用阿莫西林与克拉维酸的复方制剂是正确的，阿莫西林与克拉维酸的复方制剂可以口服，但口服的剂量有限，在比较严重的情况下可选用静脉给药，根据目前病人的情况用静脉给药有利于迅速控制感染症状，如用此药效果不佳，可根据药敏试验结果改用敏感的抗菌药物。目前临床上可供选择的抗菌药物较多。

周黎明

❖ CASE 46

A 58-year-old man presents for the evaluation of a painful rash. He says that for 3 or 4 days he had a sharp, burning pain radiating from his midback around to his left side. He thought that he was having a kidney stone. Yesterday he noticed a rash which spread in a distribution "like a line" in the same area in which he has had the pain. He is on glyburide for type II diabetes, simvastatin for high cholesterol, and lisinopril for hypertension, all of which he has been on for several years. He does have a history of having chickenpox as a child. On examination he has a low-grade fever and otherwise normal vital signs. His skin exam is remarkable for a rash in a beltlike distribution from his spine around his left flank to the midline of the abdomen. [注1] The rash consists of erythematous patches with clusters of vesicles. The remainder of his examination is normal. You make the diagnosis of herpes zoster and prescribe a course of acyclovir. [注2]

◆ **What is the mechanism of action of acyclovir?**

◆ **How is acyclovir eliminated from the body?**

ANSWERS TO CASE 46: Antiviral Agents

Summary: A 58-year-old man with herpes zoster is prescribed acyclovir.

- **Mechanism of action of acyclovir**: Purine analog that is converted to a nucleoside triphosphate that competes with the natural triphosphate substrate to inhibit the activity of viral deoxyribonucleic acid (DNA) polymerase. It is also incorporated into the growing viral DNA where it acts as a chain terminator.

- **Elimination of acyclovir**: Excreted unmetabolized via the kidney through glomerular and tubular filtration.

CLINICAL CORRELATION

Herpes zoster, also known as shingles, is caused by a reactivation of dormant varicella zoster virus. It causes a rash and frequently a painful neuropathy, usually in the distribution of a single dermatome. Acyclovir can shorten the course of symptoms of herpes zoster, although it cannot eradicate latent virus. Acyclovir is a purine analog that requires viral thymidine kinase to be converted to a monophosphate form, thus assuring that it accumulates selectively in infected cells. Host cellular enzymes then convert the monophosphate to a triphosphate form that competitively inhibits the activity of viral DNA polymerase. The triphosphate form also is incorporated into viral DNA, where it acts as a chain terminator. Acyclovir has a low oral bioavailability. It is excreted, largely unchanged, via the kidney. Valacyclovir is a prodrug form of acyclovir that has a greater oral bioavailability than acyclovir. It is rapidly and completely converted to acyclovir after absorption, resulting in higher concentrations of acyclovir.

Pharmacology of Antiviral Drugs

Objectives

1. List the specific drug classes and drugs used to treat viral disease.
2. Describe the mechanisms of action and adverse effects of antiviral drugs used to treat infections by herpes simplex virus (HSV), varicella zoster virus (VZV), and cytomegalovirus (CMV).

Discussion of Class

Viral Biology

Viruses are obligate intracellular parasites that do not have their own metabolic machinery but rather use the host's own metabolic capabilities to replicate. Antiviral medications usually attack the virus prior to cell penetration, after the virus leaves the host cell, or while the virus is active within the host cell. Nonspecific effects may be harmful to the host. Figure 46-1 shows a schematic of the viral life cycle summarized, and Table 46-1 describes specific antiviral therapies aimed at the various viral maturation steps.

There are three main types of viruses: (1) **DNA viruses** usually enter the host cell nucleus and direct the production of new viruses, (2) **RNA viruses** direct the production of new viruses, usually without entering the host cell nucleus (an exception is influenza), and (3) ribonucleic acid (**RNA**) **retro-viruses**, such as human immunodeficiency virus (HIV). Retroviruses contain an enzyme, reverse transcriptase, that makes a DNA copy of the viral RNA; the DNA copy is spliced into the host DNA and directs the production of the new viruses.

Overview of Antiviral Agents

The **three major classes of antiviral agents** are (1) **DNA polymerase inhibitors**, (2) **reverse transcriptase inhibitors**, and (3) **protease inhibitors**. It should be noted that HIV treatment usually includes the use of at least two reverse transcriptase inhibitors and one protease inhibitors. DNA polymerase inhibitors are categorized as nucleoside or nonnucleoside. Drugs may target viral nucleic acid replication such as DNA polymerase either via nucleoside (purine or pyrimidine analogs) such as acyclovir or ribavirin, or by attacking a unique viral process needed in nucleic acid synthesis such as viral pyrophosphate (nonnucleoside type).

Antiviral drugs used to treat HSV, VZV, and CMV can be classified as either nucleoside or nonnucleoside, or according to their site of action in the viral replicative cycle or according to their clinical use (see Table 46-1).

Common Antiviral Agents

Influenza. **Amantadine and rimantadine**① are primarily used against infections caused by **influenza A**. Their mechanism of action is interfering with **viral uncoating**. Both agents are fairly well absorbed orally and cause some minor central nervous system (CNS) effects (rimantadine less so) and minor gastrointestinal (GI) effects.

Herpes Virus

Acyclovir② is used against **herpes simplex virus** 1 **and 2.**③ Acyclovir, a **nucleoside DNA polymerase inhibitor**, is a deoxyguanosine triphosphate (**dGTP**) **analog** that is incorporated into the viral DNA and causes DNA chain termination. Its specificity is a result of the presence of **herpes-specific thymidine kinase**④ in infected cells, which phosphorylates acyclovir a hundred-fold more efficiently than by uninfected cells. The acyclovir triphosphate is formed in infected cells and incorporated into infected cells'DNA, and not formed in normal cells. Acyclovir can be used topically, orally for recurrent genital herpes, and intravenously for immunocompromised patients or herpes encephalitis.

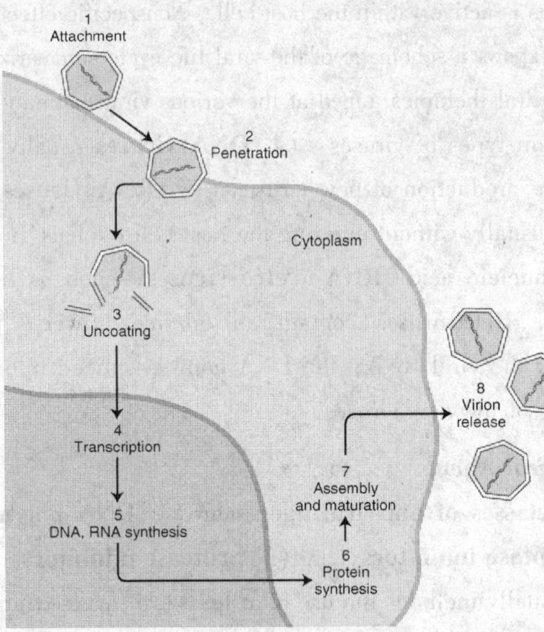

Figure 46-1. Life cycle of the virus.

Table 46-1
EXAMPLES OF ANTI-VIRAL MECHANISMS

	VIRAL LIFE CYCLE	ANTIVIRAL THERAPY	EXAMPLES
1.	Virus attaches to the cell	Gamma-globulin(binds to virus)	Hepatitis A and B
2.	Virus penetrates the cell	Gamma-globulin	
3.	Virus uncoats its nucleic acid	Amandatine	Influenza A
4a.	Synthesis of key viral enzymes such as polymerases(transcription)	Acyclovir, Ribavirin (DNA polymerase inhibitor)	Herpes simplex
4b.	Viral nucleic acid is synthesized	Zidovudine(reverse transcriptase inhibitor)	HIV
5.	Late viral structural proteins are synthesized	Indinavir(protease inhibitor)	HIV
6.	Viral proteins and particles are assembled		
7.	Viruses are released from the host cell		

Its adverse effects include headache, nausea, and rarely nephrotoxicity with IV use. **Valacyclovir**⑤ is an analog of acyclovir and is converted to acyclovir in the body. Its advantage is better bioavailability.

Penciclovir⑥ is converted to the triphosphate form and inhibits viral DNA polymerase. **Famciclovir**⑦ is converted to the active agent penciclovir in the body. Their main use is to treat **localized herpes zoster in immunocompromised**⑧ **patients**. Headache and GI effects are common. **Ganciclovir**⑨ is structurally similar to acyclovir and must be converted to the triphosphate form to be active; it competes with dGTP for incorporation into viral DNA thereby inhibiting DNA polymerase. Its primary role is against **cytomegalovirus**⑩, and is **far more effective**⑪ **than acyclovir against CMV**. Ganciclovir can induce serious **myelosuppression**⑫.

Foscarnet⑬ is a **synthetic nonnucleoside analog of pyrophosphate**⑭, and inhibits DNA polymerase or HIV reverse transcriptase by directly binding to the pyrophosphate binding site. Its use is usually for **acyclovir-resistant herpes or CMV retinitis**⑮. Significant nephrotoxicity may occur with its use.

Sorivudine⑯ is a **primidone nucleoside analog**⑰, and on being converted to the triphosphate form, it is active against herpes DNA synthesis. It is effective against **varicella zoster**⑱ and is usually well tolerated.

Idoxuridine⑲ is an **iodinated thymidine analog** that **inhibits herpes DNA synthesis**. It is used primarily topically for **herpes keratitis**⑳. Adverse effects include pain and inflammation. **Vidarabine**㉑ is an **adenosine analog**㉒ that also needs to be in its triphosphate form and blocks **herpes specific DNA polymerase**㉓. It has been used for **herpes encephalitis or zoster**㉔ **in immunocompromised individuals**, but because of its **nephrotoxicity**㉕, it has largely been supplanted by acyclovir.

Trifluridine㉖ is a **fluorinated pyrimidine nucleoside analog**㉗. Its monophosphate form inhibits thymidylate synthetase, and its triphosphate form inhibits DNA polymerase. It is active against herpes 1 and 2 and CMV, and it is used primarily against keratoconjunctivitis and recurrent keratitis.

Anti-HIV Agents

Retrovir㉘ (azidothymidine [AZT] or zidovudine [ZDV]) inhibits viral reverse transcriptase when its triphosphate form is incorporated into the nucleic acid and **blocks further DNA chain elongation**, leading to **termination of the DNA**. Also, the monophosphate form of retrovir may block deoxythymidine kinase and inhibit the production of normal dTTp. Its principal use is treating HIV infection; adverse effects include headache, **bone marrow suppression**, fever, and abdominal pain.

Didanosine㉙ is also a **nucleoside reverse transcriptase inhibitor**, primarily used as an **adjunct to retrovir**, or for those HIV patients with intolerant or unresponsive to zidovudine. **Peripheral neuropathy and pancreatic damage**[30] may be seen. **Stavudine**[31] is a thymidine nucleoside analog which inhibits HIV-1 replication. It is used in HIV patients unresponsive to other therapies.

Protease Inhibitors

Invirase or saquinavir[32] blocks HIV protease activity, rendering the virus unable to generate essential proteins and enzymes including reverse transcriptase. It is used in combination with a conventional reverse transcriptase inhibitor.

Structure

Valacyclovir (VCV), famciclovir (FCV), and valganciclovir: Ester prodrugs of, respectively, acyclovir (ACV), penciclovir (PCV), and ganciclovir (GCV).

Cidofovir (CDV): Phosphonate analog of cytidine.

Idoxuridine (IDU): Analog of thymidine.

Table 46-2

PARTIAL LISTING OF ANTIVIRAL AGENTS AND MECHANISMS OF ACTION

Nucleosides that inhibit RNA or DNA genomic replication: acyclovir (ACV), cidofovir (CDV), famciclovir (FCV), ganciclovir (GCV)/valganciclovir, penciclovir (PCV), idoxuridine (IDU), trifluridine, valacyclovir (VCV)
Nonnucleosides that inhibit RNA or DNA genomic replication: foscarnet
Nonnucleosides that inhibit transcription: interferons
Nonnucleosides that inhibit translation: fomivirsen
Nonnucleosides that inhibit uncoating: amantadine, rimantadine
Nonnucleosides that inhibit release and budding: zanamivir, oseltamivir
Other Viral Infections
Hepatitis B and C: lamivudine, adefovir, interferon alfa, and ribavirin
Influenza: amantadine and rimantadine (nonnucleosides that inhibit uncoating), zanamivir and oseltamivir (nonnucleosides that inhibit release and budding).
HIV-1: nucleoside reverse transcriptase inhibitors (NRTIs; abacavir, didanosine, lamivudine, stavudine, zalcitabine, zidovudine)
Nucleotide inhibitors (tenofovir)
Nonnucleoside reverse transcriptase inhibitors (NNRTIs; delavirdine, efavirenz, nevirapine)
Protease inhibitors (amprenavir, indinavir, nelfinavir, ritonavir, saquinavir)
Fusion inhibitors (enfuviritide)

Table 46-3

AGENTS USED TO TREAT HSV, VZV, AND CMV

(ROUTE OF ADMINISTRATION)

AGENTS	VIRAL INFECTIONS	ADVERSE EFFECTS
Acyclovir(t,o,p)	HSV, VSV	Nausea, vomiting, diarrhea, headache; parenteral administration may cause reversible neuropathy and nephropathy
Cidofovir CDV(p)	VZV, CMV	Nephrotoxicity
Famciclovir FCV(o)	HSV, VSV	Nausea, vomiting, diarrhea, headache, confusion in elderly
Ganciclovir GCV (intraocular implant, o,p)	CMV	Generally reversible myelosuppression with neutropenia and thrombocytopenia
Penciclovir PCV(t)	HSV, VSV	Well tolerated
Idoxuridine IDU(o)	HSV	Edema and burning and stinging of the eye
Valacyclovir VCV(o)	HSV, VSV	Nausea, vomiting, diarrhea, headache
Trifluridine(t)	HSV	Edema and burning and stinging of the eye
Foscarnet(p)	HSV, CMV	Reversible nephrotoxicity, hypo-or hypercalcemia and phosphatemia that may lead to neural and cardiac dysfunction; hallucinations, genital ulceration, and anemia are not uncommon
Fomivirsen(p)	CMV	Iritis, vitreitis, increased ocular pressure

t = topical, o = oral, p = parenteral

Mechanism of Action

VCV, GCV, and valganciclovir act like ACV.

IDU and FCV and the prodrug FCV, which is converted to the active agent PCV, also act like ACV except that they do not cause DNA chain termination.

Trifluridine(activated by host cell phosphorylation) and foscarnet(acts directly to inhibit viral DNA polymerase and RNA polymerase) do not require activation by viral thymidine kinase for their activity and therefore can be used to treat acyclovir-resistant viral infections.

CDV is phosphorylated to mono- and diphosphate nucleotides by cellular kinases and, therefore, accumulates in both infected and uninfected cells. As a diphosphate, CDV inhibits and serves as an alternative dCTP substrate for viral DNA polymerase, resulting in inhibition of viral DNA synthesis and termination of chain elongation.

Fomivirsen is an antisense oligonucleotide that binds to the major immediate early region 2(IE2) of CMV mRNA to prevent its translation to protein and therefore to block viral replication.

Administration

Acyclovir(ACV): Administered intravenously and orally and is used as a topical agent.

Foscarnet: Reserved to treat acyclovir-resistant viral infections and can only be administered intravenously.

Valacyclovir(VCV), famciclovir(FCV): Available only for oral use.

Ganciclovir(GCV): Administered orally; parenterally(IV); and as an intraocular, slow-release implant.

Penciclovir(PCV), trifluridine, idoxuridine(IDU): Available only for topical use.

Cidofovir: Administered parenterally with probenecid to block its active tubular secretion.

Fomivirsen: Administered by intravitreal injection.

Pharmacokinetics

Acyclovir(ACV): Low oral bioavailability.

Valacyclovir(VCV): An ester prodrug with greater oral bioavailability than acyclovir that is rapidly and completely converted to ACV after absorption.

Famciclovir(FCV), valganciclovir: Ester prodrugs that are rapidly converted by first-pass metabolism to their respective active agents, penciclovir(PCV) and ganciclovir(GCV).

Comprehension Questions

[46.1] Which of the following drugs is most likely to cause myelosuppression?

A. Famciclovir(FCV)   B. Fomivirsen

C. Ganciclovir(GCV)   D. Penciclovir(PCV)

[46.2] Which of the following drugs is a prodrug that after oral administration is converted to an active agent, penciclovir(PCV)?

A. Acyclovir(ACV)   B. Famciclovir(FCV)

C. Fomivirsen   D. Ganciclovir(GCV)

[46.3] The high levels of acyclovir(ACV) obtained in target viruses such as HSV is a result of its

A. Binding to the major immediate early region 2(IE_2) of CMV mRNA
B. Direct inhibition of viral DNA polymerase and RNA polymerase
C. Host cell enzyme conversion to triphosphate compounds
D. Monophosphorylation by viral thymidine kinase

Answers

[46.1] **C.** Ganciclovir can cause a generally reversible myelosuppression. Famciclovir can cause nausea, vomiting, diarrhea, and headache. Penciclovir is generally well tolerated. Fomivirsen causes ocular problems, including iritis, vitreitis, and increased ocular pressure.

[46.2] **B.** Famciclovir(FCV) is a diacetyl ester prodrug that after oral administration is converted to penciclovir(PCV) by first-pass metabolism. Fomivirsen is administered by intravitreal injection. Acyclovir(ACV) and ganciclovir(GCV) act directly and can be administered orally and parenterally. ACV can also be administered topically. GCV can also be administered as an intraocular implant.

[46.3] **A.** The high levels of acyclovir(ACV) obtained in target viruses such as HSV result from its monophosphorylation by viral thymidine kinase. Antiviral drugs that are activated only by host cell kinases, for example, cidofovir(CDV), will accumulate in host cells with or without viral infection. Fomivirsen is an antisense oligonucleotide that binds to the major immediate early region 2(IE_2) of CMV mRNA to prevent its translation to protein and therefore to block viral replication. Foscarnet acts directly to inhibit viral DNA polymerase and RNA polymerase.

PHARMACOLOGY PEARLS

- The primary strategy of antiviral agents is to attack a unique but vital viral enzyme or process.
- The three major types of antiviral agents include DNA polymerase inhibitors, reverse transcriptase inhibitors, and protease inhibitors.
- HIV therapy generally usually uses at least two reverse transcriptase inhibitors and one protease inhibitor.
- Didanosine is also a nucleoside reverse transcriptase inhibitor for HIV infections and is associated with peripheral neuropathy and pancreatic damage.
- Foscarnet is a synthetic nonnucleoside analog of pyrophosphate and is associated with reversible nephrotoxicity, and hypo-or hyper-calcemia and phosphatemia that may lead to neural and cardiac dysfunction. Also, hallucinations, genital ulceration, and anemia may occur.

REFERENCES

Balfour HJ. Antiviral drugs. N Engl J Med 1999; 340(16): 1255-68.

De Clercq E. Antiviral drugs: current state of the art. J Clin Virol 2001; 22(1): 73-89.

Drugs for non-HIV viral infections. Med Lett Drugs Ther 2002; 44(1123): 9-16.

词汇

1. amantadine and rimantadine[金刚烷胺和金刚乙胺]
2. acyclovir[阿昔洛韦]
3. herpes simplex virus 1 and 2[Ⅰ型和Ⅱ型疱疹病毒]
4. herpes-specific thymidine kinase[疱疹胸苷激酶]
5. valacyclovir[伐昔洛韦]
6. penciclovir[喷昔洛韦]
7. famciclovir[法昔洛韦]
8. immunocompromised[免疫缺陷的]
9. ganciclovir[更昔洛韦]
10. cytomegalovirus[巨细胞病毒]
11. effective[有效的]
12. myelosuppression[骨髓抑制]
13. foscarnet[磷甲酸钠]
14. synthetic nonnucleoside analog of pyrophosphate[合成焦磷酸酶的非核酸同系物]
15. retinitis[视网膜炎]
16. sorivudine[索利夫定]
17. primidone nucleoside analog[朴米酮核酸同系物]
18. varicella zoster[水痘带状疱疹]
19. idoxuridine[碘苷]
20. herpes keratitis[疱疹角膜炎]
21. vidarabine[阿糖腺苷]
22. adenosine analog[腺苷同系物]
23. herpes specific DNA polyherase[疱疹 DNA 多聚酶]
24. herpes encephalitis or zoster[单纯疱疹性脑炎和带状疱疹]
25. nephrotoxicity[肾毒性]
26. trifluridine[曲氟尿苷]
27. fluorinated pyrimidine nucleoside analog[氟嘧啶核苷同系物]
28. retrovir[齐夫拉定]
29. didanosine[去羟肌苷]
30. peripheral neuropathy and pancreatic damage[外周神经和胰腺的损害]
31. stavudine[司他夫定]
32. invirase or saquinavir[沙奎拉韦]

注 1

带状疱疹是由于人体感染了水痘带状疱疹病毒后而引起的一种病毒性皮肤病。病人有病损部位的发痒，疼痛和红肿热痛的炎症反应，治疗原则是对因治疗和对症治疗，对因治疗选择抗病毒药物，对症治疗可止痒，消炎止痛。

注 2

阿昔洛韦为广谱抗病毒药，体外对单纯性疱疹病毒、水痘带状疱疹病毒、巨细胞病毒等具抑制作用。药物进入疱疹病毒感染的细胞后，与脱氧核苷竞争病毒胸苷激酶或细胞激酶，药物被磷酸化成活化型阿昔洛韦三磷酸酯，然后通过二种方式抑制病毒复制：①干扰病毒DNA多聚酶，抑制病毒的复制；②在DNA多聚酶作用下，与增长的DNA链结合，引起DNA链的延伸中断。与其他抗病毒药无交叉耐药性，对病毒有特殊的亲和力，但对哺乳动物宿主细胞毒性低。阿昔洛韦能在短期内控制症状。阿昔洛韦口服生物利用度低，通常以原型通过肾脏排出体外。

点评

带状疱疹是由水豆带桩疱疹病毒所引起的急性疱疹性皮肤病。其特点是急性的粟粒至绿豆大小的丘疱疹，迅速变为水疱。皮疹形态为集簇性水疱，沿受累的周围神经带状排列，伴局部淋巴结肿痛。此病毒一般潜伏在脊髓后根神经元中。当机体抵抗力低下或劳累、感染、患肿瘤时，病毒可再次生长繁殖，并沿神经纤维移至皮肤，使受侵犯的神经和皮肤产生激烈的炎症。该患者的典型临床表现和患过水痘的历史表明其诊断无疑，治疗原则：①抗病毒治疗：阿昔洛韦是一种嘧啶类似物，阻滞病毒DNA的合成。阿昔洛韦能在短期内控制症状，尽管它不能去除潜在的病毒。阿昔洛韦口服生物利用度低，通常以原型通过肾脏排出体外。②消炎止痛：可口服消炎镇痛药，如布洛芬(芬必得)300mg口服，每日两次，可缓解部分疼痛症状，但须注意饭后服用或同时服用胃粘膜保护剂，因此类消炎止痛药有导致胃粘膜损害的副作用。③对症治疗：早期红斑水疱，可外用收敛性的药物如炉甘石洗剂，炉甘石洗剂的作用是止痒以减少病人的主观瘙痒症状；若有糜烂、坏死时，为防止皮肤的细菌感染可以0.1%利凡诺尔液作湿敷，外用抗生素软膏。

周黎明

❖ CASE 47

A 4-year-old boy is brought in by his mother because he keeps scratching a spot on his arm. His mother says that this has been going on for several days, and it appears that the spot is growing larger. No one else at home has anything similar. He has not had a fever or any systemic signs of illness. There have been no recent exposures to new foods, medications, lotions, or soaps. He attends preschool during the day. On examination of his skin you see a circular, nickel-sized ring on his right forearm. It has a red, raised border and central clearing. The remainder of his skin exam and his general physical examination are normal. You diagnose him with tinea corporis (ringworm)[注1] and prescribe topical nystatin.[注2]

◆ **What is the mechanism of action of nystatin?**

◆ **Nystatin is similar in structure and function to which other antifungal medication?**

ANSWERS TO CASE 47: Antifungal and Antiparasitic Drugs

Summary: A 4-year-old boy with tinea corporis is prescribed topical nystatin.

- **Mechanism of action of nystatin**: Creates pores in fungal membranes by binding ergosterol.
- **Nystatin is similar in structure and action to**: Amphotericin B.

CLINICAL CORRELATION

Superficial fungal infections of the skin are very common, particularly in the pediatric population. There are many topical preparations available that are effective against this problem. Nystatin is a polyene antifungal agent with similarities in structure and function to the systemic antifungal agent amphotericin B. Nystatin, which is too toxic for parenteral use, is administered topically for skin infections. It is not absorbed through the gastrointestinal (GI) tract, therefore, oral preparations are used only to treat fungal infections of the mucous membranes of the mouth or intestinal tract. Amphotericin B is given intravenously and is only used for severe, systemic fungal infections. It has significant toxicities and adverse effects. It frequently causes fever, chills, and impaired renal function. Less often it will cause anaphylactic reactions, pain, thrombocytopenia, and seizures.

Pharmacology of Antifungal and Antiparasitic Drugs

Objectives

1. List the antifungal drugs and describe their mechanisms of action, therapeutic uses, routes of administration, and adverse effects.

Discussion of Class

In addition to the pyrimidine analog, flucytosine, and the penicillium-derived antifungal agent, griseofulvin, the three major classes of antifungal agents are the polyene macrolides, azoles, and allylamines (Table 47-1).

Of all the available antifungal agents, **amphotericin B**[①] has the **broadest spectrum of activity**[②], including **activity against yeast, mycoses, and molds**[③]. It is the **drug of choice for disseminated or invasive fungal infections**[④] **in immunocompromised** patients. The **major adverse effect**[⑤] resulting from amphotericin B administration is the almost invariable **renal toxicity**[⑥] that results from decreased renal blood flow and from tubular and basement membrane destruction that may be irreversible and may require dialysis. Other adverse effects of amphotericin B relate to its intravenous infusion and include fever, chills, vomiting, hypotension, and headache, which can be ameliorated somewhat by careful monitoring and slow infusion.

The **azole antifungal agents**[7] have a **broad spectrum of activity**, including activity against **candidiasis, mycoses, and dermatophytes**[8], among many others.

Table 47-1

SELECTED ANTIFUNGAL DRUGS(ROUTE)

Polyene Macrolides	*Allylamines*
Nystatin(t,o for GI tract)	Naftifine(t)
Natamycin(t)	Terbinafine(o,t)
Amphotericin B(t,o for GI tract,p)	
Azoles	*Other Antifungal Agents*
Miconazole(t)	Flucytosine(o)
Ketoconazole(t,o)	Griseofulvin(o)
Clotrimazole(t)	
Itraconazole(o,p)	
Fluconazole(o,p)	
Voriconazole(o,p)	

t = topical, o = oral, p = parenteral

As topical agents the azoles are relatively safe. Administered orally their **most common adverse effect is GI dysfunction**[9]. Hepatic dysfunction may rarely occur. Oral azoles are **contraindicated for use with midazolam and triazolam**[10] as a consequence of potentiation of their **hypnotic and sedative effects**[11], and with 3-hydroxy-3-methylglutaryl-coenzyme A (**HMG-CoA**) **reductase inhibitors**[12] because of an **increased risk of rhabdomyolysis**[13]. **Itraconazole**[14] has been associated with **heart failure when used to treat onychomycosis**[15] and therefore **should not be used in patients with ventricular abnormalities**[16]. Monitoring patients who receive itraconazole for potential **hepatic toxicity**[17] is also highly recommended. **Voriconazole**[18] frequently causes an **acute blurring of vision**[19] with changes in color perception that resolves quickly.

The **allylamine antifungal agents**, **naftifine and terbinafine**[20], are used **topically** to treat dermatophytes. Contact with mucous membranes may lead to local irritation and erythema and should be avoided. **Terbinafine** administered orally is effective against the **onychomycosis**[21]. **Monitoring for potential hepatic toxicity**[22] **is highly recommended**.

Flucytosine[23] is active against only a **relatively restricted range of fungal infections**[24]. Because of rapid development of resistance, it is used concomitantly for its synergistic effects with other antifungal agents. The most commonly reported adverse effect is

bone marrow suppression[25], probably as a result of the **toxicity of the metabolite fluorouracil**[26], which should be continuously monitored. Other reported but less common adverse effects include reversible hepatotoxicity, enterocolitis, and hair loss.

Griseofulvin[27], the use of which is declining relative to terbinafine and itraconazole, is an effective antifungal agent that is used only **systemically**[28] to treat a very **limited range of dermatophyte infections**[29]. The most common adverse effects include **hypersensitivity**[30] (fever, skin rash, serum sickness-like syndrome) and **headache**[31]. It is **teratogenic**.

Structure

Depending on whether there are two or three nitrogen atoms in the azole ring, azole antifungal agents are subclassified, respectively, as either imidazoles (ketoconazole, clotrimazole, miconazole) or triazoles (itraconazole, fluconazole, voriconazole).

Mechanism of Action

Nystatin and amphotericin B bind to ergosterol, a major component of **fungal cell membranes**. This disrupts the stability of the cell by forming pores in the cell membrane that result in leakage of intracellular constituents. Bacteria are not susceptible to this because they lack ergosterol.

Azoles (imidazoles less so) have a greater affinity for fungal than human cytochrome P_{450} enzymes and therefore more effectively reduce the synthesis of fungal cell ergosterol than human cell cholesterol.

The allylamine antifungal agents, naftifine and terbinafine, decrease ergosterol synthesis and increase fungal membrane disruption by inhibiting the enzyme squalene epoxidase.

Flucytosine must first be transported into fungal cells via a cytosine permease and converted to 5-fluorouracil (5-FU) and then sequentially converted to 5-fluorodeoxyuridylic acid, which disrupts DNA synthesis by inhibiting thymidylate synthetase. Human cells are unable to synthesize the active flucytosine metabolites.

The mechanism of antifungal action of griseofulvin is not clearly known. It acts only on growing skin cells and has been reported to inhibit cell-wall synthesis, interfere with nucleic acid synthesis, and disrupt microtubule function, among other activities.

Administration

Amphotericin B is insoluble in water and, therefore, is generally administered as a colloidal suspension with sodium deoxycholate. Because of its poor absorption from the GI tract, amphotericin B must be given intravenously to treat systemic disease, although it is effective orally for fungal infections within the GI lumen. Likewise, nystatin is poorly absorbed but may also be used for fungal infection of the GI tract. It is too toxic for systemic use and therefore is mostly used topically to treat fungal infections of the skin and mucous membranes (e. g. , oropharyngeal thrush, vaginal candidiasis). Costly lipid formulations of amphotericin B are available for intravenous use, which reduce its nonspecific binding to cholesterol of human cell membranes and therefore lessens its potential to cause renal damage.

Griseofulvin is administered in a microparticulate form to improve absorption.

Pharmacokinetics

Amphotericin B and nystatin are poorly absorbed from the GI tract. The absorption of the azole antifungal agent, itraconazole, is reduced by antacids that block acid secretion. Through its actions on hepatic microsomal enzymes, itraconazole interacts significantly with numerous other drugs (eg. , the rifamycins, phenytoin, carbamazepine, digoxin, cyclosporine).

Comprehension Questions

[47. 1] Which of the following antifungal agents binds to ergosterol?

A. Amphotericin B B. Fluconazole
C. Flucytosine D. Terbinafine

[47. 2] Bone marrow suppression is a common adverse effect of

A. Fluconazole B. Flucytosine
C. Griseofulvin D. Terbinafine

[47. 3] Which of the following is the drug of choice for disseminated or invasive fungal infections in immunocompromised patients?

A. Amphotericin B B. Flucytosine
C. Griseofulvin D. Terbinafine

Answers

[47. 1] **A.** Amphotericin B, like nystatin, binds to ergosterol to create pores in fungal membranes. Flucytosine must first be transported into fungal cells via a cytosine permease and converted to 5-FU and then sequentially converted to 5-fluorodeoxyuridylic acid, which disrupts DNA synthesis by inhibiting thymidylate synthetase. Fluconazole binds fungal cell cytochrome P_{450} enzymes to reduce the synthesis of ergosterol. Terbinafine decrease ergosterol synthesis by inhibiting the enzyme squalene epoxidase.

[47. 2] **B.** Bone marrow suppression is a common adverse effect of flucytosine. A common adverse effect of griseofulvin is hypersensitivity (fever, skin rash, serum sickness like syndrome). Terbinafine may cause hepatic toxicity. Fluconazole causes GI dysfunction.

[47.3] **A**. Amphotericin B is the drug of choice for at least the initial treatment of disseminated or invasive fungal infections in immunocompromised patients.

PHARMACOLOGY PEARLS

❖ Itraconazole has been associated with heart failure when used to treat onychomycosis and therefore should not be used in patients with ventricular abnormalities.

❖ A common side effect of griseofulvin is hypersensitivity.

❖ Because of renal toxicity, amphotericin B is often used to initiate a clinical response before substituting a continuing maintenance dose of an azole.

REFERENCES

Groll AH, Gea-Banacloche JC, Glasmacher A, et al. Clinical pharmacology of antifungal compounds. Infection Dis Clin North Am 2003; 17(1): 159-91.

Stevens DA, Bennett JE. Antifungal agents. In: Mandell GL, Bennett JE, Dolin R, eds. Principles and practices of infectious diseases, 5th ed. New York: Churchill Livingston, 2000: 448.

词汇

1. amphotericin B[两性霉素 B]
2. broadest spectrum of activity[广谱活性]
3. activity against yeast, mycoses, and molds [抗酵母菌、真菌和霉菌]
4. invasive fungal infections[侵袭性真菌感染]
5. major adverse effect[主要的副作用]
6. renal toxicity[肾毒性]
7. azole antifungal agents[唑类抗真菌药]
8. candidiasis, mycoses, and dermatophytes[念珠菌病、真菌病、皮肤真菌]
9. GI dysfunction[胃肠道功能障碍]
10. midazolam and triazolam[咪唑类和三唑类]
11. hypnotic and sedative effects[镇静催眠作用]
12. HMG-CoA reductase inhibitors[三羟-三-甲戊二酰基辅酶还原酶抑制剂]
13. increased risk of rhabdomyolysis[增加横纹肌溶解的危险性]
14. itraconazole[伊曲康唑]
15. heart failure when used to treat onychomycosis[治疗甲癣时出现心衰]
16. ventricular abnormalities[室性异常]
17. hepatic toxicity[肝毒性]
18. voriconazole[伏立康唑]
19. acute blurring of vision[急性视力模糊]
20. allylamine antifungal agents, naftifine and terbinafine[丙稀胺类抗真菌药、奈替芬和特比萘芬]
21. onychomycosis[甲癣]
22. potential hepatic toxicity[潜在的肝脏毒性]
23. flucytosine[氟胞嘧啶]
24. relatively restricted range of fungal infections [相对控制真菌感染的范围较窄(窄谱抗

真菌)]
25. bone marrow suppression[骨髓抑制]
26. toxicity of the metabolite fluorouracil[氟尿嘧啶代谢的毒性]
27. griseofulvin[灰黄霉素]
28. systemically[系统地]
29. limited range of dermatophyte infections[限制用于皮肤感染的范围]
30. hypersensitivity[高敏性]
31. headache[头痛]

注 1

体癣：皮肤上的浅表性皮肤真菌感染。好发于颜面，颈，腰，腹，躯干及四肢等处，原发损害丘疹或小水疱，慢慢向周围扩展，中心炎症减轻伴脱屑或色素沉着，边缘微高出皮面，由丘疹或水疱连接融合在一起而呈环状。

注 2

制霉菌素是一抗真菌药，用于真菌感染的治疗，由于全身用药毒性大，仅局部用药。其结构与两性霉素相似，其作用机制相同，对多种真菌有强大抑制作用，高浓度有杀菌作用。它能选择性地与真菌细胞膜的麦角固醇相结合形成膜孔，从而增加细胞膜的通透性，导致细胞内小分子物质如电解质、氨基酸等外漏而致死。同时对哺乳动物的细胞膜类固醇也起作用，故对人体细胞毒性较大，细菌的细胞膜不含固醇类物质，故制霉菌素对细菌无效，选择性的作用于真菌。若全身用药尤其是作用于人肾小管细胞和红细胞膜上的类固醇，易引起肾损伤和红细胞膜损伤，造成严重的副作用，临床上原则上仅局部使用。

点评

体癣是由真菌引起的，凡致病性真菌寄生在人体的光滑皮肤上所引起的浅表损害统称为体癣。有经验的医生常常不用做真菌检查，即可诊断癣病，这是因为癣病的发生和皮损表现具备以下几方面共同点：①体癣常常由自身接种传染而引起，也就是说先发生手癣、脚癣、股癣、甲癣或头癣，然后由这些癣病再传染到皮肤上来，单独的体癣较少见。另外，癣病的发生与机体抵抗力强弱有关。当患有糖尿病或其他全身性疾病以及长期大量应用激素、免疫抑制剂等都会使机体免疫力下降，这时即使真菌数量很少也能引起体癣。②皮损特点：体癣初起表现为局部皮肤发生红斑、丘疹或水疱等损害。皮损周边部位炎症明显，常有活动性红斑、丘疹及水疱。制霉菌素是多烯类抗真菌药，具广谱抗真菌作用，对念珠菌属的抗菌活性高，新型隐球菌、曲菌、毛霉菌、小孢子菌、荚膜组织浆胞菌、皮炎芽生菌及皮肤癣菌通常对本品亦敏感。本品可与真菌细胞膜上的麦角固醇相结合，致细胞膜通透性的改变，以致重要细胞内容物漏失而发挥抗真菌作用。体癣或股癣在原则上以外用药治疗为宜。制霉菌素主要局部外用治疗皮肤、粘膜浅表真菌感染。口服吸收很少，注射给药毒性大，局部应用不良反应少。若皮肤出现水疱，可外用收敛性的药物如炉甘石洗剂；炉甘石洗剂的作用是止痒以减少病人的主观瘙痒症状。

周黎明

❖ CASE 48

A 66-year-old man presents for evaluation of skin growths on his face. For several years he has had scaly, rough growths on his face, forehead, and scalp. He has had individual lesions frozen off by previous physicians, but he keeps getting more and more. He has never been diagnosed with skin cancer. He has a long history of sun exposure and multiple sunburns, primarily as a consequence of working outdoors and playing golf. He takes an aspirin[注1] a day and pravastatin① for high cholesterol. He has no other significant medical history. On examination of his skin you note multiple 4-7 mm lesions on the face and scalp that are flat, pink, and scaly. They feel rough on palpation. They are all in areas that would be sun exposed. He has several on the dorsal surfaces of his hands and forearms. You diagnose him as having multiple actinic keratoses②.[注2] Along with recommending skin protection from the sun, you prescribe topical 5-fluorouracil(5-FU)③.

- **What is the mechanism of action of 5-FU?**

- **What are the adverse effects of 5-FU when given systemically?**

ANSWERS TO CASE 48: Alkylating and Antimetabolite Agents

Summary: A 66-year-old man with multiple actinic keratoses is prescribed 5-FU.

- **Mechanism of action of 5-FU**: Pyrimidine antagonist that, after a complex conversion to 5-fluoro-2′-deoxyuridine-5′-monophosphate (FdUMP), covalently inhibits thymidylate synthetase④ and thus impairs DNA synthesis.
- **Adverse effects of systemic 5-FU**: Myelosuppression⑤, nausea⑥, vomiting⑦, and hair loss.

CLINICAL CORRELATION

Actinic keratoses are premalignant skin lesions that frequently occur as a result of excessive sun exposure. Untreated, actinic keratoses may progress to become squamous cell carcinomas of the skin. Persons with multiple lesions are often treated with topical 5-FU. Systemic 5-FU is given parenterally primarily for the treatment of certain solid tumors. Systemic 5-FU is myelosuppressive and causes frequent gastrointestinal (GI) disturbances⑧ and hair loss. Topical 5-FU does not have the systemic side effects but can cause significant local redness, itching⑨, and burning of the skin.

Pharmacology of Alkylating and Antimetabolite Agents

Objectives

1. Outline the principles of cancer chemotherapy and the development of resistance to chemotherapeutic agents.
2. List the antimetabolite and alkylating chemotherapeutic agents and describe their mechanisms of action, therapeutic uses, and adverse effects.

Discussion of Class

Appropriate **cancer chemotherapy** demands a thorough understanding of the kinetics of **tumor cell growth**, including its **control and regulation**, a thorough understanding of the **pharmacological properties of available anticancer agents**, and an appreciation of the interactions between them.

Combination chemotherapy⑩ early in therapy increases the likelihood of destroying drug-resistant populations of cells that are refractory to treatment and therefore is **generally more effective than monotherapy**. To be most effective, the drugs used in combination chemotherapy should each have **therapeutic activity with different dose-limiting toxicities** and should be **administered during several cycles** of treatment **to allow recovery from acute adverse effects**.

The drugs used to treat cancer are **classified** as **alkylating agents**⑪, **anti-metabolites**⑫, **cytotoxic antibiotics**⑬, **plant alkaloids**⑭, **hormonal agents**⑮, **and miscellaneous agents**⑯ (Table 48-1). Depending on the tumor type, they are often used in combinations or as adjunct therapy to surgical and radiation procedures.

Table 48-1

SELECTED ANTICANCER DRUGS

SELECTED ANTICANCER DRUGS	TOXICITY—ACUTE & DELAYED	SELECTED INDICATIONS
Alkylating agents Cyclophosphamide Melphalan Chlorambucil Busulfan	Nausea and vomiting, GI ulceration, alopecia⑰, myelosuppression bone marrow depression (thrombocytopenia⑱, leucopenia⑲) with bleeding	*Cyclophosphamide*: Acute lymphocytic leukemia⑳, non-Hodgkin's lymphomas㉑ *Melphalan*: Multiple myeloma㉒ *Busulfan*: Chronic myelogenous leukemia㉓ *Chlorambucil*: Chronic lymphocytic leukemia
Antimetabolites Methotrexate Fluorouracil Mercaptopurine	*Methotrexate*: Diarrhea㉔, mucositis㉕, myelosuppression *Fluorouracil*: Nausea, vomiting, diarrhea, myelosuppression, neurotoxicity, head and foot syndrome *Mercaptopurine*: myelosuppression, hepatotoxicity㉖	*Methotrexate*: Acute lymphocytic leukemia *Fluorouracil*: Colorectal cancer, solid tumors of the breast, pancreas, liver, etc. *Mercaptorpurine*: Acute lymphocytic leukemia

Primary resistance㉗ to anticancer drugs is thought to occur because of some **inherent genetic characteristics of tumor cells. Acquired resistance**㉘ of tumor cells to a specific anticancer drug may occur via several different mechanisms that usually involve either **amplification or overexpression of one or more genes**. For example, resistance to methotrexate㉙ is caused by either decreased drug transport into tumor cells, a modification of the target enzyme dihydrofolate reductase (DHFR)㉚ that results in a decreased affinity for methotrexate, or an increased level of DHFR in tumor cells. Resistance to the chemotherapeutic effects of alkylating agents may develop because of decreased cell permeability, increased cell thiol content that serves as a "decoy" target for alkylation, increased activity of glutathione transferases[31], and modification of deoxyribonucleic acid (DNA) repair mechanisms. Alternatively, after exposure of a tumor cell to a number of structurally different agents, a so-called multidrug, or pleiotropic, resistance may develop to chemotherapeutic agents because of decreased uptake or retention of the drugs. This is a result of either increased expression of the constitutively expressed multidrug resistance gene (MDR-1)[32], which codes for a surface cell membrane P-glycoprotein involved in drug efflux, or by overproduction of one of a number of other multidrug resistance proteins, for example, MRP-1, that are involved in the transmembrane export of drugs. Multidrug resistance is the major form of resistance to vinca alkaloids, etoposide, paclitaxel, anthracyclines, and dactinomycin.

Other Anticancer Classes of Drugs

Cytotoxic antibiotics: Dactinomycin (actinomycin D), bleomycin, doxorubicin.

Plant alkaloids: Vinblastine, vincristine, vinorelbine, etoposide, paclitaxel, topotecan.

Hormonal agents: Steroid hormones: Megestrol acetate, hydrocortisone, prednisone.

Antiandrogens: Flutamide.

Antiestrogens: Tamoxifen.

Gonadotropic releasing hormone (GRH) agonists[33]: Goserelin acetate, leuprolide.

Aromatase inhibitors[34]: Aminoglutethimide, anastrozole, exemestane, letrozole.

Miscellaneous agents: Cisplatin, imatinib, hydroxyurea, mitotane, arsenic trioxide, procarbazine.

Mechanism of Action

Alkylating Agents

The cytotoxic effects of alkylating agents result from the transfer of their alkyl groups to numerous cellular components, most notably the bases of DNA, particularly the N7 position of guanine, which in replicating cells (G1 and S phase) results in either miscoding or strand breakage.

Antimetabolites

Methotrexate (MTX): Folic acid antagonist that binds the catalytic site of DHFR to reduce the synthesis of tetrahydrofolate that results in downstream reduction of thymidylate and an indirect inhibition of DNA synthesis as well as ribonucleic acid (RNA) and protein synthesis.

Fluorouracil (5-FU): A prodrug that is converted to FdUMP by a multistep process. FdUMP covalently forms an inhibitory ternary complex with the enzyme thymidylate synthetase and reduced folate $N^{5,10}$-methylene tetrahydrofolate, which are essential to the synthesis of thymidylate and the production of DNA. Through other metabolic conversions, 5-FU is also incorporated into DNA as 5-fluorodeoxyuridine-5′-triphosphate (FdUTP) and into RNA as 5-fluorouridine-5′-triphosphate (FUTP), which result in further inhibition of DNA function as well as inhibition of RNA processing and mRNA activity.

Mercaptopurine (6-MP)㉟: The precise mechanism of action of mercaptopurine, a modified purine, is unknown. Like the natural purines, hypoxanthine and guanine, it is converted to a nucleotide by hypoxanthine guanine phosphoribosyltransferase (HGPRT). The product, in this case 6-thioinosinic acid, inhibits purine nucleotide interconversion.

Pharmacokinetics

Cyclophosphamide㊱ is not itself cytotoxic but must first be converted by hepatic microsomal enzymes to form the cytotoxic agents phosphoramide mustard and acrolein.

Comprehension Questions

[48.1] Resistance to methotrexate is a result of

A. Increased activity of glutathione transferases

B. Increased cell thiol content

C. Modification of DNA repair mechanisms

D. Modification of the target enzyme dihydrofolate reductase (DHFR)

[48.2] Which of the following agents forms an inhibitory ternary complex with the enzyme thymidylate synthetase?

A. Cyclophosphamide B. Fluorouracil (5-FU)

C. Mercaptopurine (6-MP) D. Methotrexate (MTX)

[48.3] In general, combination cancer chemotherapy

A. Is administered during several cycles of treatment

B. Is less effective than monotherapy

C. Includes at least two drugs with similar dose-limiting toxicities

D. Includes one drug that has no inherent therapeutic activity

Answers

[48.1] **D.** Resistance to methotrexate may be a result of a modification of the target enzyme dihydrofolate reductase (DHFR). It may also be a consequence of decreased drug transport into tumor cells or an increased level of DHFR in tumor cells. Resistance to the chemotherapeutic effects of alkylating agents may develop because of decreased cell permeability; increased cell thiol content, which serves as a "decoy" target for alkylation; increased activity of glutathione transferases; and modification of DNA repair mechanisms.

[48.2] **B.** Fluorouracil(5-FU) is a prodrug that is converted to FdUMP, which covalently forms an inhibitory ternary complex with the enzyme thymidylate synthetase and reduced folate $N^{5,10}$-methylene tetrahydrofolate, both of which are essential to the synthesis of thymidylate and the production of DNA. Mercaptopurine(6-MP) is thought to inhibit purine nucleotide interconversion. Methotrexate(MTX) is a folic acid antagonist that binds the catalytic site of dihydrofolate reductase(DHFR) to reduce the synthesis of tetrahydrofolate that results in downstream reduction of thymidylate and an indirect inhibition of DNA synthesis as well as RNA and protein synthesis. The cytotoxic effects of alkylating agents like cyclophosphamide are a result of the transfer of their alkyl groups to numerous cellular components, most notably the bases of DNA that in replicating cells(G_1 and S phase) results in either miscoding or strand breakage.

[48.3] **A.** Combination chemotherapy early in therapy increases the likelihood of destroying drug-resistant populations of cells that are refractory to treatment and therefore is generally more effective than monotherapy. To be most effective, the drugs used in combination chemotherapy should each have therapeutic activity with different dose-limiting toxicities and should be administered during several cycles of treatment to allow recovery from acute adverse effect.

PHARMACOLOGY PEARLS

❖ Smaller tumors are generally more responsive to chemotherapy than larger tumors because of the increased probability of drug-resistant mutations in the larger tumors.

❖ Development of a mild leukopenia is evidence of the adequate absorption of orally administered alkylating agents.

❖ Leucovorin[37] (citrovorum factor), a folic acid analog that does not require reduction by dihydrofolate reductase, can be used to "rescue" patients from MTX overdose or high-dose MTX therapy.

REFERENCES

Chabner BA, Longo DL. Cancer chemotherapy and biotherapy, 3rd ed. Philadelphia: Lippincott Williams and Wilkins, 2001.

DeVita VT Jr, Hellman S, Rosenberg SA. Cancer: principles and practices of oncology, 5th ed. Philadelphia: Lippincott Williams and Wilkins, 1997.

Perry MD. The chemotherapy source book, 3rd ed. Baltimore: Lippincott Williams and Wilkins, 2001.

词汇

1. pravastatin[普伐他汀]
2. multiple actinic keratosis[多发性光化性角化病]
3. 5-fluorouracil(5-FU)[氟尿嘧啶]
4. thymidylate synthetase[胸苷酸合成酶]
5. myelosuppression[骨髓抑制]
6. nausea[恶心]
7. vomiting[呕吐]
8. gastrointestinal disturbances[胃肠道紊乱]
9. itching[搔痒]
10. combination chemotherapy[联合化疗]
11. alkylating agent[烷化剂]
12. antimetabolite[抗代谢物]
13. cytotoxic antibiotic[细胞毒性抗生素]
14. plant alkaloids[植物碱类]
15. hormonal agents[激素类药物]
16. miscellaneous agents[杂类药物]
17. alopecia[脱发]
18. thrombocytopenia[血小板减少(症)]
19. leucopenia[白细胞减少(症)]
20. acute lymphocytic leukemia[急性淋巴细胞白血病]
21. non-Hodgkin's lymphomas[非霍奇金淋巴瘤]
22. multiple myeloma[多发性骨髓瘤]
23. chronic myelogenous leukemia[慢性髓细胞性白血病]
24. diarrhea[腹泻]
25. mucositis[黏膜炎]
26. hepatotoxicity[肝毒性]
27. Primary resistance[原发性耐药性]
28. acquired resistance[获得性耐药性]
29. methotrexate[甲氨蝶呤]
30. dihydrofolate reductase(DHFR)[二氢叶酸还原酶]
31. glutathione transferase[谷胱甘肽转移酶]
32. multidrug resistance gene(MDR-1)[多药耐药性基因]
33. gonadotropic releasing hormone(GRH) agonists[促性腺激素释放激素激动剂]
34. aromatase inhibitors [芳香化酶抑制剂]
35. mercaptopurine(6-MP)[巯嘌呤]
36. cyclophosphamide[环磷酰胺]
37. leucovorin[甲酰四氢叶酸]

注 1

阿司匹林，又称乙酰水杨酸是最为常用的水杨酸类非甾体抗炎药(NSAIDs)。主要用于解热镇痛，抗炎，抗风湿，抗血栓形成。普伐他汀，是一种具有亲水性的竞争性 3-羟-3-甲-戊二酰辅酶 A(HMG CoA)还原酶抑制剂，能高度选择性地抑制肝脏内源性胆固醇的合成，降低血浆总胆固醇(TC)和低密度脂蛋白-胆固醇(LDL-C)水平，也能降低甘油三酯(TG)和增加高密度脂蛋白(HDL)水平。

注 2

光化性角化病主要因过度光照所致，避免光照对于治疗至关重要。局部应用5-FU是治疗光化性角化病的标准药物疗法，对于能耐受者有效率高达90%以上。

点评

本病例是典型的光化性角化病。患者是老年男性，有长期阳光暴晒史，病变部位都位于面部、前额、头皮、手背和前臂背面等暴露部位，病灶大小为4～7mm，呈多发性，且为扁平，粉红色，鳞状，触感粗糙，这些都是光化性角化病的典型症状。多发性病变可用5-FU局部给药来治疗，可以避免全身给药引起的骨髓抑制、胃肠功能失调、脱发等不良反应，但也会有局部红肿、发痒、皮肤灼伤等副作用。5-FU是一种化疗药物，由于耐药性问题，可以考虑采用0.5% 5-FU(研究表明0.5% 5-FU较5% 5-FU对病变部位的靶向性更强,且耐受性更好,两者疗效相似)，也可采用新型氟尿嘧啶微海绵给药制剂(耐受性较传统制剂更好)。光化性角化病可以发展为鳞状细胞癌，其发生率约为0.25%～1%。因为癌前病变与癌变两者的界限不易确定，且鳞癌的早期发现对治疗有重要意义，建议做病理鉴别诊断。

邵碧云　陈红专

❖ CASE 49

A 60-year-old woman presents to her oncologist for follow-up of her metastatic ovarian cancer. She was diagnosed approximately a year ago. Initial treatment included surgery and a cisplatin-based chemotherapy regimen. [注1] Unfortunately, she was recently diagnosed with recurrent disease. She currently takes only promethazine as needed for nausea and a combination of hydrocodone and acetaminophen as needed for pain. On examination she appears comfortable. She has a thin growth of hair on her scalp. Her abdomen has a well-healed surgical scar but is otherwise unremarkable. The remainder of her examination is normal. She is diagnosed with recurrent metastatic ovarian cancer[①] and placed on a chemotherapeutic regimen that includes paclitaxel. [注2]

◆ **What is the mechanism of action of paclitaxel?**

◆ **What are the common adverse reactions seen with paclitaxel?**

ANSWERS TO CASE 49: Plant Anticancer Alkaloids

Summary: A 60-year-old woman with recurrent metastatic ovarian cancer is being treated with combination chemotherapy including paclitaxel.

- **Mechanism of action of paclitaxel**: Promotes formation and inhibits disassembly of stable microtubules[2], resulting in inhibition of mitosis.
- **Adverse effects of paclitaxel**: Myelosuppression, peripheral neuropathy, gastrointestinal side effects.

CLINICAL CORRELATION

Paclitaxel is a chemical derived from bark of the Pacific yew tree. Its chemotherapeutic effect is based on its ability to inhibit mitosis. Its mechanism of action is to promote the formation of and inhibit the disassembly of stable microtubules in the M phase of cell division. Paclitaxel is used for the treatment of metastatic ovarian, breast, and small cell lung cancers. It is metabolized in the liver and excreted in the bile. Myelosuppression and peripheral neuropathy are often dose-limiting toxicities, and gastrointestinal (GI) side effects and hair loss are common.

Pharmacology of Plant Anticancer Alkaloids

Objectives

1. List the plant alkaloids used as cancer chemotherapeutic agents and describe their mechanisms of action, therapeutic uses, and adverse effects.

Definitions

Microtubules: Structures composed of tubulin polymers that are critical components of the cell cytoskeleton and the mitotic spindle.

Topoisomerases[3] (I and II): Nuclear enzymes that cleave and unwind deoxyribonucleic acid (DNA) to relieve torsional stress. They are necessary for DNA replication and ribonucleic acid (RNA) transcription. Topoisomerase II is also necessary for mitosis.

Discussion of Class

Table 49-1 describes selected anticancer drugs. See also Case 48.

Structure

Vinblastine and vincristine are derived from the periwinkle plant (*Vinca rosea*). Vinorelbine is a semisynthetic vinca alkaloid.

Table 49-1

SELECTED ANTICANCER DRUGS

(MAY BE COMBINED WITH OTHER ANTICANCER AGENTS)

AGENT	SELECTED INDICATIONS	SELECTED TOXICITY (ACUTE AND DELAYED)
Vinblastine	Non-Hodgkin's lymphomas[4], Hodgkin's disease[5], breast cancer	Nausea and vomiting, myelosuppression, neurotoxicity, alopecia
Vincristine	Acute lymphocytic leukemia[6], non-Hodgkin's lymphomas, Hodgkin's disease, multiple myeloma[7]	Neurotoxicity is dose-limiting. GI dysfunction, myelosuppression, muscular-skeletal disorders, aberrant antidiuretic hormone secretion(SIADH)
Vinorelbine	Non-small cell lung cancer, breast cancer	Myelosuppression is dose-limiting. Nausea and vomiting, GI dysfunction, neurotoxicity, SIADH
Paclitaxel	Breast cancer and a wide variety of other solid tumors	Myelosuppression is dose-limiting. Nausea and vomiting, hypotension, arrhythmias, neurotoxicity
Etoposide	Testicular and ovarian germ cell cancers, lung cancers, acute lymphoblastic leukemia	Myelosuppression is dose-limiting. Nausea and vomiting, mucositis, hypotension

Paclitaxel is a complex diterpene derived from the Western and European yew (*Taxus brevifolia and Taxus baccata*).

Etoposide is a semisynthetic podophyllotoxin, an extract from the Mandrake root (*Mandragora officinarum*) or May apple root (*Podophyllum peltatum*).

Mechanism of Action

Vinca alkaloids[8] (vinblastine, vincristine, vinorelbine): Bind tubulin to terminate microtubule assembly and cause cell arrest in metaphase (M) by blocking mitosis and chromosomal aggregation and causing mitotic spindle dissolution.

Taxanes[9] (paclitaxel)[10]: Bind to microtubules resulting in their stabilization and in an enhancement of aberrant tubulin polymerization that result in cytotoxicity, including mitotic arrest.

Epipodophyllotoxins[11] (etoposide): Reversibly complex with the enzyme topoisomerase II that results in double-stranded DNA strand breakage.

Administration

Hypersensitivity to paclitaxel can be reduced by premedication with dexamethasone[12] and histamine H_1- and H_2-receptor blockers[13].

Pharmacokinetics

Vinca alkaloid hepatic metabolism is decreased by L-asparaginase[14].

Paclitaxel is metabolized extensively by hepatic P450 enzymes[15] (CYP450 3A4) with potential, therefore, of drug-drug interactions[16]. Dose reduction is necessary for patients with liver dysfunction.

Etoposide is 95 percent plasma protein bound. Dose reduction is necessary for patients with renal dysfunction.

Comprehension Questions

[49.1] Which of the following classes of cancer chemotherapeutic agents binds tubulin and causes arrest of cells in metaphase?

A. Alkylating agents
B. Antimetabolites
C. Taxanes
D. Vinca alkaloids

[49.2] Premedication with dexamethasone, and histamine H_1-and H_2-receptor blockers, is often used to reduce hypersensitivity to which of the following drugs?

A. Etoposide
B. Paclitaxel
C. Vinblastine
D. Vincristine

[49.3] Neurotoxicity is dose-limiting for which of the following drugs?

A. Etoposide
B. Methotrexate
C. Paclitaxel
D. Vincristine

Answers

[49.1] **D.** Vinca alkaloids (vinblastine, vincristine, vinorelbine) bind tubulin to terminate microtubule assembly and cause cell arrest in metaphase (M) by blocking mitosis and chromosomal aggregation and causing mitotic spindle dissolution. Alkylating agents form covalent bonds with adjacent guanine residues and inhibit DNA replication and transcription. Antimetabolites compete with naturally occurring compounds for binding sites on enzymes or else become incorporated into DNA or RNA to interfere with cell growth and division. Taxanes (paclitaxel) binds to microtubules resulting in their stabilization and in an enhancement of aberrant tubulin polymerization that result in cytotoxicity, including mitotic arrest.

[49.2] **B**. Hypersensitivity to paclitaxel can be reduced by premedication with dexamethasone, and histamine H_1- and H_2-receptor blockers.

[49.3] **D**. Neurotoxicity is dose-limiting for vincristine. Myelosuppression is dose-limiting for paclitaxel, etoposide, and methotrexate.

PHARMACOLOGY PEARLS

❖ The plant anticancer alkaloids act on the microtubules, during the mitosis (M) phase of the cell cycle.

❖ The vinca alkaloids cause sensory and motor toxicities with the following order of activity: vincristine is greater than vinblastine is greater than vinorelbine.

❖ Neurotoxicity is dose-limiting for vincristine, whereas myelosuppression is dose-limiting for paclitaxel, etoposide, and methotrexate.

REFERENCE

Abal M, Andreu JM, Barasoain I. Taxanes: microtubules and centrosome targets, and cell cycle dependent mechanism of action. Curr Cancer Drug Targets 2003; 3(3): 193-203.

词汇

1. recurrent metastatic ovarian cancer[复发性转移性卵巢癌]
2. microtubule[微管]
3. topoisomerase[拓扑异构酶]
4. non-Hodgkin's lymphoma[非霍奇金淋巴瘤]
5. Hodgkin's disease[霍奇金病]
6. acute lymphocytic leukemia[急性淋巴细胞白血病]
7. multiple myeloma[多发性骨髓瘤]
8. vinca alkaloids[长春碱类]
9. taxanes[紫杉烷类]
10. paclitaxel[紫杉醇]
11. epipodophyllotoxins[鬼臼毒素类]
12. dexamethasone[地塞米松]
13. histamine H_1-and H_2-receptor blockers[组胺 H_1 和 H_2 受体阻断剂]
14. L-asparaginase[天冬酰胺酶]
15. hepatic P450 enzymes(CYP450 3A4)[肝细胞色素 P450 酶]
16. drug-drug interaction[药物相互作用]

注 1

目前，卵巢癌以手术加术后顺铂联合化疗为主要治疗方式。

注 2

① 转移性卵巢癌复发率很高。

② 转移性卵巢癌复发的诊断依据不够充分，只有临床症状，并没有生化和影像指标的证实。

点评

本病例有明确的卵巢癌病史，且为转移性，复发的可能性很高。卵巢癌的临床分期与生存率密切相关，组织学类别和病理分级与预后有直接关系，癌细胞的分化程度和生物学特性也与预后相关，这些都应于诊断时明确，以利于治疗方案的选择。目前，对复发性卵巢癌的诊断方法敏感性和特异性不高，常用血清 CA125 的检测。一般认为血清 CA125 水平增高（>100U/ml或成倍增加），临床检查或影像学检查发现可测量的病灶和/或出现腹水等症状时，可考虑复发；如果检测结果不明确，临床高度怀疑有复发的病例，还需进一步做 MRI 或 PET/CT 等以明确诊断。本例患者只有恶心、疼痛、脱发等症状，并没有腹水及其他指标的异常，诊断为复发，依据不够充分，应做进一步检测。一旦确诊，可考虑采用铂剂和紫杉醇联合化疗，因为患者是顺铂化疗后一年复发，属于铂敏感型（研究表明，对铂剂敏感的复发性卵巢癌再用铂剂治疗的有效率可高达 50%~60%）。由于患者年龄大，卵巢癌又为转移性，故不考虑采用再减瘤手术，而只进行化疗。

邵碧云　陈红专

❖ CASE 50

A 62-year-old woman presents for the evaluation of a breast lump. She noticed the lump in her left breast about 3 months ago but didn't come in because she "hates doctors." She denies pain, nipple discharge, or weight loss. Her last mammogram was 3 years ago. She stopped having menstrual periods at the age of 50. She is on no medications and has no significant medical history. On examination she is anxious, but her general examination is normal. Breast examination reveals a hard, 2 cm mass in the upper, outer quadrant of her left breast and several small lymph nodes in the left axilla.[注1] A fine needle aspiration of the mass confirms the diagnosis of breast carcinoma.[①] Further workup does not reveal distant metastases. She subsequently undergoes a modified radical mastectomy and lymph node dissection. Pathology studies of the tumor reveal it to be estrogen-receptor positive, and she has microscopic metastases in the lymph nodes. She is started on tamoxifen[②].[注2]

◆ **What is the mechanism of action of tamoxifen?**

◆ **What are the side effects commonly associated with tamoxifen?**

ANSWERS TO CASE 50: Steroid Hormones and Antagonists

Summary: A 62-year-old woman with estrogen receptor positive breast cancer is begun on tamoxifen therapy.

- **Mechanism of action of tamoxifen**: Competitive inhibitor of estrogen receptors.
- **Common adverse effects**: Nausea, vomiting, hot flashes.

CLINICAL CORRELATION

Tamoxifen is a competitive inhibitor of estrogen binding to both isoforms of the estrogen receptor. This inhibits estrogen-dependent synthesis and autocrine growth-promoting actions of beta-transforming growth factor. Its primary use is as a chemotherapeutic agent in women with metastatic, estrogen-receptor positive breast cancer. It is also used to reduce the incidence of breast cancer development in women who are at high risk for developing breast cancer as a consequence of genetic factors and family history. As an antiestrogen, tamoxifen causes menopausal side effects, predominantly hot flashes and vaginal dryness. It can cause menstrual irregularities in premenopausal women. Tamoxifen has an estrogen agonistic effect on other parts of the body. It may simulate the effect of unopposed estrogen on the endometrium, resulting in an increased risk of endometrial carcinoma. Similarly, tamoxifen, like estrogen, increases the risk of thromboembolic disease.

Pharmacology of Antiestrogens

Definitions

Selective estrogen receptor modulators (**SERMs**)[3] are compounds that display a range of agonist-to-antagonist actions in a tissue-selective manner.

Objectives

1. Know the steroid hormone antagonists used in chemotherapy, their mechanisms of action, therapeutic uses, and adverse effects.

Discussion of Class

Many breast cancers depend on the **proproliferative signals**[4] produced by estrogens to support their growth. Similarly, the vast majority of **prostate cancers** depend on the effects of **androgens** to support their growth. This has given rise to a class of anticancer agents that interfere with the action of estrogens or androgens in particular tissues. The **SERMs** are a relatively new class of compounds that have been developed in large part because of the understanding of the details of the molecular functioning of the estrogen receptor. There are **two forms of the estrogen receptor**⑤ (ER; see also Case 40) ER_{α} and ER_{β}, which are derived from separate chromosomes and have overlapping but distinct functions in a cell and promoter-dependent manner. Both ERs are weakly bound to the promoter/regulatory regions of genes that contain a particular deoxyribonucleic acid (DNA) sequence, the estrogen response element (ERE)⑥. Binding of agonist, for example, 17β-estradiol, causes a significant and important change in the conformation of ER. This concept of ligand-mediated changes in receptor conformation is the key to the mechanism of action of the SERMs. The change in ER conformation causes ER to dimerize (ER_{α}/ER_{α}, ER_{β}/ER_{β} or heterodimers of ER_{α}/ER_{β}) and to bind more strongly to the ERE. One particular portion of the receptor, helix 12, is positioned and available to interact with other proteins called coactivators. Coactivators recruit other proteins of the ribonucleic acid (RNA) polymerase complex to the target gene (s) and produce the increase in transcription. Ligands that are not pure agonists cause a different conformation of ER and these different conformations can interact with different coactivators. Estrogen antagonists cause a conformational shift in ER that facilitates the interaction with corepressors, proteins that reduce transcriptional activity from target genes. The effect of a given drug will depend on the nature of the compound, the ratio of ER_{α}/ER_{β}, and the particular repertoire of coactivators and co-repressors present in any given cell.

The **pharmacologic goal in the development of SERMs is to produce estrogenic actions in those tissues where it would be beneficial** (e. g., bone, brain, liver) and to have either **no activity or antagonist activity in tissues such as the endometrium or the breast where estrogenic activity** (e. g. proproliferative signals and increased risk of cancer) **might be deleterious**.

There are **three SERMs approved for use, tamoxifen, toremifene**⑦, **and raloxifene**⑧; several more SERMs are in various stages of clinical trials. **Tamoxifen** is a **triphenylethylene** derived from the estrogen agonist **diethylstilbestrol**. It binds to both ER_{α} and ER_{β}. Tamoxifen has antiestrogenic, estrogenic or mixed activity depending on the tissue and the target gene. Tamoxifen is an estrogen **antagonist in human breast** and ER positive breast cancer cells. However it has **agonist activity in the uterus** and stimulates proliferation in the endometrium. It has **estrogen agonist activity in the liver** where it causes a **decrease in total cholesterol and low-density lipoprotein (LDL)**⑨ **but does not increase triglycerides**⑩ **or high-density lipoprotein (HDL)**⑪. Tamoxifen is **antiresorptive in bone**. Tamoxifen is very useful in the treatment of breast cancer. It is used alone or in combination with other agents for treatment of advanced breast cancer in ER-positive tumors and is indicated for both early and advanced cancer in women of all ages. Response rates are about 50 percent in tumors that are ER positive and nearly 70 percent in ER and progestin-receptor (PR)⑫ positive tumors; response in ER-negative tumors is less than 10 percent. Tamoxifen reduces the risk of recurrence by about 50 percent. It is also approved for primary prevention in women at high risk of breast cancer; in clinical trials it caused a 50 percent reduction in invasive breast cancer and a 47 percent reduction in noninvasive cancers. **Treatment should be discontinued after 5 years because of the development of drugresistant tumors.** The adverse effects of tamoxifen include hot-flashes, nausea, and vaginal bleeding; more serious adverse effects include a two- to threefold increase in the risk of endometrial cancer and a twofold increase in the risk if thromboembolemic disease. It may cause gastrointestinal (GI) disturbances.

Tamoxifen is administered orally and a major metabolite produced in the liver is 4-OH tamoxifen which has a 25- to 50-fold higher affinity for ER and ER_{β}. Peak blood levels are attained 4-7 hours after administration. Tamoxifen is **metabolized by the hepatic cytochrome P450 system**[13] **and excreted in the feces. Toremifene** is similar structurally to tamoxifen, with a chlorine substitution in one ring structure. It has the same indications and effects as tamoxifen.

Raloxifene (see Case 40) is a benzothiophene that has been polyhydroxylated. Raloxifene has estrogen agonist activity in bone and inhibits resorption. It is indicated for the **treatment and prevention of osteoporosis**[14].

Like SERMs, **progestin receptor modulators** (**PRMs**)[15] and **androgen receptor modulators** (**ARMs**)[16], which would have tissue-selective hormonal actions, are in clinical development.

Aromatase Inhibitors

Estrogens produced locally, that is, within a tissue, may play a significant role in breast cancer. This has greatly stimulated interest in the use of aromatase inhibitors to selectively block the production of estrogens. Current agents include both **steroidal** [e. g., **formestane** and **exemestane**] and **nonsteroidal agents** [e. g., anastrozole, letrozole, and vorozole][17]. The **steroidal, or type 1 agents**, are **substrate analogs** that act as **inhibitors and irreversibly inactivate the enzyme**, while the **nonsteroidal, or type 2 agents, interact reversibly with the heme group in the cytochrome P_{450} moiety. Exemestane, letrozole, and anastrozole** are currently indicated for the treatment of breast cancer.

These agents may be used as first-line treatment of breast cancer or as second-line drugs after tamoxifen. They are **highly efficacious**, but unlike tamoxifen they **do not increase the risk of uterine cancer or venous thromboembolism**. Because they dramatically reduce circulating as well as local levels of estrogens, they **do produce hot flashes**, and there is concern about their long-term effects on bone and plasma lipid profiles. **Aromatase inhibitors**[18] **are under investigation for the prevention of breast cancer.**

Comprehension Questions

[50.1] A woman entering your cancer clinic is concerned about her chance of developing breast cancer. Her mother died of the disease, and her sister has been diagnosed with the disease. A breast exam is negative. Which of the following might be used prophylactically in this woman?

A. Clomiphene
B. Leuprolide
C. Progesterone
D. Tamoxifen

[50.2] As compared to 17β-estradiol, SERMs:

A. Are active orally
B. Are antagonists is all tissues
C. Have tissue-specific effects
D. More potent than 17β-estradiol

[50.3] A 44-year-old woman has developed breast cancer and is asked to participate in a clinical trial. She will be given formestane for 3 years. Which of the following are accurate statements about this medication?

A. It reversibly antagonizes the enzyme responsible for estrogen production.
B. It is a SERM similar to tamoxifen.
C. It is a nonsteroidal medication.
D. The patient will likely experience significant hot flashes.

Answers

[50.1] **D**. Tamoxifen may be used in woman at high risk to develop breast cancer. Leuprolide and clomiphene have antiestrogenic activities but are not used prophylactically in women at high risk of breast cancer. Progesterone may cause proliferation and cancer in the breast.

[50.2] **C**. SERMs are agonists at estrogen receptors in some but not all tissues.

[50.3] **D**. Formestane is a steroidal aromatase inhibitor that irreversibly inactivates the aromatase. Patients generally have significant hot flushes because of the low estrogen levels.

PHARMACOLOGY PEARLS

- ❖ Tamoxifen reduces the risk of hormonally responsive breast cancer recurrence by about 50 percent.
- ❖ Tamoxifen treatment should be discontinued after 5 years to avoid the development of drug-resistant breast tumors or uterine cancer.
- ❖ Aromatase inhibitors are highly efficacious, but unlike tamoxifen they do not increase the risk of uterine cancer or venous thromboembolism.

REFERENCES

Rutqvist LE. Adjuvant endocrine therapy. Best Pract Res Clin Endocrinol Metab 2004; 18-95.

Wickerham DL. Tamoxifen's impact as a preventive agent in clinical practice and an update on the STAR trial. Recent Results Cancer Res 2003; 163: 87-95.

词汇

1. breast carcinoma[乳腺癌]
2. tamoxifen[他莫昔芬]
3. selective estrogen receptor modulators(SERMs)[选择性雌激素受体调节剂]
4. proproliferative signals[促增殖信号]
5. estrogen receptor[雌激素受体]
6. estrogen response element(ERE)[雌激素反应元件]
7. toremifene[托瑞米芬]
8. raloxifene[雷洛昔芬]
9. low-density lipoprotein(LDL)[低密度脂蛋白]
10. triglycerides[甘油三酯]
11. high-density lipoprotein(HDL)[高密度脂蛋白]
12. progestin-receptor(PR)[孕激素受体]
13. hepatic cytochrome P-450 system[肝细胞色素 P450 系统]
14. osteoporosis[骨质疏松症]
15. progestin receptor modulators(PRMs)[孕激素受体调节剂]
16. androgen receptor modulators(ARMs)[雄激素受体调节剂]
17. steroidal and nonsteroidal agents[甾体和非甾体类药物]
18. aromatase inhibitors[芳香化酶抑制剂]

注 1

腋窝淋巴结肿大对诊断乳腺癌有很大意义。

注 2

对于未发现远处转移且为单个病灶的乳腺癌患者，考虑手术治疗为首选。

点评

本病例是确诊的乳腺癌。患者自行发现乳房肿块，但未及时就诊，一定程度上延误了治疗时机。幸而，尚未发现远处转移，且肿块为单个，因此采用手术切除局部乳房及扫除周围淋巴结治疗(国外多项研究证实保留乳房治疗与根治性乳房切除术比较,两组的无瘤生存率和无复发生存率与总生存率均无统计学差异,因而保留乳房治疗已成为西方国家Ⅰ、Ⅱ期乳腺癌的主要治疗方式)。由于患者已绝经，且肿瘤为雌激素阳性，因此术后内分泌治疗可行。可给予他莫昔芬，剂量为10~20mg/次，每日2次，持续用药1~2年或长达3~5年，无效时应更换第二线抗雌激素药物，这种治疗可以延缓肿瘤复发时间并提高生存率。但由于患者已发生腋窝淋巴结转移，应考虑加用化疗。

邵碧云　陈红专

❖ CASE 51

A 22-year-old man is brought to the emergency room unresponsive and in respiratory distress[①]. He was found unconscious[②] at home next to a suicide[③] note and an empty bottle of methanol[④]. A brief history from an accompanying family member is significant for the patient having depression, but he is not currently on any medications. On examination he is not responsive to verbal stimuli but has pupillary[⑤] and pain responses, and he is tachypneic and tachycardic[⑥] (rapid respiratory and heart rates). His lungs are clear. You quickly institute supportive measures, intubate the patient, and send blood tests that confirm a profound anion-gap metabolic acidosis[⑦].[注1] No other drugs are found in his system. You diagnose him with an acute methanol overdose, start him on IV fluids, sodium bicarbonate[⑧], and an IV infusion of ethanol.[注2]

◆ **What enzyme metabolizes methanol**?

◆ **Why is ethanol used to treat methanol toxicity**?

ANSWERS TO CASE 51: Solvent[9] Toxicities

Summary: A 22-year-old man with methanol poisoning is being treated with intravenous ethanol.

- **Enzyme that metabolizes methanol**: Alcohol dehydrogenase[10].
- **Reason for use of ethanol in methanol poisoning**: Competes for metabolism by alcohol dehydrogenase to reduce the production of toxic metabolites of methanol.

CLINICAL CORRELATION

The toxicity of methanol is primarily mediated by its metabolites. Methanol is metabolized by alcohol dehydrogenase to formaldehyde and subsequently to formic acid[11], the most likely cause of major organ toxicity. Formic acid inhibits cytochrome oxidase[12] activity, resulting in tissue hypoxia[13] and lactic acid production. The metabolic acidosis that occurs in methanol overdose is a result of the combination of formic acid and lactic acid that is produced. The most characteristic symptom in methanol poisoning is visual disturbances[14] with blurred vision and a sense of "being in a snowstorm". Isopropyl alcohol[15] and ethylene glycol[16] similarly are metabolized by alcohol dehydrogenase to toxic metabolites. Unfortunately, the toxic metabolites of all of these solvents can cause permanent neurologic damage[17], blindness[18], coma[19], and death. In these clinical settings ethanol can be used therapeutically. It is given by continuous IV infusion to compete for metabolism by alcohol dehydrogenase. This can help to reduce the ongoing production of toxins. Sodium bicarbonate can be given to help correct the metabolic acidosis.

Pharmacology of Solvent Toxicity

Objectives

1. Outline the basic principles of toxicology, including the dose-response relationship and risk and duration of exposure to toxins.
2. List the classes of solvent toxins and describe how exposure occurs and the effects of exposure.

Definitions

Toxicology: Study of the deleterious effects of chemical, biological, and physical substances, including their deleterious effects on the human body.

Xenobiotics[20]: Deleterious foreign substances.

Toxicokinetics: Study of the absorption, distribution, metabolism, and elimination of xenobiotics.

Discussion of Class

In considering the human toxicity of xenobiotics, it is important to keep in mind the following general principles:

The **toxicokinetics of xenobiotics** is equivalent to the pharmacokinetics described for drugs used as therapeutic agents.

Exposure to toxic substances is generally either **occupational** or **environmental** (air, soil, water, etc.).

Certain xenobiotics (e.g., acids, alkali, strong reducing and oxidizing agents, detergents㉑) **cause nonspecific damage** to tissues by altering proteins, nucleic acids, lipids, and other macromolecules that are integral to cell structure and integrity.

Biotransformation of **chemical toxicants** may result in formation of **reactive metabolites** or the production of **free radicals**㉒ **and reactive oxygen** that form covalent bonds㉓ with proteins, nucleic acids and lipids to disrupt cell function.

For many xenobiotics, a **dose-response relationship** for toxicity cannot be directly determined from human data but rather must be based on data derived strictly from **animal studies**.

In addition to decreasing or eliminating exposure, management of the poisoned patient is supportive and depends on the specific tissue or organ or tissue involved (Table 51-1).

Table 51-1

SOLVENT CLASSIFICATION AND TOXICITY

SELECTED SOLVENT CLASSES[1]	SELECTED TOXICITY
Aliphatic alcohols (e.g., methanol)	See above
Aliphatic hydrocarbons㉔ (e.g., hexane㉕)	CNS depression, sensorimotor disturbances㉖
Glycols and glycol ethers (ethylene glycol, propylene glycol㉗, etc.)	CNS depression, renal and hepatic toxicity
Halogenated aliphatic hydrocarbons㉘ (e.g., chloroform, carbon tetrachloride, trichloroethylene㉙, tetrachloroethylene, 1,1,1-trichloroethane㉚)	CNS depression, impaired memory, *Tetrachloroethylene*: Peripheral neuropathy *Carbon tetrachloride* (acute or chronic exposure): hepatic injury *Chloroform*, *carbon tetrachloride*, *Trichloroethylene*: Renal injury Carcinogenicity in animals (certain halogenated hydrocarbons).
Aromatic hydrocarbons㉛ (e.g., benzene, toluene㉜)	*Benzene*: CNS depression that may result in ataxia, vertigo, and coma. Chronic exposure can result in severe bone marrow depression㉝ and possibly leukemia㉞. *Toluene*: CNS depressant that acutely can cause ataxia at low exposure and at high exposure lead rapidly to loss of consciousness. The effects of chronic exposure are uncertain.

[1] These agents are used as industrial solvents, as cleaning agents, in synthesis of other chemicals, or as components of personal and household products.

Comprehension Questions

[51.1] Which of the following is the most characteristic symptom in methanol poisoning?

A. Carcinogenicity B. Hepatic injury

C. Renal injury D. Visual disturbances

[51.2] The most likely cause of organ toxicity from methanol is

A. Formaldehyde B. Formic acid

C. Lactic acid D. Methanol

[51.3] Severe bone marrow depression is most likely to result from exposure to which of the following solvents?

A. Benzene B. Ethylene glycol

C. Hexane D. Toluene

Answers

[51.1] **D.** The most characteristic symptom in methanol poisoning is visual disturbances. Hepatic injury, renal injury, and potential carcinogenicity are more characteristic of the halogenated aliphatic hydrocarbons.

[51.2] **B.** Methanol is metabolized by alcohol dehydrogenase to formaldehyde, which is then metabolized to formic acid, the most likely cause of methanol's organ toxicity. Formic acid inhibition of cytochrome oxidase activity results in tissue hypoxia with the production of lactic acid, which with formic acid can result in metabolic acidosis.

[51.3] **A.** Chronic exposure to benzene can result in bone marrow depression. Exposure to toluene results in central nervous system (CNS) depression. The effects of chronic exposure to toluene are uncertain. Hexane is more likely to cause CNS depression and sensorimotor disturbances. Ethylene glycol is likely to cause CNS disturbances and renal disturbances.

PHARMACOLOGY PEARLS

- ❖ Toxicity from the solvents commonly affect the central nervous system, causing sedation or CNS depression.
- ❖ Exposure to carbon tetrachloride can lead to hepatic toxicity.
- ❖ Chronic exposure to benzene may lead to bone marrow depression and possibly leukemia.

REFERENCES

Haddad LM, Shannon MW, Winchester JF. Clinical management of poisoning and drug overdose, 3rd ed. Philadelphia: Saunders, 1998.

Klassen CD, ed. Casarett and Doull's toxicology, the basic science of poisons, 6th ed. New York: McGraw Professional, 2001.

Rom WM, ed. Environmental and occupational medicine, 3rd ed. Philadelphia: Lippincott-Raven, 1998.

Toxnet: http://toxnet. nlm. nih. gov, 2004.

词汇

1. respiratory distress[呼吸窘迫]
2. unconscious[不省人事]
3. suicide[自杀]
4. methanol[甲醇]
5. pupillary[瞳孔的]
6. tachycardic[心跳过速的]
7. anion-gap metabolic acidosis[离子间隙型代谢性酸中毒]
8. sodium bicarbonate[碳酸氢钠]
9. solvent[溶剂]
10. alcohol dehydrogenase[乙醇脱氢酶]
11. formic acid[甲酸;蚁酸]
12. cytochrome oxidase [细胞色素氧化酶]
13. tissue hypoxia[组织缺氧]
14. visual disturbances[视觉屏障]
15. isopropyl alcohol[异丙醇]
16. ethyleneglycol[已二醇]
17. neurologic damage. [神经损害]
18. blindness[失明]
19. coma[昏迷]
20. xenobiotics[非生物物质]
21. detergents[去污剂]
22. free radicals[自由基]
23. covalent bond[共价键]
24. aliphatic hydrocarbons[脂肪烷]
25. hexan[已烷]
26. sensorrimotor disturbance[感觉运动障碍]
27. propylene glycol[丙二醇]
28. halogenated aliphatic hydrocarbons[卤代脂肪烃]
29. trichloroethylene[三氯乙烯]
30. 1,1,1-trichloroethane[1,1,1-三氯乙烷]
31. aromatic hydrocarbons[芳香烃]
32. toluene[甲苯]
33. bone marrow depression[骨髓抑制]
34. leukemia[白血病]

注 1

甲醇可通过呼吸道、消化道和皮肤吸收，吸收后可分布于机体各组织，脑脊液、泪、胆汁、尿液中浓度较高，骨髓、脂肪中含量最低。在体内经肝微粒体酶、乙醇脱氢酶、过氧化氢酶缓慢地氧化为 CO_2 和 H_2O。肺、肾、胃肠粘膜则可缓慢地排泄未被氧化的甲醇。因为甲醇是中等毒类物质，除具有显著的麻醉作用外，可损害眼、中枢神经系统、消化道，皮肤接触可引起脱脂和轻度皮炎，对视神经的损害最为严重，当饮用 5 ~ 10ml · kg^{-1} 时就可出现严重中毒，10ml · kg^{-1} 以上可致失明，100 ~ 250ml · kg^{-1} 时可能致死，这是由其中间氧化代谢产物甲酸或甲醛的作用造成，另外，甲醇还具有致突变作用和生殖毒性作用，可致子代肌肉骨骼、心血管系统和泌尿系统发育异常。

注 2

口服甲醇中毒患者，通常以1%碳酸氢钠溶液洗胃，硫酸镁导泻，并可根据血气分析或二氧化碳结合的测定，及早给予患者碳酸氢钠溶液以纠正酸中毒。还可给予酶竞争剂乙醇，通常以10%葡萄糖溶液将乙醇稀释成5%的浓度，缓慢静脉滴注。

点评

甲醇的急性中毒往往是当吸入大量的甲醇蒸气或误作乙醇或掺杂有甲醇的酒类被饮用后8~36小时发生。主要受损靶器官是中枢神经系统、视神经和视网膜，临床表现为：常有头痛、眩晕、肌无力、恶心、呕吐、烦躁不安、视力模糊和失眠等，严重者可发生帕金森综合征、谵妄、意识模糊、昏迷、甚至死亡。视神经受损后，可表现眼前黑影、闪光感、视物模糊、畏光、复视、眼球痛、严重视力下降，可致双目失明。慢性中毒系长期接触低浓度甲醇所致，可出现头痛、眩晕、眼颤、恶心、呕吐、视力减退、视野缺损、视神经萎缩、最后导致失明。这些临床症状与血中甲醇代谢产物甲酸的含量直接相关。甲醇中毒的救治除洗胃和给予碳酸氢钠溶液纠正酸中毒外，乙醇作为竞争底物——醇脱氢酶的亲和力较甲醇强100倍，故采用乙醇解毒是有效的，但在治疗中血液中乙醇的浓度应控制在1.0g·L^{-1}最为合适，先给负荷量（0.6g·kg^{-1}体重），然后给10.0g·h^{-1}的维持量，但此时若血中甲醇含量大于15.6mmol·L^{-1}或甲酸含量大于4.34mmol·L^{-1}时，并伴有代谢性酸中毒和严重视力障碍时的患者，应及早进行血液透析或腹膜透析，加速毒物排泄，不但可以挽救生命，还可减少后遗症，当然在解救中还可采用大剂量B族维生素及血管扩张药进行支持和对症治疗，必要时可给予糖皮质激素，以保护视神经，促进其恢复。

包定元

❖ CASE 52

A woman brings her 5-year-old son in for evaluation. 注1 He has had progressive difficulty walking in the past few months and has seemed irritable. He has also seemed quite tired. He has vomited on one or two occasions. His past medical history is unremarkable. He was born after an uncomplicated, full-term pregnancy①. He has had all of his vaccines② and had achieved all of his developmental milestones for his age. He lives with his parents in a home that was built in the 1920s, which they have been renovating. On examination, he is somewhat restless but cooperative. His conjunctiva③ and mucous membranes are pale. Neurologic exam is significant for an ataxic gait④ (clumsiness). His general examination is otherwise unremarkable. A complete blood count (CBC) shows him to be anemic. A serum lead level is markedly elevated. 注2 You admit him to the hospital and start him on succimer⑤.

◆ **How does chronic lead exposure cause anemia⑥?**

◆ **What is the mechanism of action of succimer?**

ANSWERS TO CASE 52: Heavy Metal[7] Poisoning

Summary: A 5-year-old boy with lead toxicity is admitted to the hospital and started on succimer.

- **Mechanism of lead induced anemia**: Inhibition of δ-aminolevulinic acid dehydratase[8], which blocks the conversion of δ-aminolevulinic acid to porphobilinogen[9], disrupting hemoglobin synthesis.
- **Mechanism of action of succimer**: Chelation[10] of lead causing increased lead excretion in the urine.

CLINICAL CORRELATION

Most lead toxicity in children is a result of gastrointestinal (GI) ingestion. Children absorb a greater portion of ingested lead than adults do. The source of this lead is often from lead-based paint that was widely used before the 1970s. Inorganic lead[11] binds to hemoglobin and distributes to soft tissues, including the brain. It later accumulates in the bone, from which it eliminated very slowly. Lead produces anemia via the inhibition of the enzyme δ-aminolevulinic acid dehydratase, which converts δ-aminolevulinic acid to porphobilinogen. This interrupts the pathway of synthesis of hemoglobin. Lead can also cause central nervous system (CNS) effects, especially in children. Common signs include vertigo[12], ataxia, headache[13], restlessness[14], and irritability[15]. Vomiting, delirium[16], and seizures may occur. Lowered IQ[17] and behavioral disturbances may be the result of childhood[18] exposure. Treatment of lead toxicity requires cessation of exposure and, in severe cases, chelation therapy. In children, succimer is frequently used. It can be administered orally. It binds to lead and increases the excretion of lead in the urine. Other drugs used for chelation include calcium disodium ethylenediaminetetraacetic acid (EDTA)[19], dimercaprol[20], and penicillamine.

Pharmacology of Heavy Metal Poisoning

Objectives

1. Discuss the general principles related to heavy metal poisoning.
2. List the common sources of heavy metal exposure and describe their mechanisms of action and their toxicities (Table 52-1).
3. List agents used for the management of heavy metal poisoning and describe their mechanisms of action.

Table 52-1

HEAVY METALS AND TOXIC EFFECTS

HEAVY METAL	TOXICITY	NOTES
Iron(Fe)	Gastrointestinal mucosa destruction, with severe gastroenteritis[21], abdominal pain, and bloody diarrhea[22], that lead to systemic absorption as transferrin[23] with subsequent endoethelial damage in the liver and kidney that can result in metabolic acidosis, coma, shock, cardiovascular collapse and death.	Exposure in children is generally by accidental ingestion of iron supplements. In adults toxicity is generally the result of repeated transfusions, inherited disorders or intentional overdosing.
Mercury(Hg)	Neurological and behavioral changes, including visual deficits, because of neuronal injury and encephalopathy[25] are among the most common adverse effects of mercury. Excitability, tremors[26] and gingivitis[27] are hallmarks of mercury toxicity. Gastrointestinal and renal injury are common with exposure to mercury salts, which can also cause severe pain and vomiting because of its corrosive[28] action on the mucosa of the mouth, pharynx, and intestine. Mercury vapor can result in severe respiratory difficulty with residual fibrosis.	Elemental[24] mercury vapor is well absorbed from the lungs. Elemental mercury in liquid form is relatively nontoxic. Inorganic mercury salts are generally ingested and when absorbed concentrate in the kidney. They have a long half-life. Organomercury compounds are absorbed readily from the GI tract. They undergo enterohepatic recycling with long half-lives. The developing nervous system is especially vulnerable to mercury exposure in utero.
Arsenic(As)	Nonspecific GI, CNS, and cardiovascular toxicity. Arsine gas can cause severe abdominal pain and, rarely, extensive hemolysis[29] with renal damage from degraded hemoglobin.	Exposure can be through ingestion or inhalation[30].
Lead(Pb)	Acute: uncommon; includes paresthesia[31], muscle weakness, hemolysis, renal damage Chronic: see Clinical Correlation; Most serious toxicity is encephalopathy that can lead to impaired learning and mental retardation[32], especially in children.	See Clinical Correlation. Crosses placental barrier and can cause in utero damage leading to impaired CNS development.

Discussion of Class

The general principles related to heavy metal toxicity are the following:

Exposure to heavy metals may be **acute or chronic**, generally through accidental occupational or environmental exposure.

Most, if not all, heavy metals **interact with SH groups** and perhaps other functional groups of cell proteins to cause their toxicity.

Multiple organ systems may be affected but particularly the **CNS, liver, kidney, and respiratory and immune systems.**

Management of metal poisoning involves **removal of the source, decontamination**, and **supportive treatment for symptoms**. In addition, **metal chelators** can be used to remove or prevent metal binding to important cell constituents (Table 52-2). The major chelators interact with the same functional groups as the heavy metals to form complexes which can then be eliminated from the body. With the exception of **deferoxamine**[33], their selectivity is relatively poor in that they **also bind important endogenous divalent cations**[34], **notably Ca^{2+}.**

Table 52-2
HEAVY METAL CHELATORS

HEAVY METAL CHELATORS	PRIMARY METALS CHELATED	NOTES
Dimercaprol	Mercury, Arsenic Hg, As	Administered parenterally; Avoid in iron or cadmium poisoning because complex is extremely hepatotoxic; Avoid with methylmercury poisoning because it facilitates entry into the CNS
EDTA	Lead Pb	Administered parenterally; Chronic treatment requires "off" periods to allow redistribution out of bone
Deferoxamine	Iron, Aluminum Fe, Al	Administered parenterally
Penicillamine Trientine	Copper Cu, adjunct for Pb, Hg	Administered orally; Used to chelate excess copper in Wilson's disease[35]; May result in allergic reaction
Succimer	Lead Pb in children; adjunct for Hg, As	Administered orally; Causes GI disturbances and rash

Comprehension Questions

[52.1] Which of the following heavy metal chelators is used as a primary treatment for mercury poisoning?

A. Dimercaprol B. EDTA C. Penicillamine D. Succimer

[52.2] Gastrointestinal mucosa destruction, with severe gastroenteritis, abdominal pain, and bloody diarrhea are characteristic symptoms of poisoning from which of the following heavy metals?

A. Arsenic B. Elemental liquid mercury

C. Iron D. Lead

[52.3] Lead-induced anemia is a result of inhibition of which of the following enzymes?

A. Aldehyde dehydrogenase B. Cytochrome oxidase

C. δ-aminolevulinic acid dehydratase D. Monoamine oxidase

Answers

[52.1] **A**. Dimercaprol is used as a primary heavy metal chelator for treatment of mercury poisoning. EDTA and succimer are used for lead poisoning. Penicillamine is used to treat copper poisoning. EDTA and penicillamine are used as adjuncts to treat mercury poisoning.

[52.2] **C**. Iron poisoning causes characteristic gastrointestinal mucosa destruction, with severe gastroenteritis, abdominal pain, and bloody diarrhea. Elemental liquid mercury is relatively nontoxic. A nonspecific GI, CNS, and cardiovascular toxicity is caused by arsenic. The most serious (chronic) toxicity from lead poisoning is encephalopathy.

[52.3] **C**. Lead produces anemia via the inhibition of the enzyme δ-aminolevulinic acid dehydratase, which converts-aminolevulinic acid to porphobilinogen. This interrupts the pathway of synthesis of hemoglobin.

PHARMACOLOGY PEARLS

❖ Iron toxicity can lead to gastroenteritis, liver, and kidney damage and, if severe enough, death.

❖ The most common manifestations of mercury poisoning are the neuronal toxicity such as visual deficits.

❖ Lead poisoning is most worrisome in the developing fetus or children and can lead to mental retardation.

REFERENCES

Klassen CD, ed. Casarett and Doull's toxicology, the basic science of poisons, 6th ed. New York: McGraw Professional, 2001.

Rom WM, ed. Environmental and occupational medicine, 3rd ed. Philadelphia: Lippincott-Raven, 1998.

Toxnet: http: //toxnet. nlm. nih. gov

词汇

1. full-term pregnancy[足月妊娠]
2. vaccine[疫苗]
3. conjunctiva[结膜]
4. ataxic gait[共济失调步态]
5. succimer[琥巯酸]
6. anaemia[贫血]
7. heavy metal[重金属]
8. δ-aminolevulinic acid dehydrase[氨基-δ-酮戊酸脱水酶]
9. porphobilinogen[胆色素原]
10. chelation[螯合]
11. inorganic lead[无机铅]
12. vertigo[眩晕]
13. headache[头痛]
14. restlessness[坐立不安]
15. irritability[易怒,应激性]
16. delirium[谵妄,妄想]
17. IQ[智商,智力商数]
18. childhood[童年,儿童期]
19. calcium disodium ethylenediaminetetra acetic acid(EDTA)[依地酸二钠钙]
20. dimercaprol[二基丙醇]
21. gastroenteritis[胃肠炎]
22. bloody diarrhea[血样腹泻]
23. transferrin[转铁蛋白]
24. elemental[元素的]
25. encephalopathy[脑病]
26. tremor[震颤]
27. gingivitis[龈炎]
28. corrosive[腐蚀性的,腐蚀药]
29. hemolysis[溶血]
30. inhalation[吸入]
31. paresthesia[异感症]
32. mental retardation[精神发育迟缓]
33. deferoxamine[去铁胺]
34. divalent cations[二价阳离子]
35. Wilson's disease[肝豆状核变性]

注 1

为何选择 5 岁儿童中毒的病例？这是由于铅的开发利用而深入导现代人的日常生活中，从而成为威胁人类健康，尤其是儿童健康的因素之一，儿童在解剖和生理上与成人有着许多不同特点，表现在铅代谢方面亦较成人具有吸收多，排泄快，吸收储存与骨骼组织肿的铅亦较成人易向血液，组织转移。而实际受到铅损害或致中毒量也远超过成人。

注 2

琥珀酸(succimer)属琥珀酸衍生物，又称二巯丁二酸(CHEMT)，已由美国食品药品管理局批准上市，获准用于血铅含量高于4.5μg/dl的儿童与其与体内铅螯合而解毒，从而减少因铅中毒所致的疾病及死亡率。

点评

国际上关于儿童铅中毒的防治原则是：①环境干预是根本手段，即只有脱离铅污染环境，才能得到铅中毒的根本治疗。②健康教育是主要方法，这是既简便又有效的干预手段，一般认为，对无症状血铅水平为10～20μg/dl的儿童均以健康教育和环境干预的方法为主。③临床治疗是主要环节，当儿童的血铅水平在20μg/dl中度以上铅中毒者，才需要结合进行临床治疗，包括非药物和药物性驱铅，不过对于血铅水平超过45μg/dl的症状性铅中毒是在进行环境干预和健康教育的同时，需要采用药物驱铅，琥巯酸属竞争性解毒药，以其含有的活泼巯基(-SH)竞争夺取已有细胞和酶结合的铅，促进铅与细胞解离，并与铅结合成为可溶性的，无毒铅化合物随尿排泄，而达到解毒目的。治疗中也可采用其他的驱铅药，如依地酸二钠钙，二巯丁二酸。

包定元

SECTION Ⅲ

Listing of Cases

Listing by Case Number

Listing by Medication Class(Alphabetical)

LISTING BY CASE NUMBER
案例列表(按案例序号)

LISTING BY MEDICATION(ALPHABETICAL)
案例列表按药物字母顺序

CASE#	MEDICATIONS DISCUSSED	DISEASE	PAGE #
41	Adrenal cortex, drugs related to 作用于肾上腺的药	Cushing disease 库欣病	341
6	Adrenoreceptor antagonist 肾上腺素受体拮抗剂	Myocardial infarction 心肌梗塞	53
48	Alkylating and antimetabolite agents 烷化和抗代谢药	Actinic keratosis(skin lesions) 光化性角化病	411
11	Antiarrhythmic agents 抗心律不齐药	Cardiac Arrhythmia 心律失常	93
45	Antibacterial agents 抗菌药	Pneumococcal pneumonia 肺炎球菌性肺炎	381
15	Antidepressant drugs 抗抑郁药	Depression 抑郁症	131
31	Antiemetics 止吐药	Emesis(chemotherapy) 呕吐化疗	259
18	Antiepileptic agents 抗癫痫药	Epilepsy 癫痫症	153
47	Antifungal and antiprotozoal agents 抗真菌药和抗原虫药	Tinea corporis(ringworm) 癣	403
24	Antihistamines 抗组胺药	Allergic rhinitis 过敏性鼻炎	207
12	Antihypertensive agents 抗高血压药	Hypertension 高血压	103
17	Antiparkinsonian agents 抗帕金森药	Parkinson disease 帕金森病	145
14	Antipsychotic drugs 抗精神病药	Schizophrenia 精神分裂症	123
46	Antiviral agents 抗病毒药	Herpes zoster 带状疱疹	391
37	Asthmatic medications 治哮喘药	Asthma 哮喘	303
20	Benzodiazepines 苯二氮革类	Benzodiazepine overdose 地西泮过量	175
44	Calcium homeostatis, agents affecting 影响钙恒定的药	Osteoporosis 骨质疏松症	371
10	Congestive heart failure agents 充血性心力衰竭药	Congestive heart failure 充血性心力衰竭	83